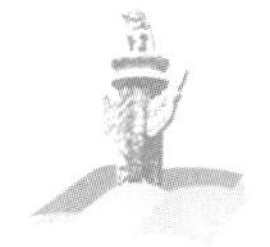

An Intensively Compiled Practical English-Chinese Library of Traditional Chinese Medicine

(英汉对照)精编实用中医文库

Chief General Compilers CHEN Kaixian LI Qizhong(Executive) HE Xinghai

总主编 陈凯先 李其忠(执行) 何星海

Chief General Translators SHI Jianrong HU Hongyi XU Yao(Executive)

总主译 施建蓉 胡鸿毅 徐 瑶(执行)

Gynecology of Traditional Chinese Medicine

中医妇科学

Chief Compiler ZHANG Tingting

Chief Translator ZHU Jianmin

主编 张婷婷

主译 诸建民

上海浦江教育出版社(原上海中医药大学出版社)

Shanghai Pujiang Education Press (Former Shanghai University of TCM Press)

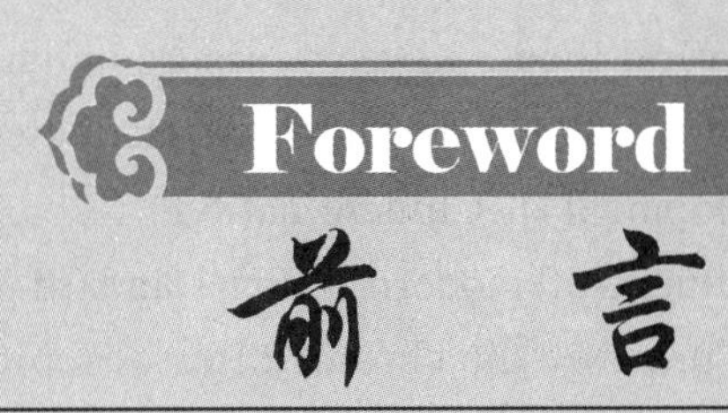

Foreword
前言

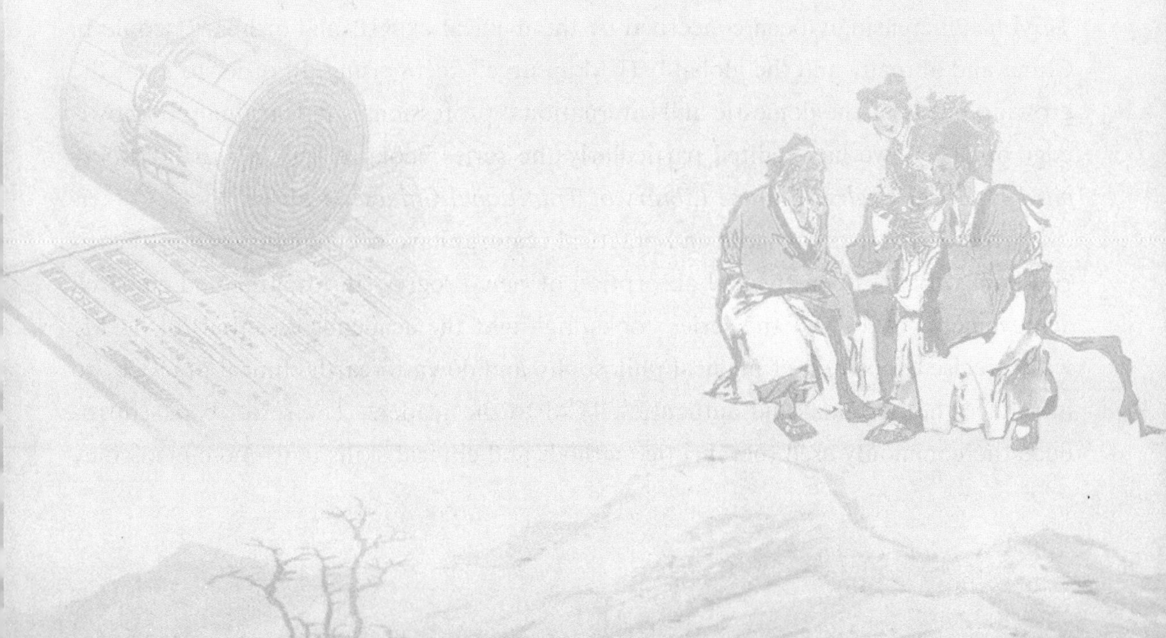

With the traditional medical philosophy and clinical experience as the principal body, the science of Traditional Chinese Medicine (TCM) is a comprehensive subject to study the rules of life activities and the disease prevention, diagnosis, treatment, rehabilitation as well as healthcare. The science of TCM has a long history of development and belongs to a summary of experiences that Chinese nation has fought against diseases for over several thousand years, is also an important component part of Chinese outstanding traditional culture and has contributed greatly to the healthcare undertaking and development of Chinese nation.

By increasing enhancement of modern living standard, change of living modes and acceleration of ageing process, the chronic diseases represented by tumors, cardiovascular diseases and diabetes become gradually the important factors in impacting the health of mankind, but TCM presents the better therapeutic effects. Nowadays, the modern medical mode of "society-psychology-biology" has been advocated in medical science, changing from the medical idea of "disease treatment" to "health promotion". The more and more patients in China and abroad have chosen natural and low side-effect Chinese herbal medicine for their problems. With the changes in medicine modes and in spectrum of diseases in the recent several dozens of years, TCM has increasingly been concerned by the medical experts and ordinary people in China and abroad, and the global " TCM upsurge" keeps rising. In order to meet the growing needs of the domestic and international professionals in learning the knowledge of TCM, we have edited particularly the series books of *An Intensively Compiled Practical English-Chinese Library of Traditional Chinese Medicine*.

The scientific, systematic and practical features have been emphasized in the series books. Based upon the full absorption of new progress in teaching and research achievements of TCM , the series books highlight the academic essentials of TCM, with precise exposition of medical philosophy and down-to-earth clinical practice, to introduce the "original and authentic" TCM to the readers. The series books introduce the commonly used therapeutic methods and clinical skills in Chinese medicine, by the clinically encountered and frequently seen diseases and the relevant ailments predominantly effective by Chinese medical therapies.By studying the series books, the readers can learn the knowledge and techniques of TCM on gradual progress and become proficient gradually in TCM.

The series books highlight "the precise features in three aspects"—capable in authors, refined in contents and accurate in translation. The majority of the authors of the series books are senior experts from the related faculties of Shanghai University of Traditional Chinese Medicine. The translator team is composed of the senior teachers with plentiful expertise in translation of TCM from international education college and foreign language center of Shanghai University of Traditional Chinese Medicine. In order to meet the needs of the readers in China and abroad, the basic and clinical core contents are selected and the latest research achievements are consulted based upon the principle "to seek its essentials but its completion" in the series books.

The series books can satisfy the beginners with certain knowledge of English language in studying TCM systematically and can also be used as the textbooks for education of TCM and pharmacy for foreign students. We sincerely hope the publication of the series books plays its promoting role for TCM going to the world.

Editors

June, 2017

中医学是以传统医学理论与实践经验为主体，研究人体生命活动规律和疾病预防、诊断、治疗、康复以及保健的一门综合性学科。中医学历史悠久，源远流长，是中华民族几千年来同疾病作斗争的经验总结，也是中国传统文化的重要组成部分，长期以来为中国人民的健康保健事业和民族繁衍作出了巨大的贡献。

随着现代生活水平的不断提高、生活方式的改变以及老龄化进程的加快，以肿瘤、心血管疾病和糖尿病等为代表的慢性病日渐成为影响人类健康的重要因素，而中医药显示了良好的治疗效果。当今的医学倡导“社会—心理—生物”的现代医学模式，医学理念从“疾病治疗”向“健康促进”转变，国内外越来越多的患者选择天然、毒副作用低的中医药治疗疾病。近几十年来，随着医学模式的转变和疾病谱的改变，中医学日益引起越来越多的海内外医学专家和普通民众的关注，全球性的“中医热”正在持续升温。为了满足海内外人士日益高涨的学习中医学知识的需求，我们特地编撰了《（英汉对照）精编实用中医文库》丛书。

本丛书注重“三性”——科学性、系统性、实用性。丛书在充分吸取近年中医教学、科研进展的基础上，突出中医学术精华，理论阐述准确、临床切合实际，向读者介绍“原汁原味”的中医学；丛书介绍中医学常用的治疗方法和临床技能，所涉及的病证均为临床常见病、多发病和中医优势病种。丛书的 13 个分册涵盖了中医基础与临床的主干课程，通过阅读本丛书，读者可以由浅入深、循序渐进地学习中医药知识和技能。

本丛书突出“三精”——作者精干、内容精炼、翻译精准。丛书的中文作者绝大部分为上海中医药大学各相关教研室的资深专家，翻译团队由上海中医药大学国际教育学院和外语中心具有丰富的中医药学翻译经验的骨干教师组成。为了适合海内外读者的需求，丛书本着“求其精而不求其全”的原则，选取了基础和临床的核心内容，翻译上参考了最新的研究成果。

本丛书既可满足具有一定英语水平的初学中医者系统学习中医所用，也可供中医药留学生教育作为教材使用，衷心希望本丛书的出版在中医药走向海外进程中发挥应有的推动作用。

编者

2017 年 6 月

Note for Compilation

编写说明

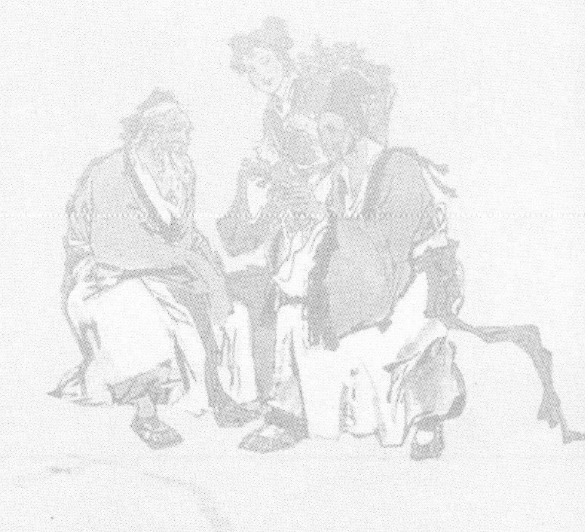

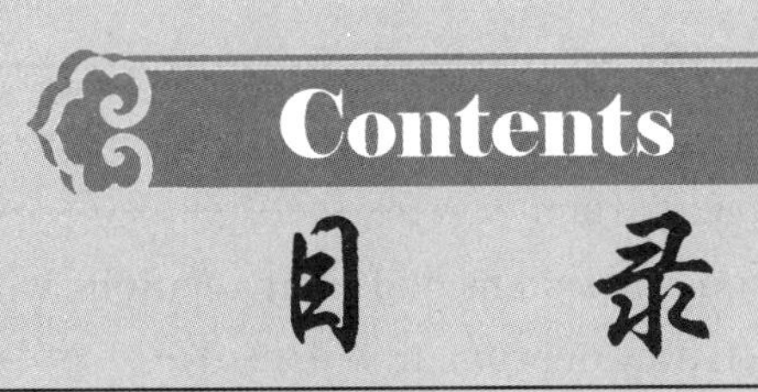
Contents
目录

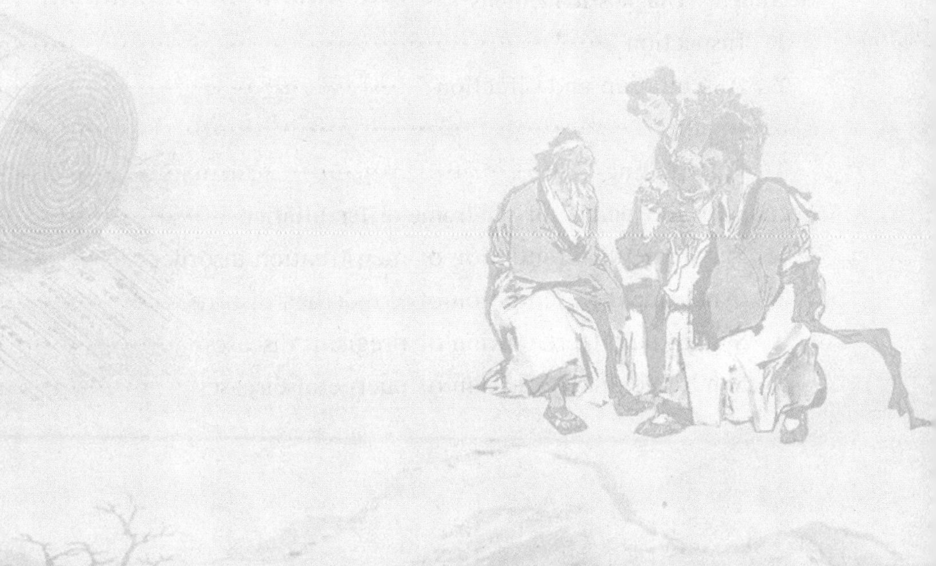

General Introduction

总 论

Therapeutic Modalities

各 论

Ceneral Introduction

总 论

Chapter 1 Physiological and pathological characteristics of women

第 1 章 女性的生理、病理特点

By TCM theories, Gynecology of TCM is a clinical specialty to understand the anatomy, the physiological and pathological characteristics, to study the diagnostic and therapeutic principles and specific diseases related to women. Through a long history of 2000 years of practice and improvement, gynecology of TCM has developed to unique theories, diagnostic and therapeutic methods. Because women have physiological characteristics of menstruation, pregnancy, delivery and child-feeding, disorders in menstruation, leucorrhea, pregnancy and delivery may often be induced. Based on the cognition of uterus, menstruation, pregnancy, delivery and child-feeding as well as their relation with the viscera, meridians, qi and blood, gynecology of TCM studies the pathological characteristics of women disease and the principles for prevention and clinical treatment.

中医妇科学是运用中医学的理论，认识女性的解剖、生理与病因病机特点，研究妇科疾病诊疗规律，防治妇女特有疾病的一门临床学科。在两千多年漫长的历史发展过程中，经历代医家的不懈努力与临床实践，中医妇科学形成了一个较为完整、系统的理论体系和诊治方略。由于女性具有月经、胎孕、产育、哺乳等方面的生理特点，常可导致经、带、胎、产等的异常而产生妇科疾病。中医妇科学是通过认识子宫、月经、胎孕、产育、哺乳等与脏腑、经络、气血的关系，研究女性的病理特征，探索妇科疾病的特点及其防治规律。

Section 1 Physiological characteristics

第1节 生理特点

1 Uterus

The uterus is located in the pelvis, like an upside down pear, posterior to the bladder and anterior to the rectum with its lower opening connected to vagina, and is the most important female reproductive organ. By the bifurcation on the top of uterus, it is the internal genital organ which produces and transports ovum. Similar to fallopian tubes and oviduct, situated in left and right lower abdomen, it is a proper female reproductive organ. The uterus is responsible for menstruation, fetusand reproductive-related functions: secreting leukorrhea, promoting labor, draining lochia and other physiological functions.

Under physiological conditions, the uterus is to store essence and blood for menstruation and conception of fetus, demonstrating the "storage" function of the zang organs; and to discharge menstruation or deliver baby, manifesting the "excretion" function of the fu organs. That is why it is called "extraordinary organ" in *Inner Canon* (Nei Jing). Such physiological functions of the uterus are closely related to meridians, viscera, qi and blood. Firstly, The uterus is connected with the heart and kidney through meridians. The heart governs blood and the kidney stores essence. Only when the heart blood is sufficient and kidney essence is abundant, can blood

1 胞宫

胞宫即子宫，又称女子胞、子肠、子户、子脏、子处等，是女性最重要的生殖脏器。其位置在小腹的正中，在不受孕的情况下，呈倒置的梨形，腔状器官，居于膀胱之后，直肠之前，下口连接阴道；上有两歧，乃产生和输送卵子的内生殖脏器，位于左右少腹，类似于输卵管和卵巢，是女性特有的生殖器官。胞宫的主要作用是行月经和孕育胎儿的生殖功能，并由此派生出与生殖相关的泌带液、促分娩、排恶露等生理功能。

在生理状态下，子宫的功能活动，平时蓄积经血，为月经的来潮或为胚胎的孕育奠定应有的物质基础，表现了脏"藏"的功能；而在行经期排出月经，或在分娩时娩出胎儿，又表现了腑的"泻"的功能；由于有这种双重的功能，故《内经》称之为"奇恒之府"。子宫的这些生理功能与脏腑、经络、气血密切相关。首先，因为子宫在经络上与心肾相通，而心主血、肾

and essence flow into the uterus for the preparation of menstruation and pregnancy. Besides, the uterus is also closely related to Thoroughfare Vessel, Conception Vessel, Governor Vessel and Belt Vessel, and also is communicated with the twelve meridians and Zangfu organs via those extraordinary meridians. In particular, the uterus is closely related to the Thoroughfare Vessel and Conception Vessel. The Thoroughfare Vessel is a sea of blood, and the Conception Vessel governs the fetus. When females reach the age of about 14, the Conception Vessel opens to flow smoothly and the Thoroughfare Vessel flourishes, and sea of blood becomes full and sufficient to fill into the uterus, so as to accomplish its functions in producing menses and breeding fetus.

藏精，若心血、肾精充足，通过经脉注入胞中，才具备产生月经、胎孕的主要条件。此外，子宫还与奇经中的冲、任、督、带等经脉有密切联系，并通过这些经脉与十二经及脏腑相通。尤其与冲、任二脉密切。冲为血海，任主胞胎，女子到十四岁左右，任脉通，太冲脉盛，血海满盈，下注胞宫，从而完成其行月经和孕育胎儿的生理作用。

2　Menstruation

Menstruation refers to regular and periodic uterine bleeding in women at a certain age. Normal menstruation occurs once a month. But sometimes under normal conditions, menstruation may occur once every other month known as bimonthly menstruation or once three months known as tri-monthly menstruation, or even once a year known as yearly menstruation. If menstruation never occurs in the whole life of a woman who can still conceive, it is called latent menstruation. Menstruation may occur regularly in the early months of pregnancy without affecting the fetus, it is called menstruation in pregnancy. Such changes in menstruation are regarded as normal phenomena, not morbid.

2　月经

月经是女性在一定年龄阶段内有规律、周期性的子宫出血现象。因其一般以一个阴历月为一个周期，经常不变，信而有期，故称之为“月经”，又称为“月事”“月使”“月水”“月候”“月信”“经水”。正常的月经是每月一行，但个别妇女身体无特殊不适而定期两个月来潮一次者，古人称为“并月”；3 个月一潮者称为“居经”，亦名“季经”；一年一行者称为“避年”；终生不潮而能受孕者称为“暗经”；妊娠早期仍按周期有少量阴道流血，但无损于胎儿者，称为“激经”，亦称“盛胎”或“垢胎”。这些都属于生理上的个别现象，不属于病态。

Menstruation is a normal physiological phenomenon while uterus is acted on by viscera, meridians, qi and blood. Blood is the main ingredients of menstruation, and is engendered by viscera. The generation and operation of blood are adjusted by qi and blood reaches the uterus through meridians. Rooted in viscera, qi and blood are the essential substances that generate menstruation. The heart governs blood, the liver stores blood and the spleen controls blood. The stomach governs the acceptance and decomposition of water and grain, and shares the same source of the production and transformation with the spleen. The kidney stores essence and essence is the basis to generate qi and blood. The lung governs qi of body, assembles the hundred meridians and transforms the nutrient substances. If the viscera are healthy, qi and blood are sufficient, meridians are smooth, menstruation remains regular. Otherwise, disease occurs.

月经的产生，是脏腑经络气血作用于胞宫的正常生理现象。月经的成分，主要是血，血为脏腑所生化，而血的生成、统摄运行，有赖于气的生化与调节，通过经脉才能达到胞宫。气血是产生月经的最根本的物质，来源于脏腑，心主血，肝藏血，脾统血；胃主受纳，腐熟水谷，与脾同为生化之源；肾藏精，精又为气血生成之本；肺主一身之气，朝百脉而输精微。脏腑无病，气血充足，经脉畅通，月经也就正常。反之就会成为疾病。

Exuberance and harmony of qi and blood are important conditions to generate menstruation. The sufficiency of kidney qi plays a leading role in generating menstruation. Kidney qi is the key to physiological development of women all through the life. In *Canon of Medicine* (Nei Jing), the rules between the condition of the kidney qi and the growth, adulthood and senility of females are explained in three phases. ① Growth and development phase: At the age of 7, female is gradually rich in kidney qi, the reproductive organs begin to grow and teeth change starts. At the age of 14, the reproductive substance has well developed, Conception Vessel is smooth in circulation, Thoroughfare Vessel is in predomination, menstruation occurs regularly and

气血充盛与和调是月经产生的重要条件，肾气的充盛起着主导作用。《内经》将肾气的盛衰与女性生长壮老的规律分为三个时期进行了阐述。①生长发育期：指出女性在 7 岁以后，肾气逐渐充盛，促使生殖器官开始发育，同时更换乳牙。14 岁左右，天癸开始成熟。由于天癸的作用，使任脉畅通，冲脉充盛，随之月经便开始初潮，具备了受孕生育的能力。②壮盛期：指出女性 21 岁肾气充盛已渐趋成熟，到 28 岁左

erence of sour taste, nausea and vomiting, which are physiological changes and usually disappear in three months. At the mid-term of pregnancy, since blood accumulates in the uterus to nourish the fetus, it is already deficient during pregnancy. Hemorrhage during delivery further worsens blood deficiency. Asthenia of yin fails to keep yang inside and leads to leakage of yang, bringing about such symptoms as slight fever, aversion to cold and spontaneous sweating which will disappear automatically after yin and yang are balanced. At the end of pregnancy, the fetus enlarges and fetal position moves down. The head of fetus oppresses bladder and rectum, causing frequent urine and constipation. Pregnant women feel prolapsing and distending sensation in the waist and lower abdomen and have a call of nature. Some pregnant women have liquid from vagina or discharge a small amount of blood, which is a parturient sign.

迫膀胱和直肠，引起尿意频数，大便易于秘结，孕妇自觉腰腹阵阵作痛，下腹部坠胀而有便意，有的见有液体自阴道流出，或排出少量血水，这是已届临产的征兆。

The breasts are obviously enlarged, the nipple and areola of mamma get darker usually after 8 weeks of pregnancy. After delivery, essence of grain and water ascend with Thoroughfare Vessel and Yangming qi (breasts belong to the stomach meridian of Foot-Yangming). And then there will be secretion of milk and no menstruation during breast feeding period.

通常在妊娠 8 周后乳房会明显增大隆起，乳头乳晕着色加深。分娩以后，水谷之精微随冲脉与阳明之气上行(乳房属足阳明胃经)，产妇就有乳汁分泌。故哺乳期一般不来月经。

5 Viscera, qi, blood, meridians and their relations with physiological activities of women

5 脏腑、气血、经络与女性生理的关系

5.1 Viscera

5.1 脏腑

Physiologically the viscera in women mainly function to produce essence and transform qi and blood. The heart governs the blood, the liver stores

在女性生理方面，脏腑的作用主要是生精化气化血。其中心主血，肝藏血，脾

the blood, the spleen commands the blood and is also the source of the blood; the lung controls qi and qi moves the blood; the kidney stores the essence, and the essence and blood share the same origin. The Zang-organs and Fu-organs, interiorly and exteriorly related to each other, together control the production, storage and regulation of the essence, qi and blood, also closely related to menstruation, leukorrhea, pregnancy and childbirth. Among the Zang-organs and Fu-organs, the kidney, liver and spleen (stomach) are the most important ones.

统血,又是血的生化之源;肺主气,气运血;肾藏精,精血又同源;腑与脏为表里,同司精、气、血的生化、贮存、统摄、调节等,与经、带、胎、产均有密切关系,其中又以肾、肝、脾(胃)的作用更为重要。

5. 1. 1 Kidney

The main function of kidney lies in kidney qi, which is composed of kidney yin and kidney yang and depend on and restrain each other. They are the key factor for maintaining yin and yang of body and other viscera. It is said in *Jing-Yue's Complete Compendium* (Jing Yue Quan Shu) that viscera yin and viscera yang are only produced by kidney. The exuberance and debilitation of kidney qi are directly related to physical development and reproduction of woman. When kidney qi becomes exuberant, the reproductive essence in the kidney will be fully developed, the Conception Vessel will transport qi freely and the Thoroughfare Vessel will be abundant in content. Under such a condition, menstruation occurs regularly and pregnancy is possible.

The kidney is connected with uterine collaterals. After pregnancy, the fetus in the uterus depends on the nourishment of kidney yin and warmth of kidney yang to develop normally. Therefore, the kidney plays a vital role in the embryonic development.

5. 1. 1 肾

肾的主要功能体现为肾气,包括肾阴和肾阳。肾阴亦称真阴、元阴,肾阳亦称元阳、真阳,二者相互依存,相互制约,是维持机体及其他脏腑阴阳的本源。《景岳全书》谓:“五藏之阴气,非此不能滋,五藏之阳气,非此不能发。”故肾气的盛衰,与人体的生长发育、衰老和生殖能力有直接关系。女性在肾气盛后,肾中所藏先天之精逐渐成熟,任脉乃通,冲脉乃盛,月事以时下,而能受孕生子。

肾又系胞,胞宫络脉与肾相连通,故能维系胞胎;受孕之后,胚胎在子宫中须依赖肾阴的滋养和肾阳的温煦才能正常发育。因此,肾对胚胎的发育也起着极其重要的作用。

The kidney also governs water as well as opening and closing activities of stomach. If the kidney is abundant in qi and normal in closing and opening, yin fluid will constantly flow into the Conception and Belt Vessels to lubricate the vagina and produce physiological leukorrhea.

肾还主水，司胃关开阖，肾气充沛，开阖有度，则阴液不断输于任、带二脉，津液常润于阴道，成为生理性白带。

5.1.2　Liver

The liver stores blood and governs distribution and conveyance of qi and blood, pertaining to yin physically and to yang functionally. Blood stored in the liver nourishes all viscera and skeleton and also flows into the Thoroughfare Vessel. That is why it is said that "the liver governs the Thoroughfare Vessel" and "the liver is the congenital base of life for women". The liver also plays an important role in the production of menstruation. The storage, circulation and regulation of blood in the liver depend on the distribution and conveyance of liver qi. Only when the distribution and conveyance functions of the liver is normal can sufficient blood flow into the uterus regularly. Besides, the liver meridian starts from the big toe and moves upwards along the inner line of the lower limbs to the genitals and lower abdomen, connected with the liver, gallbladder and diaphragm, distributing over the hypochondria and rib-side, finally reaching the vertex. Liver qi is also significant in distributing and conveying gastrosplenic qi and bile. The normal distribution and conveyance functions of liver qi are prerequisite to the reception and digestion of food by the stomach, the normal transformation and production of essence by the spleen, smooth transportation of bile from the gallbladder and constant production of qi and blood. The dysfunction of the liver in distribu-

5.1.2　肝

肝藏血，主疏泄，体阴而用阳。肝所藏之血，营养脏腑百骸，下注于冲脉，冲为血海，肝为血脏，故又有"肝司血海"和"女子以肝为先天"之说。女性的月经生理依赖于肝的作用，肝主条达疏泄，肝血的贮存、流通、调节须赖肝气的疏泄作用，肝疏泄功能正常，血海满溢如期。另外，足厥阴肝经由足大趾经下肢内侧上行，绕前阴，抵少腹，夹胃属肝，络胆，上贯膈，布胁肋（在此经过乳头）……上至巅，与胆、胃、乳房均由一定关系。肝气还有疏泄脾胃和胆汁的功能。肝气疏达，则胃的受纳、腐熟，脾的运化、散精，胆汁的输出正常，则气血的生化有源。若肝失疏泄，可以影响脾、胃、胆的正常功能，而发生脘闷、纳呆、腹胀、便溏、胁痛、口苦等肝脾、肝胃、肝胆失调的证候。由于肝的经脉经过乳头、少腹、阴部等部位，因此，肝气的疏泄和肝血畅旺，与

tion and conveyance affects the normal functions of the spleen, stomach and gallbladder, leading to epigastric oppression, hypochondriac pain, bitter taste in the mouth, anorexia, abdominal distension and loose stool which are commonly encountered in gynecology. Since the liver meridian distributes over the breasts, lower abdomen and genitals, the functions of liver qi and the conditions of liver blood are closely related to states of lactation and the nourishment of the genitals.

乳汁的通调和阴部的滋养也有密切关联。

5.1.3 Spleen (Stomach)

The spleen and the stomach function to transform and transport water and grain, distribute the nutrient substances, known as the postnatal base of life and the source of qi and blood. Menstruation, nourishment of the fetus and production of milk all depend on the spleen and stomach to transform and transport food nutrients to nourish qi and blood. The spleen also controls blood to flow inside the meridians. Normal functions of the spleen ensure normal production, transportation and command of blood, indispensable to menstruation, pregnancy, delivery and breast-feeding.

The spleen also governs the distribution of body fluid and transformation of water and dampness. Normal functions of the spleen will maintain normal distribution and conveyance of body fluid, to nourish the muscles, luster the skin, lubricate the joints, moisten the orifices, and to produce thc moist lcukorrhea to moisten the vigina frequently in women. On the contrary, dysfunction of the spleen affects the distribution and conveyance of body fluid, leading to the production of phlegm due to accumulation of fluid and morbid leukorrhagia due to infusion of

5.1.3 脾(胃)

脾主运化水谷,输布精微,为后天之本,气血生化之源。经之能行,胎之得养,乳之所化,无不赖脾之运化水谷,生养气血的功能。脾统血、摄血,血能正常运行于脉内,而不至流散,赖脾气之统摄。脾气健运,则血的生化、运行、统摄有常,这是女性月经、胎产、哺乳等生理变化所需的条件。

脾主输布津液,运化水湿。如脾气健运,则津液输布正常,能养肌肉,泽皮肤,濡关节,润孔窍,女性能白带津液常润以滑泽阴道。反之,脾失健运,则津液失于输布,聚而为湿为痰;下注任带,为带下证。

fluid into the Conception and Belt Vessels.

The stomach, a fu organ characterized by sufficient qi and blood, governs reception and digestion of food and manages blood and qi production with the spleen. The stomach meridian moves downward to meet with the Thoroughfare Vessel at the Path of Qi. That is to say why the thoroughfare vessel is affiliated to yangming. Only when food and water in the stomach are sufficient, can blood in the Thoroughfare Vessel and uterus be full enough to produce menstruation. Thus, the stomach also plays an important role in menstruation. Since the stomach meridian distributes downwards through the middle line of breast, the stomach influences the production of milk. So only when stomach qi is sufficient, can blood and qi be abundant and the production of milk be constant.

胃主受纳腐熟水谷，为水谷之海，与脾同司气血生化之源，又为多气多血之腑。足阳明经下行，与冲脉会于气街，故有“冲脉隶于阳明”之说，胃中水谷盛，则冲脉之血亦盛，血海满盈，月事以时下。因此，胃在月经的正常来潮上也有重要的作用。而且，胃的经脉在胸部经乳中线下行，故乳房属胃所司，乳汁的分泌与胃气的作用也有密切关系。胃气充盛，则气血充足，乳汁分泌旺盛。

5.1.4 Heart and lung

Both the heart and the lung are located in the upper energizer, the former controls blood and the latter governs qi, both playing an important role in the transportation, circulation and regulation of blood. Menstruation, pregnancy, delivery and lactation in women are all related to qi and blood. The heart governs blood and vessels, the propelling of which depends on heart qi. Sufficiency of heart blood and smooth circulation of heart qi will enable blood to flow into the uterus to produce menstruation. The lung governs qi, connecting with all meridians and distributing food nutrients down to the uterus to influence menstruation.

The heart governs the mind. The liver storesblood. The spleen controls contemplation and the kidney stores willpower. The functions of these

5.1.4 心与肺

主血与主气，均居上焦，在血的输布、运行、调节方面均有重要作用。妇女的经、孕、产、乳，无不与气血相关。心主血，其充在血脉，即心有推动血液在经脉内运行的作用。心的这种功能全赖心气，若心血旺盛，心气宣通，血脉流畅，则月事如常。肺主气，朝百脉而输精微，如雾露之溉，下达胞宫而参与月经的生理活动。

此外，由于心主神明，肝主藏血，脾主思虑，肾主藏志，这些脏腑功能及其精神

viscera and normal mental activities are also importantly influential to the regulation of menstruation.

活动的正常与否，对月经的调节也有至关重要的影响。

Apart from direct influence on menstruation, leukorrhea, fetus and delivery, the kidney, liver, spleen, heart and lung depend upon and restrain each other by their inter-promoting, inter-acting, inter-restraining and inter-transforming relationship, and by the extensive connection of the meridian system unite the viscera, qi, blood and meridians into an integrity to maintain and regulate the physiological functions of women.

肾、肝、脾、心、肺五脏，除了与经、带、胎、产有直接作用外，还通过其生克制化的联系，互相依存，互相制约，并借助于经络系统的广泛联系，使脏腑、气血、经络构成一个有机的整体，共同维持和调节女性的生理功能。

5.2 Qi and blood

5.2 气血

Blood is fundamental for women. Menstruation is transformed from blood. In pregnancy blood is needed to nourish the fetus. After childbirth, blood is transformed into milk to foster the infant. So, it is clear that blood plays an important role in menstruation, pregnancy, childbirth and lactation. Blood depends on qi to produce, circulate and control, while qi relies on blood to nourish and protect. That is why it is said that qi is the commander of blood and blood is the mother of qi.

女性以血为本，月经为血所化生，妊娠需血以养胎，胎儿娩出后，血化为乳，以供养婴儿。可见血在经、孕、产、乳方面均有重要作用。血依赖气的生化、运行和统摄，气又要依靠血的营养和固护，相互依存，不可分离，故有气为血帅，血为气母之说。

5.3 Meridians

5.3 经络

Meridians refer to the pathways through which qi and blood flow. The meridians of the human body are composed of the regular meridians, extraordinary meridians, divergent meridians, collaterals and muscular regions. The meridians that are closely related to the physiological activities of woman arc the Thoroughfare, Conception, Governor and Belt Vessels in the eight extraordinary meridians.

经络又称经脉，是运行气血的通路。人体的经络，由正经、奇经、经别、络脉、经筋等构成，其中与女性生理有密切的联系的，是奇经中的冲、任、督、带四脉。

The Thoroughfare Vessel, Conception Vessel, Governor Vessel and Belt Vessel are the main component part in the eight extraordinary meridians.

冲、任、督、带是奇经八脉的重要组成部分。奇经在人体的作用，既能贮存十二

The functions of the extraordinary meridians in the human body are to store the qi and blood transported by the twelve meridians and to regulate qi and blood for nourishing the twelve meridians and viscera. Among the Thoroughfare, Conception, Governor and Belt Vessels, the Thoroughfare and Conception Vessels are most important in the physiological functions of the reproductive system of women.

经脉所运行的气血，又能随时加以调节，以供十二经脉和脏腑活动之需。而冲、任、督、带四脉，与女性生殖功能有密切关系，其中又以冲、任二脉最为重要。

5.3.1 The Thoroughfare Vessel

The Thoroughfare Vessel originates from the uterus and moves together with the kidney meridian to the lower abdomen and upward along the navel. It is the region where qi and blood converge, that is why it is called "sea of the twelve meridians", "sea of blood" and "sea of five zang and six fu organs". When woman is well developed, the Thoroughfare Vessel will be abundant in content and qi and blood from the viscera will flow into the uterus to produce menstruation. The Thoroughfare Vessel moves upward to connect with the stomach meridian at Qichong (ST 30). So it also governs the production of milk. It is obvious that the Thoroughfare Vessel is closely related to menstruation, pregnancy and lactation in women.

5.3.1 冲脉

起于胞中，并足少阴肾经，经下腹部，夹脐上行，为十二经气血汇聚之所，故被称之为"十二经之海""血海"，又称为"五脏六腑之海"。女性在身体发育成熟后，冲脉太盛，脏腑气血下注血海，血海满溢而为月经。冲脉上行出于足阳明经的气冲穴，与胃的经脉相通，同司乳汁的生化。因此，冲脉在女性的生理中，与月经、妊娠、乳汁生化等均有密切关系。

5.3.2 The Conception Vessel

The Conception Vessel starts from the uterus, moving out from perineum and going upward along the middle line of abdomen to connect with all yin meridians on its pathway, the key of in meridian, termed "sea of yin meridians". The Conception Vessel governs essence, blood and body fluid of the human body. It is the base of pregnancy. That is why it governs pregnancy. The smooth circulation of qi and blood in the Conception Vessel, in combination

5.3.2 任脉

与冲脉同起于胞中，出于会阴，上至前阴沿腹部正中线上行，在循行过程中与各阴经相联系，为阴脉之总纲，故称"阴脉之海"。人体的精、血、津、液，都属任脉总司，又为妊养之本，故主胎孕。任脉通畅，与冲脉相协同，能导致月经来潮和受孕

with the Thoroughfare Vessel, is responsible for menstruation and pregnancy.

育胎。

5.3.3 The Governor Vessel

The Governor Vessel also starts from the uterus, moving out from the perineum and going posteriorly upward along the middle line of the spine to the vertex. On its pathway, it links with the spinal cord, brain and all yang meridians. So it is called "the sea of yang meridians". Its branch moves anteriorly and posteriorly from the genitals. The anterior branch is connected with the Conception Vessel from Changqiang (GV 1) and the posterior branch is connected with the kidney meridian at the end of sacrum and continues to move upward in the spine. The Thoroughfare, Conception and Governor Vessels all start from the uterus, the Thoroughfare Vessel is the sea of blood and the Conception Vessel governs uterus and fetus. The Governor Vessel controls all yang meridians and the Conception Vessel controls all yin meridians, communicating with yin and yang, regulating qi and blood, to maintain normal conditions of menstruation, pregnancy, delivery and lactation.

5.3.3 督脉

亦起于胞中，出于会阴，向后循脊柱正中线上行，至巅顶。在循行过程中，与脊髓、脑与各阳经经脉联系，是阳经经脉的总纲，又称"阳脉之海"。其别络循阴器而分行前后，前行者自长强走任脉与任脉并，其后行者在骶首端与少阴会，并脊里上行，其气通于肾。冲、任、督三脉皆起于胞中，冲为血海、任主胞胎，又主一身之阴，督主一身之阳，沟通阴阳，调摄气血，共同正常维持经、孕、产、乳。

5.3.4 The Belt Vessel

The Belt Vessel starts from the hypochondria and moves around the waist like a belt. Its function is to control the meridians moving upward and downward so as to strengthen the connections of meridians. It is significantly related to the Thoroughfare, Conception and Governor Vessels which all start from the uterus, together constituting a system in direct relation with the physiological functions of woman. Such a system, in cooperation with the activities of the viscera, not only influences menstrua-

5.3.4 带脉

起于季肋之端，环绕腰部一周，如带束腰，故称为带脉。它的作用是约束全身上走下行的经脉，加强经脉间的联系。其中与冲、任、督三脉的联系更为密切。带脉与冲、任、督三脉相通，而三脉皆出于胞中，这样就使冲、任、督、带四脉共同构成与女性生理功能有直接关系的一个系统。

menstruation, profuse menorrhea, metrorrhagia and metrostaxis, reddish leukorrhea, uterine bleeding during pregnancy and lochiorrhea and so on. Because of yin-blood depletion, vacuity heat harassing the inner body, some women's liver wind stirs internally, or extreme heat engendering wind resulting in their epilepsy in pregnancy and so on.

内动，或热极生风而发生妊娠痫证等。

1.1.3 Dampness

Dampness is either exogenous or endogenous. Exogenous dampness has something to do with climate environment, such as staying in wet environment, walking in the rain or working in water for a long time; the main cause of endogenous dampness is spleen and stomach weakness, abnormal moving and transforming function, water-damp collecting internally, spreading Conception and Belt Vessels. This diseases of damp nature are mostly caused by endogenous dampnese clinically.

Dampness is a pathogenic factor of yin nature. It is heavy, turbid, greasy and stagnant by nature, difficult to be eliminated, tending to stagnate qi. Dampness tends to mix up with other pathogenic factors. It may mix up with heat or transform into heat due to stagnation, leading to damp-heat; it may mix up with cold and produce cold-dampness; it may accumulate into phlegm and cause phlegm-dampness. If damp-heat attacks qi and blood or damages the Thoroughfare and Conception Vessels, it will lead to profuse menorrhea, metrorrhagia and metrostaxis as well as lochiorrhea; when it attacks the Conception and Belt Vessels or the liver meridian, it may lead to leukorrhagia and pudendal pruritus. If cold-dampness attacks the Thoroughfare and Conception Vessels, it stagnates qi and

1.1.3 湿

有外湿和内湿之分。外湿与气候环境有关，如久处雾露潮湿之地，长时间冒雨涉水，或水中劳作过久；内湿则多因脾胃功能虚弱，运化功能失常，水湿内停，浸淫任、带二脉。湿邪致病临床上以内湿为多。

湿为阴邪，其性重浊黏腻缠绵，易于阻滞气机，日久难去，易从热化、寒化，或湿聚成痰或兼感邪毒成湿毒。如积久化热，则为湿热；与寒相结，则为寒湿；湿聚生痰，则为痰湿，如湿热搏于气血或伤于冲任，则可发生月经过多、崩漏、恶露不绝；伤于任带或肝经，则可发生带下、阴痒。寒湿伤及冲任，凝滞气血，可导致痛经、闭经、不孕；痰湿阻滞冲任，则引起闭经、带下、不孕等。

blood, leading to dysmenorrhea, amenorrhea and sterility. When phlegm-dampness stagnates in the Thoroughfare and Conception Vessels, it may lead to amenorrhea, leukorrhea and sterility, etc.

Wind is the leading factor in causing diseases. Wind is either endogenous or exogenous. Exogenous wind, one of the six exogenous pathogenic factors, often combines with other pathogenic factors to cause diseases, such as wind-cold and wind-heat. Wind pertains to yang and tends to change. In gynecology, wind often mixes up with cold to damage the Thoroughfare and Conception Vessels and causes various diseases. Clinically gynecological diseases due to wind and cold attacking qi and blood as well as damaging the Thoroughfare and Conception Vessels are also commonly encountered. Endogenous wind refers to a series of symptoms during the course of a disease, such as tremor of limbs, convulsion, dizziness, distorted face, coma and abnormal sensation of skin that are caused by dysfunction of the viscera, adverse flow of qi and blood or deficiency of liver blood. Such symptoms are known as interior disturbance of liver wind, interior stirring of wind or generation of wind due to blood asthenia, often presenting dizziness during pregnancy, premonitory signs of eclampsia gravidarum and eclampsia gravidarum as well as numbness of limbs and formication on the skin and pudendal pruritus during menopause.

其他如风为百病之长，有外风和内风之分。外风为六淫之一，常与其他病邪结合而致病，如风寒、风热等。风邪在妇科致病，常与寒邪相结合，损伤冲任而为病。临床上由于风寒搏于气血，损伤冲任，引起的妇科病亦属常见。内风，是指病变中出现的肢体震颤、抽搐、眩晕、口眼㖞斜、昏厥以及皮肤感觉异常等一类证候，是疾病发展过程中脏腑功能失调、气血逆乱或肝血亏虚所引起的，称为肝风内动、风气内动或血虚生风。常见妊娠眩晕、先兆子痫、绝经期诸证出现的肢体发麻、皮肤蚁行感、阴痒等。

1.2 Damage by seven emotional factors

Seven emotions refer to joy, anger, anxiety, contemplation, sorrow, fright and terror, and are human spiritual and emotional changes which reflect objective external things. Excessive changes of sev-

1.2 内伤七情

七情是指喜、怒、忧、思、悲、恐、惊，是人体对客观外界事物反映的精神情志变化。若突然、强烈、长期的刺

properly rest but also take appropriate activities and avoid over leisure, because over leisure affects the circulation of qi and blood and gives rise to the occurrence of various diseases. And therefore to do some proper physical work is beneficial to health.

逸则气血运行不畅，也易产生疾病。因此，在不影响健康的情况下，参加一定的劳动，对身体是有益的。

1.3.3 Frequent loss of pregnancy and birth

1.3.3 孕产屡殒

Frequent and excessive birth or sexual activity during menstruation or after delivery tends to consume qi and blood, impair the liver and kidney as well as damage the Thoroughfare and Conception Vessels, consequently leading to menstruation disorders, leukorrhea problems, abortion, premature delivery and prolapse of uterus. Early marriage, pregnancy, labor and abortion not only impairs the physique of gravida, but also affects the healthy development of the next generation. So proper sexual life and family planning are important measures for preventing woman diseases.

妇女生育过多、过频，或经期产后不禁性生活，易耗伤气血，伤及肝肾，损伤冲任，是引起月经病、带下病、流产、早产、子宫脱垂等的原因之一。特别是早婚、孕产堕胎，不仅影响产妇的体质，而且影响下一代的健康成长。所以，适度、适时地过好性生活，节制产育，也是预防妇产科病的重要措施。

In addition, various ovulation-inducing drugs of human assisted reproductive technology have different degrees of impact to endocrine environments and can lead to qi-blood and yin-yang disharmony, resulting in irregular menstruation.

另外，人类辅助生殖中各种促排卵药对人体内分泌环境有不同程度的影响，可导致人体气血失和、阴阳失衡出现月经不调。

2 Pathogenesis

2 病机

Menstruation, pregnancy, delivery, lactation and leukorrhea are all related to the viscera and meridians. Thus, visceral dysfunction, disorder of qi and blood, as well as damage to the Thoroughfare Vessel, Conception Vessel, Governor Vessel and Belt Vessel due to invasion of pathogenic factors may all lead to gynecological diseases.

女性的经、孕、产、乳、带，与脏腑、经络相关。因此，致病因素的侵袭而导致脏腑功能的失常，气血的失调，或冲、任、督、带的损伤，都可以发生妇科疾病。

2.1 Dysfunction of the viscera

2.1 脏腑功能失常

Blood, essential to the health of woman, is

女性以血为本。血生化

transformed by the spleen and stomach, governed by the heart, stored in the liver, drained by kidney and distributed by the lung to the whole body. The disorder of one viscus or the attack of any pathogenic factors on the viscera may lead to woman diseases.

于脾胃，总属于心，储藏于肝，宣布于肺，施泄于肾。如某一脏或腑的功能失常，或某种致病因素影响脏腑功能，都可以引起妇科疾病。

The kidney is essential to life, the base of primordial qi and connected with the uterine collaterals. Insufficiency of kidney qi or asthenia of kidney yin or declination of kidney yang inevitably affects Thoroughfare and Conception Vessels and leads to woman diseases. Deficiency of kidney yin and asthenia of both essence and blood cause delayed menstruation, scanty menstruation or amenorrhea. Relative hyperactivity of asthenia fire will drive blood to flow abnormally, eventually resulting in early menstruation, profuse menstruation, metrorrhagia and metrostaxis, threatened abortion and fetal irritability. Blood dryness due to heat may bring about amenorrhea. Insufficiency of kidney yang will lead to interior exuberance of cold, giving rise to sterility, leukorrhagia, abortion and premature delivery, etc.

肾为生命之本，元气之根，胞脉又系于肾。如肾气不足，或肾阴亏损，或肾阳衰微，均能影响冲任而发生妇科疾病。肾阴不足，精血双亏，则可导致月经后期、经量过少或闭经；或虚火偏亢，热迫血行，可导致月经先期、经量过多、崩漏、胎漏和胎动不安等病；热灼血枯，又可引起闭经。肾阳不足，阴寒内盛，可导致不孕、带下、流产、早产等妊娠疾病。

The liver prefers free action and detests stagnation. Liver qi stagnation may lead to delayed menstruation, irregular menstruation, dysmenorrhea, amenorrhea and various symptoms before menstruation. Deficiency of liver yin and hyperactivity of liver yang generate endogenous wind and lead to eclampsia gravidarum. Impairment of the liver by anger and upflaming of stagnant fire may drive liver qi to flow adversely upward and lead to hematemesis and epistaxis. Attack of liver qi on the stomach may bring about morning sickness.

肝性喜条达而恶抑郁，如肝郁气结，可发生月经后期、月经先后无定期、痛经、闭经、经前期诸证等；肝阴不足，肝阳偏亢，肝风内动，可引起子痫；怒气伤肝，郁火上炎，肝气上逆，血随气逆，可发生经行吐衄；肝气犯胃，胃失和降，可引起妊娠恶阻。

The spleen (stomach) is the source of transformation and commands blood. Impairment of the spleen and stomach and insufficiency in transforming source may result in delayed menstruation, scanty menstruation, amenorrhea, sterility and hypogalactia. Asthenia of spleen qi in its commanding ability may cause abnormal circulation of blood and lead to profuse menstruation and metrorrhagia and metrostaxis. Sinking of gastrosplenic qi may result in prolapse of the uterus. Failure of spleen yang in transporting nutrient substances may give rise to dampness accumulation, fluid retention, production of phlegm and downward migration of dampness, in turn, leading to leukorrhagia. Retention of fluid in the muscular interstices causes edema during pregnancy. Accumulation of dampness into phlegm obstructs the Thoroughfare and Conception Vessels and leads to amenorrhea and sterility.

脾(胃),为生化之源,又主统血。脾胃损伤,化源不足,可导致月经后期、经量过少、闭经、不孕、乳汁缺乏等病证;脾气虚弱,统摄无权,致使血不循经,则可发生月经过多、崩漏等病;中气下陷,则可发生子宫脱垂;脾阳不运,不能输布精微,则聚湿、停水、生痰;湿邪下注任带,则可发生带下;水停肌腠,可发生妊娠水肿;湿聚生痰,阻滞冲任,则可导致闭经、不孕等病证。

Besides, the heart governs blood. Overstrain of the heart may lead to deficiency of heart yin, hyperactivity of heart fire and consumption of blood by fire and heat, eventually resulting in amenorrhea. Asthenia of pulmonary qi or obstruction of pulmonary qi affects blood circulation and causes amenorrhea.

此外,心主血,如因劳心过度,致心阴不足,心火偏亢,火热耗血,可致闭经。肺主气,贯心脉而运血。如肺气虚损,或气不宣通,亦能影响血的运行而致闭经。

Since there exist relations of mutual promotion, restraint and dependence among the viscera, the disorder of one viscus may involve the others. For example, liver is being promoted by the kidney, so kidney disease may involve the liver. Similarly the kidney is being promoted by the lung, the disorder of the lung will involve the kidney, leading to disorder simultaneously involving the liver and kidney as well as the lung and kidney. Besides, there exists a

由于脏腑之间有五行生克制化的相互依存、相互制约的关系,因而在某一脏或腑受病时,由于这种联系而相互影响。例如,因肝为肾之子,肾病可以通过相生的关系而影响到肝;同样,肾为肺之子,肺病亦可以通过相生的关系而影响到肾,形成

mutual promoting relationship between yin and yang among the zangfu-organs. Because of such a relationship, the disorder of one zang-organ or fu-organ may affect the other. For example, failure of kidney-yang in warming spleen-yang and failure of kidney-yin in coordinating with heart-yin may result in simultaneous disorder of the spleen and kidney as well as the heart and kidney. The disorders of viscera caused by other individual organs also follow such an order. Such an interaction among the viscera is different in principal and secondary symptoms, so the pathological conditions may vary from one disease to another.

肝肾、肺肾同病。此外，脏腑之间还有阴阳水火相承相济的关系，也可以在某脏或腑受病时，由于这种联系而相互影响。如脾可因肾阳不温脾阳、心可因肾阴不得上济心阴而为脾肾、心肾同病。其他各脏以此类推。脏腑之间的影响还有标本缓急，其具体病理则随有关病症而有不同。

Apart from the influence of mutual promotion and restraint among the viscera, visceral dysfunction may be gradually transmitted and change during the course of a disease. For example, improper diet, overstrain or impairment of the spleen by excessive contemplation may affect the functions of the spleen in its abilities of transformation, transportation and distribution, leading to abdominal fullness, epigastric distress, loose stool and severe palpitation followed by poor appetite. Asthenia of both the spleen and stomach, insufficiency of transformation and emptiness in the sea of blood, eventually resulting in amenorrhea. If both the spleen and stomach are deficient, the lung fails in its nourishing ability, qi is exhausted in the upper body, and essence is deficient in the lower body, the problems arc critical. The disorder or dysfunction of any viscus will consequently result in abnormal changes in menstruation, leukorrhea, pregnancy and delivery. However, the disorder or dysfunction of viscera that is most likely to cause woman diseases is that of the kidney,

脏腑功能失常，除有生克制化关系之外，还能在发病过程中逐步传变。例如，饮食劳倦或忧思伤脾，使运化、输布功能失常，始则腹满便溏，食少脘闷，继则心悸怔忡，脾胃俱虚，化源不足，血海无余，则月经不行；脾胃皆虚，肺失滋养，气竭于上，精亏于下，病则危矣。任何一脏或一腑的功能失常，最终都有可能造成经、带、孕、产的病态，但是关系最为密切的，最易或较常导致妇科疾病的是肾、肝、脾三脏的功能失常。

heart, liver and spleen.

2.2 Disorder of qi and blood

Blood is essential to woman and is easy to be consumed during menstruation, pregnancy, delivery and breastfeeding, eventually leading to relative hyperactivity of qi due to deficiency of blood. So the invasion of pathogenic factors is likely to affect qi and blood and cause diseases. For example, invasion of exogenous pathogenic heat or excessive intake of pungent and hot foods tends to generate heat, the struggle between heat and blood drives blood to flow abnormally and lead to such problems as early menstruation, profuse menstruation, metrorrhagia and metrostaxis, hematemesis and epistaxis during menstruation, abortion and puerperal fever. Invasion of exogenous pathogenic cold or excessive intake of cold and uncooked foods generates cold, the struggle between cold and blood coagulates blood and leads to delayed menstruation, dysmenorrhea, amenorrhea, puerperal abdominal pain, abdominal mass and sterility, etc. Invasion of exogenous pathogenic dampness, or dampness due to spleen asthenia, accumulation of dampness into phlegm and struggle between damp-heat and blood in the meridians and collaterals may bring about leukorrhagia, amenorrhea and sterility, etc. Transformation of heat from dampness retention and struggle between accumulated damp-heat and blood may result in profuse menstruation, yellowish vaginal discharge and multi-colored vaginal discharge. Dampness accumulation and fluid retention in the muscular interstices may cause edema during menstruation. Besides, blood asthenia due to prolonged duration of disease, dysfunction of the viscera and insufficiency of trans-

2.2 气血失调

女性以血为本，经、孕、产、乳期间又易于耗血，致使其处于血不足而气偏盛的状态。因此一旦遭受病邪的侵袭，气血容易受损而为病，如外感热邪或过食辛热容易生热，热搏于血，迫血妄行，可致月经先期、经量过多、崩漏、经行吐衄、流产、产后发热等。外感寒邪或过食生冷寒凉，寒搏于血，血为寒凝，运行不畅，可致月经后期、痛经、闭经、产后腹痛、癥瘕、不孕等。外感湿邪，或脾虚生湿，湿聚生痰，湿痰与血相结，阻滞经脉，可为白带、闭经、不孕等；或湿郁化热，湿热蕴结，与血相搏，可致月经过多、黄带、赤白带；湿聚水停，浸渍肌腠，可致妊娠水肿。另外，久病或多产伤血，或脏腑功能失常，生化之源不足而致血虚，可引起月经后期、经量过少、痛经、闭经、不孕、乳汁缺乏等，都是血分病变所常见的。

formation may give rise to delayed menstruation, scanty menstruation, dysmenorrhea, amenorrhea, sterility and hypogalactia, etc.

Other factors responsible for profuse menstruation, metrorrhagia and metrostaxis as well as hematemesis and epistaxis are consumption of qi by pathogenic heat and abnormal flow of blood due to leakage of qi caused by heat. Invasion of pathogenic cold stagnates qi and blood, consequently leading to oligomenorrhea, dysmenorrhea and amenorrhea. Invasion of pathogenic dampness prevents qi from normal flowing and results in swelling and distension during pregnancy.

其他如热邪伤气，热则气泄，气泄则血亦随之而泄，可致月经过多、崩漏、经行吐衄。寒邪伤气，寒则气收，气收则闭而不通，血亦随之阻滞，可致月经量少、痛经、闭经。湿邪伤气，阻滞气机，亦可致妊娠肿胀等。

Seven emotional factors often cause upward flow of qi, slack flow of qi, exhaustion of qi, sinking of qi, disorder of qi, stagnation of qi and consumption of qi, and impair the viscera and cause various woman diseases. Qi commands and controls blood. Consumption of qi due to prolonged illness or overstrain leads to profuse menstruation, early menstruation, metrorrhagia and metrostaxis as well as abortion. If qi collapses due to deficiency and fails to hold the viscera in the original position, it may induce prolapse of the uterus and other problems.

七情所伤，常导致气上、气缓、气消、气下、气乱、气结、气耗等，损伤脏腑功能，亦可引起妇科疾病。气又帅血、摄血。如久病或劳倦伤气，可致月经过多、月经提前、崩漏、流产；如气虚下陷，不能升举内在脏器，可致子宫脱垂等病证。

2.3 Impairment of the thoroughfare, conception, governor and belt vessels

2.3 冲、任、督、带损伤

Impairment of the Thoroughfare, Conception and Governor Vessels is the main pathological change in gynecological diseases. The Thoroughfare Vessel is the sea of blood and is closely related to menstruation. The Conception Vessel is responsible for providing nutrition during pregnancy and is closely related to pregnancy. The Governor Vessel governs yang and is connected with the Conception

冲、任、督、带的损伤，是妇科病的主要病理变化，冲为血海，与月经关系密切相关。任主妊养，与孕育密切相关。督司诸阳，与任脉循环往复，共同维持脉气阴阳的相对平衡，与孕育亦有关系。带脉约束诸脉，与冲、

Vessel. Altogether they maintain a relative balance between yin and yang and are responsible for pregnancy. The Belt Vessel manages all the meridians and regulates the reproductive system together with the Thoroughfare, Conception and Governor Vessels. The disorder of the Thoroughfare Vessel may lead to irregular menstruation, metrorrhagia and metrostaxis, amenorrhea and abortion. The disorder of the Conception Vessel may result in leukorrhagia due to downward migration of fluid, sterility due to malnutrition during pregnancy and abdominal mass due to stagnation of qi and blood. The disorder of the Governor Vessel may affect the function of yang-qi and cause sterility. The disorder of the Belt Vessel may bring about leukorrhagia and prolapse of the uterus. The impairment of these meridians may be direct or indirect.

任、督共同调节生殖系统的功能。冲脉受病，血海蓄溢失常，可发生月经失调、崩漏、闭经、流产等。任脉受病，或致阴液不固而为带下，或妊养失司而为不孕，或气血积滞而为癥瘕。督脉为病，阳气失调，可致不孕。带脉为病，约束无权，可致带下、子宫脱垂等。导致这些经脉损伤的原因，可为间接损伤，也可为直接损伤。

Indirect impairment is caused by disorder of the viscera, qi or blood. For example, insufficiency of kidney qi and deficiency of the Thoroughfare Vessel may lead to primary amenorrhea. Migration of dampness due to spleen asthenia into the Conception and Belt Vessels may result in leukorrhea and pudendal pruritus. Weakness of the Thoroughfare and Conception Vessels due to qi asthenia and sinking may bring about profuse menstruation, metrorrhagia and metrostaxis as well as prolapse of the uterus. Abnormal flow of blood due to heat and weakness of the Thoroughfare and Conception Vessels may cause profuse menstruation, metrorrhagia and metrostaxis, etc.

由脏腑或气血功能失常，影响冲、任、督、带功能的，为间接损伤。如肾气未充，冲任未盛，可致原发性闭经；脾虚生湿，湿注任带，任带不固，可致带下、阴痒；气虚下陷，冲任不固，可致月经过多、崩漏、子宫脱垂；血热妄行，冲任不固，可致月经过多、崩漏等病证。

Improper sterilization during delivery, abortion and vaginal operation, or lack of proper care or sexual activity during menstruation and after delivery

由于分娩、流产或阴道手术时消毒不严，或经期、产后不洁，或不禁房事，以致病

may lead to invasion of pathogenic factors into the uterus and result in such problems as irregular menstruation, dysmenorrhea, puerperal fever, lochiorrhea, leukorrhea, abdominal mass and sterility, as the direct impairment of the Thoroughfare and Conception Vessels. Generally speaking, only direct or indirect impairment of the Thoroughfare, Conception, Governor and Belt Vessels, especially the Thoroughfare and Conception Vessels, can lead to disorders of menstruation, leukorrhagia, pregnancy and delivery.

邪乘虚侵袭,发生诸如月经不调、痛经、产后发热、恶露不尽、带下、癥瘕、不孕等,均可视为冲任的直接损伤。一般来说,只有在直接或间接损伤冲、任、督、带,特别是损伤冲、任二脉的情况下,才会发生经、带、胎、产等妇女特有的疾病。

Though the diseases caused by dysfunction of the viscera, disorders of qi and blood as well as impairment of the Thoroughfare, Conception, Governor and Belt Vessels are different in pathogenesis, they also affect each other in pathogenesis. So in the analysis of diseases, it is necessary to determine which organs or meridians are invaded by pathogenic factors and whether qi or blood is impaired, and also to analyze the interaction between them. Such a comprehensive analysis is essential to recognizing the nature and giving proper treatment in accordance with the pathological change.

脏腑功能失常,气血失调,冲、任、督、带损伤,虽各有不同的病机,但它们之间又可互相影响。因此,无论病变起于任何经脉、任何脏腑,还是在气、在血,其病理反应总是有关联的。所以在分析病情的时候,既要了解病邪侵入何经何脉,病变在何脏何腑,是伤气还是伤血,更要了解它们的相互关系,才能从复杂的证候中抓住实质,视病情转变,遵从病证而进行治疗。

Chapter 2 Diagnostic methods, key points for syndrome differentiation and therapeutical principles of gynecological diseases

第2章 妇科疾病的中医诊断方法、辨证要点与治疗原则

Generally, the diagnostic methods for gynecological diseases are similar to those for the diseases in internal medicine, by using the four diagnostic methods and syndrome differentiation. The general conditions of the patient are studied first with the four diagnostic methods. Then the cause and location of disease, the relation between the pathogenic factors and healthy qi as well as the development and variation of the principal and secondary aspects of disease can be figured out by analysis and judgement of the changes in menstruation, leucorrhea, fetus and labor, with the relavant concepts of pathogenic factors, Zangfu organs, qi and blood, meridians and pathogenesis, in order to make correct diagnosis. The diagnosis and syndrome differentiation in gynecology mainly focus on the aspects of menstruation, leukorrhea, pregnancy and delivery of child.

妇科病的诊断方法一般与内科相同，运用四诊和辨证，但又有一定的特点。总的来说，就是通过四诊掌握疾病的全部征象，然后运用有关病因、脏腑、气血、经络、病机等概念，结合经、带、胎、产的变化进行分析、判断，寻找出疾病的病因、病位和正邪消长、标本传变等变化，做出正确的诊断。妇科病的四诊和辨证，着重于有关经、带、胎、产的四诊和辨证特点。

Section 1 Diagnostic methods

第1节 诊断方法

1 Inspection

1.1 Complexion

Pale or bright-whitish complexion indicates qi asthenia or yang asthenia. Sallow complexion indicates blood asthenia or spleen asthenia. Grayish complexion or blackish periorbit indicates decline of kidney qi. Blackish spots on the forehead, nose bridge and upper lip are known as pregnant macules, not pathological.

1.2 Lips and tongue

Bright-reddish color indicates asthenia heat. Light-reddish color indicates blood asthenia. Purplish color or petechiae on the tongue indicates blood stasis; and light, tender and blackish color indicates yang asthenia.

1.3 Menstruation, leukorrhea and lochia

Cares should be taken to differentiate the changes in the quantity, color and nature.

2 Auscultation and olfaction

It includes listening to sound and smelling odors. Listening to voice is the same as that in the other clinical specialties. To smell odor is mainly for understanding the special odor of menses, leukorrhea and lochia, so as to confirm what the patient has described.

3 Inquiry

Inquiry in gynecology includes the following aspects.

3.1 Inquiry for age

Age should be inquired at patient's first visit.

1 望诊

1.1 面色

苍白或㿠白为气虚或阳虚;萎黄为血虚或脾虚;灰暗或眶暗多为肾气虚衰。妊娠期前额、鼻柱、上唇出现暗色斑点,称妊娠斑,不是病态。

1.2 唇、舌

色鲜红为虚热,淡红为血虚,紫暗或舌有瘀点为内有瘀血,舌淡胖为阳虚。

1.3 月经、白带及恶露

应注意量、色、质的改变。

2 闻诊

闻诊包括听声音和嗅气味。听声音与临床各科相同。嗅气味主要是了解月经、白带、恶露的特殊臭气。用以证实患者自述的情况。

3 问诊

妇科问诊必须包括以下内容。

3.1 问年龄

初诊时首先要问年龄。

Women in different ages are different in the physiological conditions and pathogenesis. Dysmenorrhea, metrorrhagia and metrostaxis are frequently-occurring diseases in adolescent women. Women in childbearing age may suffer from pelvic inflammatory diseases more likely. Menopause syndrome is a frequently-occurring disease in perimenopausal women.

不同年龄的妇女，生理状况亦有不同，发病机制也各异，青少年妇女多发痛经、崩漏，育龄妇女多发盆腔炎性疾病、不孕症，围绝经期妇女多发绝经综合征等。

3.2 Inquiry for menstruation

Inquiry for menstruation includes age of menarche, cycle, duration, quantity, color and nature of menstruation, whether there is blood clot and foul odor, whether there are such symptoms like distension and pain in the lower abdomen, waist and sacrum, chest and hypochondria as well as breast before and during menstruation, the date of last menstruation and the date of menstruation before the last period in necessity, whether there are dizziness, lassitude, nausea, vomiting and partiality in food as well as distension and pain in the waist, sacrum and lower abdomen in the case of amenorrhea.

3.2 问月经

必须问初潮年龄、周期、经期、经量、经色及经质，有无血块及异味。经前、经期、经后有无下腹、腰骶、胸胁、乳房作胀或疼痛，有无经期以外的出血，末次月经的日期，必要时应追询末次月经的前一次月经的日期。如系停经，应问停经时间，有无头晕、倦怠、恶心、呕吐、择食等症状以及腰骶、下腹胀痛等伴随症状。

3.3 Inquiry for leukorrhea

Inquiry for leukorrhea includes quantity, color, thick or thin texture and odor of leukorrhea.

3.3 问白带

应问白带的多少、颜色、质清或稠、有无臭气等。

3.4 Inquiry for pregnancy and delivery

Inquiry for pregnancy and delivery includes whether there are pregnancy, delivery, abortion (including artificial abortion), times of delivery, the last deliver and abortion date, whether there are dystocia, operation, massive postpartum hemorrhage, lactation after delivery, puerperal fever and abdominal pain as well as the quantity, color, nature and odor of lochia, whether there is contraception and what kind of measures are taken, months

3.4 问胎孕

已婚妇女，应问是否妊娠、生育、流产（包括人工流产）和分娩次数，末次分娩及流产的日期。有无难产和手术史，有无产后大出血，产后有无乳汁，产后有无发热、腹痛以及恶露的量、色、气味等。是否采取避孕措施以及采用何种避孕方法。如是孕

or weeks of pregnancy and morning sickness as well as whether there are symptoms of edema, dizziness and headache in inquiring a pregnant woman.

妇应问妊娠月份或周数，恶阻情况，有无水肿、头晕、头痛等症状。

3.5 Inquiry for postpartum conditions

Inquiry for postpartum conditions includes whether the delivery is normal, bleeding amount during delivery, lochia amount, abdominal pain and whether bowel movement is smooth.

3.5 问产后

应问生产情况是否正常，产时出血多少，恶露多少，小腹有无胀痛，大便是否通畅。

3.6 Inquiry for life, occupation, hobby and family information

Inquiry for life, occupation, hobby and family information have reference value to the analysis of state of illness.

3.6 问生活、职业、嗜好以及家庭情况

充分了解对分析病情有参考价值。

4 Pulse taking

Normal pulse in woman is usually feebler and softer than that in man. In menstruation, leukorrhagia, pregnancy and delivery, there are some special pulse conditions.

4 切诊

女性正常脉通常弱于男性，脉象略沉静而柔软。在经、带、胎、产期间，也有一些常见的特殊脉象。

4.1 Menstruation pulse

Before or during menstruation, if pulse in the *cun* region is floating and full or floating and slippery without the symptoms of fever, headache and bitter taste in the mouth, it is normal pulse in menstruation. If the pulse is taut and rapid or slippery, rapid and powerful, it indicates accumulation of heat in the Thoroughfare and Conception Vessels, usually seen in early menstruation, profuse menstruation and metrorrhagia and metrostaxis. Deep and slow or thready and slow pulse indicates interior cold due to yang asthenia and insufficiency of the Thoroughfare and Conception Vessels, usually seen in delayed menstruation and scanty menstruation. Thready and scattered pulse indicates interior heat

4.1 月经脉

在月经将来或行经期，出现无身热、头痛、口苦等外感或里热现象，而寸脉浮洪或浮滑，是经期的常脉。如脉见弦数或滑数有力，常为冲任蕴热，可见月经先期、经量过多、崩漏等症；沉迟或细迟，常为阳虚内寒，冲任不足，可见月经后期、经量过少；脉细而散，多为阴虚内热，可见于月经量多、漏下淋漓；脉细而涩，多为肝肾两虚，精血不足，可见于经量过少、痛经；脉弦而涩，则为气

due to yin asthenia, usually seen in profuse menstruation and dripping vaginal bleeding. Thready and unsmooth pulse indicates asthenia of both the liver and kidney as well as deficiency of essence and blood, often seen in scanty menstruation and dysmenorrhea. Taut and unsmooth pulse indicates qi stagnation and blood stasis, frequently seen in delayed menstruation or dysmenorrhea. Thready and unsmooth pulse in amenorrhea without pregnancy indicates blood asthenia. Slippery and uneven pulse signifies blood sthenia and qi stagnation.

滞血瘀，可见于月经后期或痛经。经闭不行，若证实非孕，脉细而涩，多为血虚不足；脉滑而断续不匀，多为血实气滞。

4.2 Leukorrhea pulse

Profuse leukorrhea with taut and slippery or deep, rapid and forceful pulse may indicate internal accumulation of damp-heat. Slippery and powerful pulse may signify interior retention of phlegm-dampness. Deep and slow or weak pulse over the *chi* region on both hands may suggest insufficiency of kidney yang. Soft and slow pulse may be the sign of downward migration of pathogenic dampness due to spleen asthenia.

4.2 带下脉

白带过多，脉弦滑或沉数有力，应考虑湿热内蕴；滑大有力，要注意痰湿内停；两尺沉迟或微弱，多见肾阳不足；脉濡而缓，为脾虚湿邪下注。

4.3 Pregnancy pulse

Preference for sour taste and vomiting 2 or 3 months after amenorrhea, accompanied by moderate pulse conditions over the six regions, or with slippery *chi* pulse or slippery *cun* pulse, may suggest pregnancy. After pregnancy, deep and thready or short and unsmooth pulse over the six regions or weak pulse over the *chi* region may indicate deficiency of qi and blood or insufficiency of kidney qi, and cares should be taken to prevent abortion. Shanghai doctor He Shixi described his experiences of pregnancy pulse: Loose *cun* pulse, powerful *chi* pulse pulsing at fingers, taut, rapid and slippery

4.3 妊娠脉

停经二三月，思酸作呕，六脉平和，或尺脉滑利，或寸脉滑动，为有孕的脉象。怀孕以后，六脉沉细或短涩，或尺脉微弱，多为气血亏虚或肾气不足，应防流产。上海医家何时希描述对妊脉的体会：寸脉浮“动”、尺脉“搏”指，三部脉“弦”“数”“滑”，为常见的胎脉。如果微细无力，生气萧条，便是母体气血不足的症状，必须及早治疗，

pulse at three positions are common pregnancy pulse. Thready and weak qi is the symptom of maternal insufficiency of qi and blood, and it must be treated as early as possible lest affecting the growth of futus. For consistent thready, weak, short, deep and unsmooth pulse, atrophied fetus should be prevented. For deep, firm, faint and thready pulse, dead fetus should be prevented.

以免对胎儿成长有碍。若始终细弱短小脉,沉涩不畅,毫无活泼流利之象者,须防胎萎,若见沉、牢、微、细,须防死胎。

4.4 Pulse after delivery

The pulse just after delivery is usually short and immediately turning into moderate and smooth due to sudden asthenia of blood and predomination of yang-qi. If the pulse under such a condition is large, or accompanied by fever and headache, it indicates failed restoration of yin blood or invasion of exogenous pathogenic factors.

In general, the data collected by using the four diagnostic methods should be comprehensively analyzed in combination with color, pulse and syndrome in clinical treatment. For some special cases, syndrome differentiation has to be made according to the conditions of the pulse other than the syndrome or vice versa. These must be carefully judged in the clinical treatment.

4.4 产后脉

新产之初,因阴血骤虚,阳气偏盛,脉可偏数,但多短暂,后即转为缓和平脉。如反见大数,或兼有身热、头痛,常示阴血未复或感受外邪。

总之,在临证时,通常都应四诊合参,色、脉、证结合起来分析,但个别情况,也不排除舍脉从证或舍证从脉的辨证分析,而这些都应当在临证时仔细权衡。

Section 2 Key points for syndrome differentiation

第 2 节 辨证要点

1 Syndrome differentiation of menstruation disorders

The menstrual situations should be analyzed in accordance with the period, amount, color, quality

1 月经病的辨证

月经情况,应着重月经的期、量、色、质、气味以及下

breath or weak pulse is due to asthenia of both qi and blood. Vaginal bleeding accompanied by aching and weakness of loins and prolapsing sensation in the lower abdomen is due to kidney asthenia. Deep-red blood or accompanied by dysphoria, dry mouth and slippery-rapid pulse is due to blood heat. Morning sickness, vomiting, anorexia or slow, slippery and weak pulse are due to asthenia of spleen and stomach qi. Vomiting of bitter fluid or sour fluid, or accompanied by taut and slippery pulse is due to adverse flow of liver and stomach qi. Vomiting of sputum or saliva, distension or accompanied by soft and slippery pulse is due to retention of phlegm-dampness in the middle energizer. Edema or lassitude or epigastric distension, or accompanied by deep, slippery and weak pulse, is due to spleen asthenia. Aching in loins and sacrum or aversion to cold as well as deep or slow pulse are due to insufficiency of kidney yang. Dizziness, headache, blurred vision, chest distress and vomiting in the late stage of pregnancy are premonitory signs of eclampsia gravidarum and measures should be taken to prevent eclampsia gravidarum.

心烦口干或色红，脉滑数者，属血热。妊娠恶阻，呕吐厌食或脉缓滑无力者，多为脾胃气虚；呕吐苦水或酸水，或伴脉弦滑者，多为肝胃气逆；呕吐痰涎，作胀或兼脉濡滑者，为痰湿中阻。妊娠水肿或倦怠或脘胀，或兼脉沉滑无力者，属脾虚；兼见腰骶酸痛或畏寒怯冷，脉或沉迟者，属肾阳不足。妊娠晚期，出现头晕、头痛、眼花、胸闷作呕等，为先兆子痫，应积极处理，预防发展为子痫。

4　Syndrome differentiation of puerperal diseases

In the ancient times there were so called “three examinations” of puerperal diseases. The first is to examine whether there is pain in the lower abdomen, so as to decide whether there is lochiostasis. The second is to examine whether defecation is smooth, in order to make sure whether body fluid is sufficient or deficient. The third is to examine whether lactation is smooth or not and whether appetite is normal or abnormal for the purpose to check wheth-

4　产后病的辨证

凡孕妇产后，古有“三审”之说：一审下腹痛与不痛，以辨有无恶露停滞；二审大便通与不通，以验津液的盛衰；三审乳汁行与不行以及饮食多少，以查胃气的强弱。另外，还应注意恶露的量、色、质、气味，以及有无发热等。如恶露量多、秽臭，下

er gastric qi is sufficient or deficient. Besides, cares should be taken to examine the quantity, texture, color and odor of lochia as well as whether there is fever. Profuse lochia with foul odor, aggravated lower abdominal pain, or even fever, headache, thirst, reddish tongue with yellowish fur and full and rapid pulse are the signs of virulent heat invading the uterus and damaging the Thoroughfare and Conception Vessels. Scanty lochia lingering for days with purplish color and blood clot as well as aggravated lower abdominal pain are signs of blood stasis. Light-colored and thin lochia indicates insufficiency of qi and blood. Lack of milk after delivery, distension, hardness and pain of breast as well as poor appetite are signs of liver qi stagnation. Softness of breasts without distending pain and scanty and thin milk are due to asthenia of qi and blood.

腹疼痛拒按，甚或身热、头痛、渴欲饮冷、舌红、苔黄、脉洪数者，多为热毒直犯胞宫，损伤冲任。量少而多日不净，色紫暗，有小血块，下腹痛而拒按，多为瘀血停滞；色淡质清，多为气血不足。产后乳少，乳房胀硬而痛，胸胁胀满，胃纳不佳，多为肝气郁滞。如乳房柔软，无胀痛，乳汁少儿清稀，多为气血虚弱。

The characteristics of syndrome differentiation above are described according to the commonly encountered symptoms of menstruation, leukorrhagia, pregnancy and childbirth. In clinical application, syndrome differentiation must be done in view of the physical condition, vitality, complexion, pulse and general symptoms of the patient, with the four diagnostic methods and eight principles; and by synthetic analysis of the cause, viscera, qi, blood and meridians, in order to make precise conclusion.

以上辨证特点，是根据经、带、胎、产的常见证候来叙述的。临床应用时，还应结合患者的形、气、色、脉以及全身症状，运用四诊八纲的方法，通过对病因、脏腑、气血、经络等基本理论综合分析，做出准确的辨证结论。

Sectiom 3 Therapeutic principles for gynecological diseases

第3节 治疗原则

The therapeutic methods for gynecological dis-

妇科疾病的治法，与临

eases are basically the same as those for the diseases of other clinical specialties. Pathologically, the gynecological diseases are mainly related to the kidney, liver, spleen, stomach, qi and blood as well as the Thoroughfare and Conception Vessels. In terms of the causes, the gynecological diseases are usually caused by cold, heat, dampness and emotional factors. So therapeutically, it is necessary to differentiate between the exterior and interior, cold and heat, asthenia and sthenia as well as yin and yang in order to figure out whether the disease in question is due to the disorder of the kidney, liver, spleen, heart or qi and blood, and after the treatment by syndrome differentiation and actual situation for achieving the anticipated effects. Now, the commonly-used therapy modalities for the gynecological diseases are introduced in the following.

床其他各科基本相同，但由于妇科病的特殊病理反应主要集中在肾、肝、脾胃和气血、冲任等方面，而病因又以寒、热、湿及七情内伤等为多见，因此在治法上，也应根据四诊八纲，分清表里、寒热、虚实、阴阳，着重辨其属肾、属肝、属脾、属心和在气、在血，并按标本缓急进行辨证论治，方能收到应有的效果。现将妇科的集中常用治法介绍于下。

1　Regulating qi and blood

In the treatment of the gynecological diseases, the stress is focused on blood. Blood follows qi to flow, because menstruation, pregnancy, delivery and breast-feeding tend to consume blood and damage qi, eventually leading to dysfunction of qi and blood and further inducing the gynecological diseases. Blood is fundamental for women. So to regulate qi and blood is one of the main therapeutic methods used to treat the gynecological diseases. In syndrome differentiation, it must be necessary to figure out whether the diseases involves qi or blood and whether they are of cold or heat, or of asthenia or sthenia, as a basis to establish the methods. Qi and blood are mutually dependent and unseparable. Therefore, blood must be regulated simultaneously

1　调理气血

妇科病着重在血，血随气行，由于经、孕、产、乳易耗血伤气，使气血失调而引起疾病，妇女以血为本，因此调理气血为治疗妇科病的一个重要治法。惟在辨证时，必须分清病之在气、主血，属寒、属热，属虚、属实，以为立法的依据。气与血相互依存，不可分割，故调气必兼理血，理血必兼调气，但应各有侧重。病在气者，以调气为主，佐以理血，虚者补之，滞者行之，并佐以养血或活血。病在血者，以理血为主，并佐

in the regulation of qi, and qi must be regulated simultaneously in the regulation of blood, in particular stress respectively. If the disease mainly involves qi, the treatment focuses on regulating of qi, supplemented by balancing blood. The asthenia syndrome is treated by reinforcing therapy and the stagnation syndrome is treated by promoting therapy with the supplementation of nourishing blood or activating blood. If the disease mainly involves blood, the treatment mainly concentrates on regulating of blood with the supplementation of harmonizing qi. Blood asthenia syndrome is treated by supplementing blood and nourishing blood. Blood stasis is treated by activating blood and resolving stasis. Blood heat is treated by clearing away heat and cooling blood. Blood cold is treated by warming meridians to disperse cold. Massive bleeding or continuous bleeding is treated by astringing blood to stop bleeding. If diseases involve both qi and blood, they should be treated by proper application of the therapeutic methods mentioned above. For the asthenia of both qi and blood, it should be treated by nourishing both qi and blood. For the disorder of qi asthenia and blood stasis, it can be treated by supplementing qi, combined with by activating blood and resolving stasis. For the disorder of blood asthenia and qi stagnation, it may be treated by supplementing blood, combined with by regulating qi and dredging stagnancy. In such a way, the supplementation of asthenia will not lead to stagnation of pathogenic factors and the attack on pathogenic factors will not damage qi.

以调气,血虚者补血养血,血瘀者活血祛瘀,血热者清热凉血,血寒者温经散寒,出血多或日久不止者固涩止血。若气血同病,则宜参考上述方法,适当配合运用。如气血两虚者,则宜气血双补;气虚血瘀者,则宜于补气中佐以活血祛瘀;血虚气滞者,又当在补血中佐以理气行滞。如此,补虚而不致滞邪,攻邪也不致伤正,总之,以气血充盛和畅为度。

2 Harmonizing the stomach and fortifying the spleen

The spleen is the postnatal base of life and the source of qi and blood. The spleen manages transformation and transportation as well as commanding blood. The stomach that is internally and externally in relation with the spleen governs reception of food and is an organ with sufficient qi and blood. The Thoroughfare Vessel also pertains to Yangming meridian. Normal functions of the spleen and stomach in woman ensure sufficient blood in the uterus for normal menstruation and pregnancy. Dysfunction of the spleen and stomach, weakness in reception, transformation and transportation, may lead to either insufficiency of the source for transformation, or failure in commanding blood, or retention of dampness, which may further impair the Thoroughfare and Conception Vessels and lead to such disorders as irregular menstruation, metrorrhagia and metrostaxis, amenorrhea, leukorrhagia, morning sickness, edema during pregnancy and prolapse of uterus. So strengthening the spleen and harmonizing the stomach is also one of the important therapeutic methods in treating the gynecological diseases. Such a treatment is especially important for the treatment of menopausal syndrome in the aged women whose kidney qi has declined and both qi and blood have become asthenic. Since these women mainly depend on food nutrients, spleen-invigorating therapy for promoting transformation is essential to them. The general therapeutic principles are nourishing therapy for the asthenia syndrome, circulating therapy for the stagnation syndrome, warming therapy for

2 和胃健脾

脾为后天之本，气血生化之源，脾主运化，又主统摄；与之互为表里的胃又主受纳，为多气多血之腑，而冲脉又隶属于阳明。女性脾胃功能强健，则血海满而月经如期，胎孕正常；脾胃失调，受纳运化功能减弱，或致生化之源不足，或统摄无权，或水湿停滞，若进而损及冲任，则可导致月经失调、崩漏、闭经、带下、妊娠恶阻、妊娠水肿、子宫脱垂等病，故健脾和胃为妇科病的重要治法。尤其是绝经期女性在经断前后，肾气已衰，气血俱虚，全赖水谷滋养，此时补脾以资化源，就显得尤为重要。但具体治法，应本虚者补之、滞者行之、寒者温之、热者清之、陷者升之、逆者平之等施治原则，同时还应注意温寒无过于辛燥，清热无过于苦寒，养阴无过于滋腻，以免辛燥伤阴、滋腻伤阳或苦寒克伐而重伤脾胃。

the cold syndrome, clearing therapy for the heat syndrome, elevating therapy for the sinking syndrome and soothing therapy for the adverse syndrome. Cares should be taken to avoid using warming therapy with excessive acrid and dry herbs to treat cold syndrome, clearing therapy with excessive herbs of bitter taste and cold nature to treat heat syndrome and nourishing therapy with excessive tonic herbs to nourish yin lest yin be consumed by acridness and dryness, yang be damaged by tonic elements and the spleen be restrained by herbs of bitter taste and cold nature. Such errors in using herbs will all seriously impair the spleen and stomach.

The functions of the stomach and spleen in reception, digestion, transformation and transportation are in close relation with the conveyance of liver qi and warming function of kidney yang. Failure of the liver in conveyance and dispersion may affect the functions of the spleen in transformation and transportation and the function of the stomach in reception, leading to chest oppression, vomiting, epigastric and abdominal distension and hypochondriac distension and pain due to disharmony between the liver and spleen or disharmony between the liver and stomach. Such dysfunctions are commonly seen in irregular menstruation and morning sickness. Such disorders should be treated by soothing the liver, regulating the spleen or suppressing the liver and harmonizing the stomach. If fire in *Mingmen* (gate of life) declines and fails to warm the spleen to promote transformation and transportation, leading to diarrhea and edema during menstruation and edema during pregnancy or thin leukorrhagia, they should be treated by warming and

脾胃的受纳、腐熟、运化功能，与肝气的疏泄和肾阳的温煦作用有密切关系。如肝失疏泄，可以影响脾的运化或胃的受纳，出现胸闷纳呆、呕吐、脘腹作胀、两胁胀痛等肝脾不和或肝胃不和的症状，这在月经失调、妊娠恶阻中也是常见的。对此，又须疏肝理脾或抑肝和胃。再如命门火衰，不能暖脾以助运化，或有经行泄泻、经行浮肿，妊娠水肿或带下清稀者，又宜温补脾肾法。

nourishing the spleen and kidney.

The spleen and the heart are closely related to each other. The heart governs blood and the spleen produces blood, both of which depend on the spleen to transform and transport food nutrients. The function of heart yang in transporting blood in the meridians relies on the spleen qi to command. Insufficiency of transformation may lead to deficiency of heart blood, resulting in palpitation, insomnia, or scanty menstruation and amenorrhea. Failure of the spleen in commanding blood may lead to profuse menstruation, metrorrhagia and metrostaxis, which consume blood, and cause palpitation and insomnia. So asthenia of both the spleen and the heart is common in disorders of menstruation and should be treated by nourishing both the heart and the spleen.

脾与心也有密切联系。心主血，脾生血，赖脾之运化水谷精微；而心阳之运血行于脉中，亦须赖脾气之统摄。若化源不足，致心血衰少，发生怔忡、不寐，或见经少、经闭。若统摄无权，或致经多、崩漏，耗伤阴血，亦可见心悸失眠。故月经病心脾两虚者并非少见。对此，则又当治以补益心脾法。

3 Supplement kidney qi

The kidney is the prenatal base of life, source of reproduction and connected with the Thoroughfare and Conception Vessels. Only when kidney qi is sufficient in women, can menstruation come, the Conception Vessel be free in circulation and the Thoroughfare Vessel keep predominant. Such a condition is also essential to the physiological activities of menstruation, pregnancy, delivery and breastfeeding. Insufficiency of kidney qi or consumption of kidney yin or decline of kidney yang or asthenia of both yin and yang will prevent *Tiangui* from occurring or lead to senility and disturbance of the Thoroughfare and Conception Vessels, consequently resulting in disorders related to menstruation, leukorrhea, pregnancy, delivery and lactation. So kidney-invigorating method is the basic therapeu-

3 补益肾气

肾为先天之本，天癸之源，又主藏精气，是机体生长发育的动力。冲任之脉皆系于肾，女性肾气充沛，然后天癸至，任脉通，冲脉盛，才有经、孕、产、乳的生理功能活动。如肾气不足，或肾阴亏耗，或肾阳衰少，或阴阳俱虚，不能协调充盛，以致天癸不至或早竭，冲、任通盛失调，就能导致经、带、胎、产、乳等方面的疾病。所以，补肾应为妇科的根本治法，特别对肾气未充的青年女子尤为重要。其补益方法，则应根据病情，酌选温肾助阳、滋

tic method in treating the gynecological diseases, especially for the treatment of young woman whose kidney qi is not sufficient yet. In the application of kidney-invigorating methods, it is necessary to choose the methods of warming kidney to reinforce yang, nourishing kidney to enrich yin, fostering yin to suppress yang or nourishing both yin and yang according to the pathological conditions.

肾养阴、育阴潜阳、阴阳双补等法。

The kidney and the liver are all located in the lower energizer. The kidney essence and liver blood share the same origin. So kidney yin deficiency can nourish liver yin and prevent liver yang from becoming hyperactive. Liver blood and kidney essence are closely related to menstruation, pregnancy, delivery and breast-feeding. Clinically deficiency of kidney yin may lead to asthenia of both liver and kidney yin, eventually resulting in irregular menstruation or even amenorrhea and menopausal syndrome. Deficiency of kidney yin fails to nourish wood and leads to hyperactivity of liver fire, consequently bringing about profuse menstruation, metrorrhagia and metrostaxis, or even dizziness during menstruation due to liver yang transforming into wind. Failure of the liver to convey and disperse may lead to consumption of yin by stagnant fire with the involvement of the kidney, frequently resulting in liver stagnation and kidney asthenia, which bring about scanty menstruation, delayed menstruation, amenorrhea and dysmenorrhea. Such disorders should be treated by regulating both the liver and the kidney.

肾与肝同居下焦，肾精与肝血有乙癸同源、相互资生的关系，由于有这种“精血同源”“肝肾同源”的相互联系，所以肾阴虚可以滋养肝阴，使肝阳不至于亢奋。肝血、肾精与经、孕、产、乳有直接关系，临床上有因肾阴不足，导致肝肾阴虚，或见月经不调，乃至闭经，或经断前后诸证；或因肾阴不足，水不涵木，致肝火偏旺，见月经过多、崩漏，甚而肝阳化风，出现经行眩晕；亦有因肝失疏泄，郁火伤及肾阴而致肝郁肾虚，常见月经过少、月经后期、闭经、痛经等，这些均宜肝肾共同进行调治。

The kidney and heart also have a relationship of mutual coordination. The heart fire interacts downward with the kidney to warm and nourish kid-

肾与心也有相互协调的关系，心火下交于肾，以温养肾阳，肾水上济与心，以滋养

ney yang. The kidney water connects upward with the heart to enrich and nourish heart yin. The kidney yang and kidney yin move up and down mutually and keep a relative balance. The kidney yin depletion and heart fire preponderance may lead to vexation, palpitation, insomnia, flushed cheeks, tidal heat sensation and night sweating due to fire hyperactivity of yin deficiency and non-interaction of the heart and kidney. These symptoms are frequently seen in metrorrhagia and metrostaxis, amenorrhea and menopausal syndrome. Such disorders could be treated clinically by the methods of enriching yin and reducing fire.

心阴。在正常情况下，肾阳和肾阴相互升降，上下交通，保持相对平衡，也即是所谓的“水火既济”，从而达到“阴平阳秘”。如肾阴亏损，或心火炽盛，就会出现阴虚火旺的心烦、怔忡、失眠、潮红、潮热、盗汗等心肾不交证候，这在崩漏、闭经、经断前后诸证中经常见到。临证可以选用滋阴降火、交通心肾的方法。

4　Regulating and coursing the liver

The liver is significant in storing blood, controlling blood sea, maintaining close contact with the Thoroughfare Vessel and managing conveyance and dispersion. The liver physically pertains to yin and functionally to yang. It prefers free action and detests stagnation. Dysfunction of the liver in conveyance, or stagnation of qi transforming into fire, or stimulation of liver fire due to rage may consume liver yin and lead to hyperactivity of liver yang, or asthenia of yin and hyperactivity of yang, which will all affect the Thoroughfare Vessel and bring about such disorders as irregular menstruation, metrorrhagia and metrostaxis, dysmenorrhea, amenorrhea, morning sickness and eclampsia gravidarum. So regulation and nourishment of the liver is also one of the important therapeutic methods for the treatment of gynecological diseases. In the middle aged women, menstruation, pregnancy, delivery and breast-feeding frequently impair blood and tend

4　调肝疏肝

肝为藏血之脏，司血海，与冲脉相通，肝又主疏泄，体阴而用阳，喜条达而恶郁滞。若肝气平和，则血脉流畅，血海宁静，周身之血亦随之而安。如肝之疏泄失调，或气郁化火，或怒动肝火，使肝阴亏损，或肝阳偏亢，或阴虚阳亢，均能影响冲脉，而致月经不调、崩漏、痛经、闭经、恶阻、子痫等病症。因此，养肝疏肝亦为妇科病的重要治法之一。中年妇女由于经、孕、产、乳等数伤于血，易致肝血偏虚、肝气偏盛，平肝养肝就更为必要。具体的治疗方法应视病情而定。肝失疏泄者，宜疏之散之；肝郁化火或怒动肝火者，清之、平之、泄

to result in asthenia of liver blood and exuberance of liver qi. So regulation and nourishment of the liver is especially important for the treatment of middle-aged woman. However, in actual treatment, the therapeutic method should be selected according to the conditions of the patient. For example, failure of the liver to convey should be treated with dispersing therapy. Liver qi stagnation transforming into fire or liver fire due to rage can be treated by clearing and purgative therapy. Consumption of liver yin or deficiency of liver blood can be treated by softening and nourishing therapy. The hyperactivity of liver yang can be treated by suppressing therapy. In a word, the purpose of regulating the liver is to balance liver qi and make liver blood sufficient.

之；肝阴亏损或肝血不足者，宜柔之、养之；肝阳偏亢者，又当抑之、平潜之。总之，应使肝气平和，肝血充足，和为要。

5 Regulating the Thoroughfare and Conception Vessels

5 调理冲任

Gynecological diseases are mainly caused by impairment of the Thoroughfare and Conception Vessels. So regulating the Thoroughfare and Conception Vessels is one of the basic treatments for gynecological diseases. The treatment of gynecological disease usually is focused on the treatment of the heart, liver, kidney, spleen and stomach, though the impairment of the Thoroughfare and Conception Vessels is emphasized. This is due to the fact that qi, blood, essence and fluid in the Thoroughfare and Conception Vessels all come from the heart, liver, kidney and spleen. Obviously the kidney, liver, spleen and stomach meridians are closely related to the Thoroughfare and Conception Vessels. That is why the treatment of the kidney, liver, spleen and stomach is effective in regulating the

妇科病又多系损伤冲任而作，故调理冲任是妇科病的重要治法之一。妇科病虽很强调冲任损伤，但其治法又多重在心、肝、肾、脾、胃。这是因为冲任所受之气、血、精、液均来自于心、肝、肾、脾、胃等脏腑，而肾、肝、脾、胃之经脉与冲任二脉有紧密联系，故调治肾、肝、脾、胃大多兼有调治冲、任之法。从中药的归经来看，部分入肾、肝、脾、胃的药，能兼冲、任，尤以入肝、肾两经的药兼入冲、任者居多，所以历代医家取入肝、肾之药来调治冲、任

Thoroughfare and Conception Vessels. In view of the meridian tropism of the herbal drugs, some of the drugs entering the kidney, liver, spleen and stomach meridians also enter the Thoroughfare and Conception Vessels, especially, most drugs entering the liver and kidney meridians. That is why doctors in the past dynasties usually used drugs entering the liver and kidney meridians to treat the disorders of the thoroughfare and conception vessels. For instance, a series of the representative heral formulas to regulate, tranquilize, secure and warm up the Thoroughfare Vessel, created by Zhang Xichun, a famous medical practitioner in the modern times, in accordance with the gynecological characteristics.

之病，如近代名医张锡纯根据妇科特点，创理冲、安冲、固冲、温冲等系列代表方，专供调理冲任之用。

Therapeutic Modalities

各 论

Chapter 1 Menstruation diseases

第1章 月经病

Irregular menstruation

月经失调

Irregular menstruation refers to abnormal changes of cycle, period and quantity of menstruation, commonly-encountered menstruation disease, including early menstruation, delayed menstruation, irregular menstruation, menostaxis, profuse menstruation and scanty menstruation, etc.

月经失调是指月经周期、经期或经量的异常，是常见的月经病，包括月经先期、月经后期、月经先后无定期、经期延长、月经过多、月经过少等，可统称为月经失调。

Irregular menstruation is usually due to emotional factors, or attack by exogenous cold, heat and dampness, impairing the Thoroughfare and Conception Vessels and affecting the functions of the viscera and the balance between qi and blood as well as between yin and yang. Various pathogenic factors and physical factors affect each other, causing cold, heat, asthenia, sthenia and other changes in viscera, Thoroughfare and Conception Vessels and uterus, resulting in abnormal menstruation period and quantity due to qi and blood disorder in Thoroughfare and Conception Vessels and abnormal storage and drainage in uterus.

月经失调多由内伤七情，或外感寒、热、湿邪，以致冲、任二脉损伤，脏腑功能紊乱，气血阴阳失调而发生疾病。各种致病因素与体质因素互为影响，导致脏腑、冲任、胞宫发生寒、热、虚、实等改变，则可引起冲任气血失调，胞宫藏泻失常，表现为月经周期或经期、经量的异常。

Syndrome identification of irregular menstruation is mainly based on menstrual cycle, menstrual period, volume, color, quality, combined with gen-

月经失调的辨证，主要根据月经的周期、经期、经量、经色、经质，结合全身症

eral symptoms, tongue and pulse to identify the cold, heat, asthenia and sthenia. Generally speaking, profuse menstruation with light color and thin clear quality is mostly caused by qi asthenia. Scanty menstruation with reddish color and thin clear quality is mostly caused by blood asthenia. Scanty menstruation with bright red color and thick sticky quality is mostly caused by asthenia heat. Profuse menstruation with dark-red color and thin clear quality is mostly caused by asthenia cold. Profuse menstruation with dark-red color and clot is mostly caused by sthenia cold. Irregular menstruation with dark-purple color and clot is mostly caused by blood stasis.

状、舌脉等审其寒热虚实。一般而言，经血量多、色淡、质清稀，多为气虚；量少、色淡红、质清稀，多为血虚；经血量少、色鲜红、质黏，多为虚热；量多、色深红、质稠，多为实热；量少、色淡暗、质清稀，多为虚寒；量多，色暗红有块，多为实寒；经量多少不定，色紫暗有块，多为血瘀。

The therapeutic methods for the treatment of irregular menstruation are stressed to regulate menstruation to treat the causative factor. The specific methods are regulating qi and blood, nourishing the kidney, strengthening the spleen and soothing the liver. For the regulating of qi and blood, the key point is to differentiate whether the disorder involves qi or blood and then treat it respectively. Menstruation comes from the kidney, so nourishing the kidney qi can stabilize the uterus and supplementing the kidney is essential to the regulation of menstruation. Nourishing the spleen and stomach can promote the production of blood, and soothing the liver can promote the flow of qi. As soon as the Thoroughfare and Conception Vessels are full and sufficient with blood on time, menstruation can be normal gradually.

月经失调的治疗原则，重在调经以治本。具体有调理气血、补肾、扶脾、疏肝之法。调理气血，首先应辨清在气在血，分别论治；月经源于肾，养肾气以安血室，为调经之要；补脾胃以资血之源；疏肝以条达气机，冲、任血海按时盈满，则月经渐趋正常。

Besides, treatment should concentrate on either the root aspect or branch aspect in clinical treatment according to the occurrence of disorder before menstruation, or during menstruation or after menstrua-

此外，临证尚需按经前、经期和经后的不同，分别采取着重治标或治本的调治方法，一般以平时治本、经期治

tion. Usually routine treatment focuses on the root aspect, treatment during menstruation concentrates on the branch aspect and treatment after menstruation emphasizes on the regulation of the spleen and stomach as well as that of qi and blood. Regulation of menstruation should be done according to whether irregular menstruation occurs before or after disease. If disease occurs after irregular menstruation, the treatment should focus on the regulation of menstruation; if disease occurs before irregular menstruation, the treatment should concentrate on dealing with the disease. Moreover the treatment should be carried out according to the age of the patient. Cares should be taken not to overuse drugs of warm and dry naturein resolving stagnation, not to overuse drugs of sweet, moistening, warm and acrid nature in fortifying the spleen. In reinforcing and benefiting the kidney water, the drugs to foster the fire should be combined, in order to invigorate essence and blood for ensuring smooth menstruation.

标、经后调养脾胃气血最为常用。调经还需分清先病后病，经不调而后生病者，当先调经，先生病而后经不调者，当先治疗其病。此外，还要照顾各年龄阶段的特点进行治疗，用药还应注意开郁不宜过用香燥，健脾不宜过用甘润或辛温，补益肾水必配养火之品，使精血俱旺，月经调畅。

1 Early menstruation

Menstruation occurring 1-2 weeks earlier for 3 cycles continuously is called early menstruation. If it occurs 3-5 days earlier or just occasionally, it is not early menstruation.

Early menstruation is usually due to blood heat and qi asthenia. Blood heat is due to frequent predomination of yang, or five emotions transforming into fire by extreme emotional changes, or excessive intake of acrid and hot foods, or attack by exogenous heat, which lead to accumulation of heat in blood and the Thoroughfare and Conception Ves-

1 月经先期

月经周期提前 1～2 周，经期正常，连续 3 个周期以上，称为月经先期。若仅超前 3～5 日，或偶有提前者，一般不作先期而论。

本病以血热、气虚证多见。血热可因素体阳盛，或七情过极，五志化火，或过食辛热，或外感热邪，致血分蕴热，伏于冲任，迫血妄行；也可因素体阴虚，或纵欲无度，或大病久病，阴液耗伤，冲任

sels, driving blood to flow abnormally. It may be caused by frequent deficiency of yin or intemperance in sexual life or serious or prolonged disease, consumption of body fluid, and weakness of the Thoroughfare and Conception Vessels.

不固所致。

1.1 Key points for diagnosis

(1) Menstruation occurs 1-2 weeks earlier and continues for over 3 cycles.

(2) If accompanied by profuse discharge of menses early menstruation may lead to metrorrhagia and metrostaxis.

(3) Menstruation more than 10 days earlier with vaginal bleeding should be differentiated from intermenstrual bleeding.

(4) No organic changes in the pelvis are found in gynecologic examination.

1.1 诊断要点

（1）月经周期提前 1～2 周，连续发生 3 个周期或以上。

（2）本病若伴经量过多则可发展为崩漏。

（3）月经若提前 10 余日见有阴道出血者，应与经间期出血鉴别。

（4）妇科检查盆腔无器质性改变。

1.2 Syndrome differentiation and treatment

For early menstruation, syndrome differentiation concentrates on advanced cycle and the changes in quantity, color and texture, in combination with the conditions of general symptoms, tongue and pulse diagnosis, so as to make sure whether it is of asthenia or sthenia, or of heat syndrome. For the treatment of asthenia syndrome, the therapeutic method is either reinforcing method, or supplementing gastrosplenic qi, or strengthening kidney qi. For the treatment of heat syndrome, the therapeutic method should be clearing away heat. For the treatment of sthenic-heat, the therapeutic method is mainly clearing away heat and cooling blood. For the treatment of asthenia-heat, the therapeutic method is mainly nourishing yin and clearing away heat.

1.2 辨证论治

月经先期的辨证，重点在于周期的提前，经量、经色、经质的改变，结合全身证侯及舌脉的情况，辨其属虚、属实、属热之不同；治疗以虚则补之，或补中气，或固肾气；热则清之，实热者清热凉血为主，虚热者又当养阴清热为主。

The main pathogenesis of early menstruation is weakness of Thoroughfare and Conception Vessels due to qi asthenia and disquieted sea of blood by blood heat. Therapeutic methods are concentrated on regulating menstruation and stanching bleeding, by the supplementing or clearing technique according to pathogenesis, in order to achieve the purpose of restoration of menstrual cycle.

月经先期的主要病机是气虚冲任不固和血热血海不宁。治疗原则重在调经止血，针对病机，或补或清，达到恢复月经周期之目的。

1.2.1 Blood heat syndrome

1.2.1 血热证

(1) Syndrome of liver stagnation and blood heat

(1) 肝郁血热证

Main manifestations Early menstruation, increased or decreased quantity, purplish and sticky menses with clot, distension and pain in breasts, hypochondria and lower abdomen before menstruation as well as mental depression, restlessness, bitter taste in mouth, dry throat, red tongue with yellow fur, wiry and fast pulse.

主要证候 经行先期，经量或多或少，经色紫红，质稠有小块。经前乳房、胸胁、少腹胀满疼痛，抑郁或烦躁，口苦咽干。舌红，苔薄黄，脉弦数。

Therapeutic methods Soothing the liver and resolving stagnation, clearing away heat and regulating menstruation.

治法 疏肝解郁，清热调经。

Formulas and herbs *Moutan and Gardenia Free Wanderer Powder* (Dan Zhi Xiao Yao San) composed of 10 g of *Moutan* (Mu Dan Pi), 6 g of *Fructus Gardeniae* (Zhi Zi), 6 g of *Radix Bupleuri* (Chai Hu), 10 g of *Radix Angelicae Sinensis* (Dang Gui), 10 g of *Radix Rehmanniae Cruda* (Bai Shao), 10 g of *Rhizoma Atractylodis Macrocephalae* (Bai Zhu), 10 g of *Poriae* (Fu Ling), 6 g of *Herba Menthae* (Bo He), 3 g of Zingiberis Rhizoma Tostum (Wei Jiang) , 3 g of *Radix Glycyrrhizae* Praeparata (Zhi Gan Cao).

方药 代表方为丹栀逍遥散；常用药如牡丹皮 10 克，栀子 6 克，柴胡 6 克，当归 10 克，白芍 10 克，白术 10 克，茯苓 10 克，薄荷 6 克，煨姜 3 克，炙甘草 3 克。

Modification For profuse menstruation, *Radix Angelicae Sinensis* (Dang Gui) is deleted while

加减 若经行量多者，去当归，选加地榆、槐花以凉

Radix Sanguisorbae (Di Yu) and *Sophora Flower* (Huai Hua) are added to cool blood and stanch bleeding. For liver stagnation with stomach fire, dry mouth and tongue, *Trichosanthes Root* (Tian Hua Fen) and *Rhizoma Anemarrhenae* (Zhi Mu) are added to nourish yin and engender liquid. For menstruation with blood clot, *Radix Curcumae* (Yu Jin) is added to move qi and dissolve stasis and activate blood. For serious distension and pain in breasts and hypochondria during menstruation, *Semen Vaccariae* (Wang Bu Liu Xing), *Fructus Aurantii Immaturus* (Zhi Shi) and *Fructus Meliae Toosendan* (Chuan Lian Zi) are added to course the liver and disperse stagnation.

血止血；若肝郁挟胃火，口干舌燥者，加天花粉、知母养阴生津；经行挟血块，加郁金以行气化瘀；经行胸胁乳房胀痛较重者，加王不留行、枳实、川楝子以疏肝散结。

Shanghai doctor CAI Xiaosun's experience prescription, *Liver-Clearing and Menstruation-Regulating Prescription* (Qing Gan Tiao Jing Fang): 9 g of *Radix Angelicae Sinensis* (Dang Gui), 12 g of *Radix Rehmanniae Cruda* (Sheng Di Huang), 9 g of *Cortex Lycii Radicis* (Di Gu Pi), 9 g of *Moutan* (Mu Dan Pi), 4.5 g of *Radix Bupleuri* (Chai Hu), 9 g of *Cyperi Rhizoma Praeparatum* (Zhi Xiang Fu), 9 g of *Radix Rehmanniae Cruda* (Bai Shao), 9 g of *Radix Scutellariae* (Huang Qin), 9 g of *Rhizoma Alismatis* (Ze Xie) and 9 g of *Rhizoma Atractylodis Macrocephalae* (Bai Zhu).

上海医家蔡小荪经验方（清肝调经方）：当归 9 克，生地黄 12 克，地骨皮 9 克，牡丹皮 9 克，柴胡 4.5 克，制香附 9 克，白芍 9 克，黄芩 9 克，泽泻 9 克，白术 9 克。

(2) Syndrome of predominant yang and blood heat

（2）阳盛血热证

Main manifestations Early menstruation with profusereddish violet and sticky menses, flushed face and generalized heat, dysphoria, thirst with preference of cold drinking, yellow urine, dry feces, reddish tongue with yellow fur, and rapid pulse.

主要证候 经行提前，经血量多，色红紫，质稠。身热面赤，口渴喜冷饮，心胸烦闷，大便秘结，小便黄赤。舌红，苔黄，脉滑数。

Therapeutic methods Clearing away heat and cooling blood, nourishing yin and regulating men-

治法 清热凉血，养阴调经。

struation.

Formulas and herbs *Channel-Clearing Powder* (Qing Jing San) composed of 10 g of *Moutan* (Mu Dan Pi), 10 g of *Cortex Lycii Radicis* (Di Gu Pi), 10 g of *Radix Rehmanniae Cruda* (Bai Shao), 10 g of *Radix Rehmanniae Praeparata* (Shu Di Huang), 10 g of *Herba Artemisiae Chinghao* (Qing Hao), 10 g of *Poriae* (Fu Ling) and 10 g of *Cortex Phellodendri* (Huang Bo).

方药　代表方为清经散;常用药如牡丹皮10克,地骨皮10克,白芍10克,熟地黄10克,青蒿10克,茯苓10克,黄柏10克。

Modification For profuse menstruation during menstrual period, *Poriae* (Fu Ling) is deleted while *Radix Sanguisorbae* (Di Yu) and *Sophorae Flos* (Huai Hua) are added to cool the blood and stanch bleeding. For blood heat with stasis and clot in menstruation, *Radix Notoginseng* (San Qi), *Pollen Typhae* (Pu Huang) and *Madder* (Qian Cao) are added to dissolve stasis and stanch bleeding. For stasis due to heat with lower abdominal pain, 15 g of *Herba Leonuri* (Yi Mu Cao) and 15 g of *Pollen Typhae* (Pu Huang) (to be wrapped for decocting) are added.

加减　若时值经期经血量多者,去茯苓,酌加地榆、槐花以凉血止血;若血热挟瘀,经血有块者,选加三七、蒲黄、茜草以祛瘀止血;因热致瘀而伴少腹疼痛者,酌加益母草15克,蒲黄(包煎)15克。

Shanghai doctor TANG Xiyuan's experience prescription, *Moutan, Scutellariae Radix Fricta and Four Agents Decoction* (Dan Qin Si Wu Tang): 12 g of *Moutan* (Mu Dan Pi), 9 g of *Scutellariae Radix Fricta* (Chao Huang Qin), 10 g of *Stir-Fried Chinese Angelica* (Chao Dang Gui), 9 g of *Stir-Fried Radix Paeoniae Rubra* (Chao Chi Shao), 12 g of *Radix Rehmanniae Cruda* (Sheng Di Huang), 9 g of *Folium Mori* (Sang Ye), 9 g of *Cortex Mori Radicis* (Sang Bai Pi), 12 g of *Rhizoma Imperatae* (Bai Mao Gen), 9 g of *Radix Cyathulae* (Chuan Niu Xi) and 5 g of *Radix Glycyrrhizae* (Gan Cao).

上海医家唐锡元经验方(丹芩四物汤):牡丹皮12克,炒黄芩9克,炒当归10克,炒赤芍9克,生地黄12克,桑叶9克,桑白皮9克,白茅根12克,川牛膝9克,甘草5克。

(3) Syndrome of yin asthenia and blood heat

(3) 阴虚血热证

Main manifestations Early menstruation with scanty red and sticky menses, emaciation, tidal heat

主要证候　经行提前,经血量少,经色红赤,质稠。

with flushed cheeks, dry throat and lips, vexing heat in the five body parts, thin and red tongue with scanty fur as well as thin and rapid pulse.

形体瘦弱，潮热颧红，咽干唇燥，五心烦热。舌体瘦红，少苔，脉细数。

Therapeutic methods Enriching yin and clearing away heat, nourishing blood and regulating menstruation.

治法 滋阴清热，养血调经。

Formulas and herbs *Rehmannia and Lycium Root Bark Decoction* (Liang Di Tang) composed of 10 g of *Radix Rehmanniae Cruda* (Sheng Di Huang), 10 g of *Radix Scrophulariae* (Xuan Shen), 10 g of *Ophiopogon* (Mai Dong), 10 g of *Cortex Lycii Radicis* (Di Gu Pi), 10 g of *Colla Corii Asini* (E Jiao)(to be melted) and 10 g of *Radix Rehmanniae Cruda* (Bai Shao).

方药 代表方为两地汤；常用药如生地黄 10 克，玄参 10 克，麦冬 10 克，地骨皮 10 克，阿胶 10 克，白芍 10 克。

Modification For profuse menstruation, *Eclipta* (Han Lian Cao) and *Fructus Ligustri Lucidi* (Nü Zhen Zi) are added to enrich yin and stanch bleeding. For scanty menstruation, *Processed Radix Polygoni Multiflori* (Zhi He Shou Wu) and *Fructus Lycii* (Gou Qi Zi) are added to nourish the blood and regulate menstruation. For vexing heat in the five body parts, *Radix Cynanchi Atrati* (Bai Wei), *Testudinis Carapax et Plastrum cum Liquido Fricti* (Zhi Gui Jia) and *Radix Stellariae* (Yin Chai Hu) are added to enrich yin and clear heat.

加减 若经血量者多加旱莲草、女贞子以滋阴止血；经行量少者加制何首乌、枸杞以养血调经，五心烦热者选加白薇、炙龟甲、银柴胡以滋阴清热。

1.2.2 Qi asthenia syndrome

1.2.2 气虚证

Main manifestations Early menstruation with profuse light-colored and thin menses, fatigued spirit and lack of strength, fatigue and somnolence, shortness of breath and lazy to speak, distention in stomach and abdomen, reduced food intake and poor appetite, empty prolapsing sensation in the lower abdomen, loose stool, as well as thin and slow pulse.

主要证候 经行提前，经血量多，色淡，质清稀。神疲乏力，倦怠嗜卧，气短懒言，或脘腹胀满，食少纳呆，小腹空坠，便溏。舌淡红，苔薄白，脉缓弱。

Therapeutic methods Fortifying the spleen and boosting qi, controlling blood circulation and regulating menstruation.

治法 健脾益气，摄血调经。

Formulas and herbs *Center-Supplementing Qi-Boosting Decoction* (Bu Zhong Yi Qi Tang) composed of 10 g of *Radix Astragali* (Huang Qi), 10 g of *Radix Codonopsis Pilosulae* (Dang Shen), 6 g of *Pericarpium Citri Tangerinae* (Chen Pi), 6 g of *Rhizoma Cimicifugae* (Sheng Ma), 6 g of *Radix Bupleuri* (Chai Hu), 10 g of *Radix Angelicae Sinensis* (Dang Gui), 10 g of *Rhizoma Atractylodis Macrocephalae* (Bai Zhu) and 3 g of *Radix Glycyrrhizae* (Gan Cao).

方药 代表方为补中益气汤；常用药如黄芪10克，党参10克，陈皮6克，升麻6克，柴胡6克，当归10克，白术10克，甘草3克。

Shanghai doctor CAI Xiaosun's experience prescription, *Qi-Boosting Yin-Nourishing Decoction* (Yi Qi Yang Yin Tang): 12 g of *Stir-Fried Lu'an Codonospsis* (Chao Lu Dang), 10 g of *Stir-Fried Rhizoma Atractylodis Macrocephalae* (Chao Bai Zhu), 10 g of *Stir-Fried Radix Angelicae Sinensis* (Chao Dang Gui), 10 g of *Radix Rehmanniae Cruda* (Sheng Di Huang), 6 g of *Radix Salviae Miltiorrhizae* (Dan Shen), 10 g of *Radix Paeoniae Alba* (Bai Shao), 10 g of *Processed Plastrum Testudinis* (Zhi Gui Jia), 10 g of *Processed Fructus Ligustri Lucidi* (Shu Nü Zhen Zi), 12 g of *Ecliptae Herba* (Han Lian Cao) and 10 g of *Herba Agrimoniae* (Xian He Cao).

上海医家蔡小荪经验方(益气养阴汤)：炒路党12克，炒白术10克，炒当归10克，生地黄10克，丹参6克，白芍10克，炙龟甲10克，熟女贞10克，旱莲草12克，仙鹤草10克。

Modification For profuse and red menstruation, *Herba Agrimoniae* (Xian He Cao) and *Trachycarpi Petiolus Carbonisatus* (Zong Lü Tan) are added to astringe and stanch bleeding. For profuse and light-colored menses, *Artemisiae Argyi Folium Carbonisatum* (Ai Ye Tan) and *Zingiberis Rhizoma Praeparatum* (Pao Jiang Tan) are added to warm the channels and induce astringency. For spleen vacuity affecting the kidney, cold and pain in the lumbus and abdomen, urinary frequency, *Fructus*

加减 若经血量多而经色偏红者，加仙鹤草、棕榈炭以收涩止血；若量多而色淡者，加艾叶炭、炮姜炭以温经固涩；若脾虚及肾，腰腹冷痛，小便频数者，加益智仁、杜仲、菟丝子以补肾涩精；若心脾两虚，心悸失眠者，去柴胡、升麻，加酸枣仁、远志、大枣以宁心安神；若小腹隐痛

Alpiniae Oxyphyllae (Yi Zhi Ren), *Cortex Eucommiae* (Du Zhong) and *Semen Cuscutae* (Tu Si Zi) are added to supplement the kidney and astringe essence. For dual vacuity of the heart and spleen, heart palpitations and insomnia, *Radix Bupleuri* (Chai Hu) and *Rhizoma Cimicifugae* (Sheng Ma) are deleted while *Semen Ziziphi Spinosae* (Suan Zao Ren), *Radix Polygalae* (Yuan Zhi) and *Fructus Ziziphi Jujubae* (Da Zao) are added to quiet the heart and spirit. For dull pain in lower abdomen, *Radix Paeoniae Alba* (Bai Shao) and *Radix Glycyrrhizae* (Gan Cao) are added to relax tension and relieve pain. For thin sloppy stool, *Halloysitum Rubrum* (Chi Shi Zhi), *Granati Pericarpium* (Shi Liu Pi) and *Fructus Mume* (Wu Mei) are added to induce astringency and check diarrhea.

者，加白芍配甘草以缓急止痛；若大便溏薄者，加赤石脂、石榴皮、乌梅以固涩止泻。

1.3 Other therapeutic methods

1.3 其他疗法

1.3.1 Chinese patent drugs

1.3.1 中成药

(1) *Angelica Splenic Pills* (Gui Pi Wan): 6 g each time and three times a day, applicable to the treatment of qi asthenia syndrome.

（1）归脾丸：每次 6 克，每日 3 次，适用于气虚证。

(2) *Menses-Securing Pill* (Gu Jing Wan): 6 g each time and three times a day, applicable to the treatment of blood heat syndrome.

（2）固经丸：每次 6 克，每日 3 次，适用于血热证。

(3) *Shen Qian Menses-Securing Granules* (Shen Qian Gu Jing Ke Li): 50 g each time and twice a day, take it one week before menstruation, applicable to the treatment of early menstruation, profuse menstruation, metrorrhagia and metrostaxis due to qi and yin vacuity, heat driving the blood to flow abnormally.

（3）参茜固经颗粒：每次 50 克，每日 2 次，经前 1 周开始服用。适用于气阴两虚、热迫血行所致的月经先期、月经过多、崩漏。

1.3.2 Empirical and folk recipes

1.3.2 单验方

(1) 30 g of *Radix Rehmanniae Cruda* (Sheng Di Huang) is washed, cut into slices and decocted into

（1）生地黄 30 克，粳米 60 克，生地黄洗净后切片，煎

100 ml decoction, and then mixed up with porridge made of 60 g of *Semen Oryza Sativae* (Jing Mi) for oral taking, applicable to the treatment of heat syndrome.

熬成100毫升，粳米煮粥与汁混合，连服数日，用于热证。

(2) 15 g of *Radix Codonopsis Pilosulae* (Dang Shen), 15 g of *Radix Astragali* (Huang Qi), 20 pieces of *Fructus Ziziphi Jujubae* (Da Zao), 60 g of *Semen Nelumbinis* (Bai Lian Mi). *Radix Codonopsis Pilosulae* (Dang Shen) and *Radix Astragali* (Huang Qi) with 1, 000 mL of water are decocted into 200 mL of decoction. After removal of the residue, the decoction is added with *Fructus Ziziphi Jujubae* (Da Zao) and *Semen Nelumbinis* (Bai Lian Mi) to decoct into porridge for oral taking, one dose per day, for one week to the treatment of qi asthenia syndrome.

(2) 党参15克，黄芪15克，大枣20枚，白莲米60克，先以党参、黄芪加水1 000毫升，煎至200毫升去渣，入大枣和白莲米共煮成粥，每日1料，连用1周，用于气虚证。

2　Delayed menstruation

Delayed menstruation means that menstruation occurs over seven days later or even occurs once in 3-5 months. Occasional delayed menstruation is regarded as normal.

The pathogenesis of delayed menstruation is mainly caused by inhibited movement of qi and blood, obstruction of Thoroughfare and Conception Vessels, the sea of blood failing to be full and sufficient on time. Asthenia is either kidney asthenia or blood asthenia. Sthenia is either blood cold or qi stagnation. It may develop into amenorrhea and even affecting pregnancies. Therapeutic methods are mainly warming the meridians, nourishing and circulating blood according to patterns identified. As

2　月经后期

月经周期延后7日以上，甚至3～5个月一行，经期正常，连续出现3个月经周期以上，称为月经后期。若偶见延后，且无其他病象出现，不作后期而论。

月经后期的病机主要是气血运行不畅，冲任受阻，血海不能按时满盈。虚者有肾虚、血虚；实者有血寒、气滞。可发展为闭经，甚则可影响孕育。治疗原则是根据辨证，温经、养血、行血为主，温经则寒去，养血则血充，行血则滞通。

soon as the meridians are warmed up, cold will be gone. As soon as blood is nourished, blood will be sufficient. As soon as blood flows, stagnation will be removed.

2.1 Key points for diagnosis

2.1.1 Symptoms

menstruation occurs seven days later continuously for three cycles.

2.1.2 Examination

Gynecological examination without obvious abnormalities; other examinations such as basal temperature, hormone measurement and B ultrasound examination are helpful for diagnosis.

2.2 Syndrome differentiation and treatment

Scanty menstrual flow with light color, backache and fatigue due to kidney vacuity, scanty menstrual flow with dark color and blood clot, cold and pain in lower abdomen because of blood cold; light red menstrual flow with dull pain in hypogastrium, palpitation with reduced sleep and sallow facial complexion due to blood vacuity; scanty menstrual flow with dark color and contingent blood clot, abdominal distention and pain with distending pain in breast due to qi stagnation. According to syndrome differentiation, therapeutic principles are supplementing the asthenia, purging the sthenia, warming the cold, removing stagnation and freeing the meridians to regulate menstruation.

2.2.1 Blood asthenia syndrome

Main manifestations Delayed menstruation with scanty, light-colored and thin menses, without blood clot, lower abdominal pain with sallow yellow facial complexion, dizzy head and dim eyesight,

2.1 诊断要点

2.1.1 症状

月经经期延后 7 日以上，连续 3 个月经周期以上者。

2.1.2 检查

妇科检查，一般无明显异常；其他检查，包括基础体温、性激素测定及 B 超等检查有助于诊断。

2.2 辨证论治

经量少色淡，腰酸乏力为肾虚；经少色暗有血块，小腹冷痛为血寒；经色淡红，下腹隐痛，心悸少寐，面色萎黄为血虚；经少色暗，或有血块，下腹胀痛，乳房胀痛为气滞。治疗原则是根据辨证，虚者补之，实者泻之，寒者温之，滞者行之，疏通经脉以调经。

2.2.1 血虚证

主要证候 经行错后，量少，色淡，质稀无块。经行小腹绵绵作痛，面色萎黄，头晕眼花，心悸失眠，爪甲不

palpitation, insomnia, lusterless nails, pale tongue and thread and weak pulse.

荣。舌淡，苔薄，脉细弱。

Therapeutic methods Supplementing blood and replenishing essence, nourishing qi and regulating menstruation.

治法　补血填精，益气调经。

Formulas and herbs ① *Major Yuan (Primary) Qi-Reinforcing Decoction* (Da Bu Yuan Jian): 15 g of *Radix Codonopsis Pilosulae* (Dang Shen), 15 g of *Rhizoma Dioscoreae* (Shan Yao), 12 g of *Radix Rehmanniae Praeparata* (Shu Di Huang), 12 g of *Radix Angelicae Sinensis* (Dang Gui), 12 g of *Radix Paeoniae Alba* (Bai Shao), 10 g of *Cortex Eucommiae* (Du Zhong), 10 g of *Fructus Corni* (Shan Zhu Yu), 10 g of *Radix Salviae Miltiorrhizae* (Dan Shen), 10 g of *Rhizoma Cyperi* (Xiang Fu) and 3 g of *Radix Glycyrrhizae* (Gan Cao). ② *Ginseng Construction-Nourishing Decoction* (Ren Shen Yang Rong Tang): 12 g of *Radix Ginseng* (Ren Shen), 12 g of *Radix Astragali* (Huang Qi), 15 g of *Radix Angelicae Sinensis* (Dang Gui), 9 g of *Radix Paeoniae Alba* (Bai Shao), 12 g of *Radix Rehmanniae Praeparata* (Shu Di Huang), 6 g of *Cinnamomi Cortex Rasus* (Gui Xin), 9 g of *Pericarpium Citri Tangerinae* (Chen Pi), 9 g of *Rhizoma Atractylodis Macrocephalae* (Bai Zhu), 12 g of *Poriae* (Fu Ling), 15 g of *Fructus Schisandrae* (Wu Wei Zi), 9 g of *Radix Polygalae* (Yuan Zhi), 5 g of *Radix Glycyrrhizae* (Gan Cao), 3 slices of *Rhizoma Zingiberis Recens* (Sheng Jiang) and 5 pieces of *Fructus Ziziphi Jujubae* (Da Zao, Hong Zao).

方药　代表方：①大补元煎；常用药如党参 15 克，山药 15 克，熟地黄 12 克，当归 12 克，白芍 12 克，杜仲 10 克，山茱萸 10 克，丹参 10 克，香附 10 克，甘草 3 克。②人参养荣汤；常用药如人参 12 克，黄芪 12 克，当归 15 克，白芍 9 克，熟地黄 12 克，桂心 6 克，陈皮 9 克，白术 9 克，茯苓 12 个，五味子 15 克，远志 9 克，甘草 5 克，生姜 3 片，大枣 5 枚。

Modification For qi vacuity and lack of strength, *Astragali Radix cum Liquido Fricta* (Zhi Huang Qi) and *Rhizoma Atractylodis Macrocephalae* (Bai Zhu) are added to fortify the spleen and boost

加减　若气虚乏力者加炙黄芪、白术以健脾益气；若食少便溏证，则去当归，加砂仁、茯苓以醒脾；若兼脾肾阳

qi. For poor appetite and loose stool, *Radix Angelicae Sinensis* (Dang Gui) is deleted while *Fructus Amomi* (Sha Ren) and *Poriae* (Fu Ling) are added to arouse the spleen. For physical cold and cold limbs due to spleen-kidney yang vacuity, *Aconiti Radix Lateralis Tosta* (Pao Fu Zi) and *Rhizoma Zingiberis Praeparata* (Pao Jiang) are added to warm yang. For palpitation and insomnia, *Ziziphi Spinosi Semen Frictum* (Chao Zao Ren) and *Radix Polygalae* (Yuan Zhi) are added to nourish the heart and quiet the spirit.

虚，形寒肢冷者，加炮附子、炮姜以温阳；若心悸失眠者，加炒枣仁、远志以养心安神。

2.2.2 Kidney vacuity syndrome

Main manifestations Delayed menstruation with scanty and grayish menses, with blood clot, cold and pain in lower abdomen, aversion to cold, cold limbs, pale facial complexion, long voidings of clear urine, dark-red tong with white fur, deep-tense or deep-slow pulse.

Therapeutic methods Warming the meridians and dispersing cold, moving the blood and regulating menstruation.

Formulas and herbs *Uterus-Warming Decoction* (Wen Bao Yin): 3 g of *Aconiti Radix Lateralis Tosta* (Pao Fu Zi), 3 g of *Cortex Cinnamomi* (Rou Gui), 12 g of *Radix Morindae Officinalis* (Ba Ji Tian), 12 g of *Semen Cuscutae* (Tu Si Zi), 12 g of *Fructus Psoraleae* (Bu Gu Zhi), 12 g of *Cortex Eucommiae* (Du Zhong), 12 g of *Radix Ginseng* (Ren Shcn), 9 g of *Rhizoma Atractylodis Macrocephalae* (Bai Zhu), 12 g of *Rhizoma Dioscoreae* (Shan Yao) and 10 g of *Semen Euryales* (Qian Shi).

Shanghai doctor CAI Xiaosun's experience prescription, *Uterus-Warming and Menstruation-Regulating Prescription*

2.2.2 肾虚证

主要证候 经行错后，量少，色暗有块。小腹冷痛，畏寒肢冷，面色苍白，小便清长。舌暗红，苔白，脉沉紧或沉迟。

治法 温经散寒，行血调经。

方药 代表方为温胞饮；常用药如炮附子3克，肉桂3克，巴戟天12克，菟丝子12克，补骨脂12克，杜仲12克，人参12克，白术9克，山药12克，芡实10克。

上海医家蔡小荪经验方（温宫调经方）：炒当归10克，生熟地

(Wen Gong Tiao Jing Fang): 10 g of *Fried Chinese Angelica* (Chao Dang gui), 10 g of *Radix Rehmanniae Cruda* (Sheng Di Huang), 10 g of *Radix Rehmanniae Praeparata* (Shu Di Huang), 10 g of *Rhizoma Ligustici Chuanxiong* (Chuan Xiong), 10 g of *Radix Paeoniae Alba* (Bai Shao), 3 g of *Ramulus Cinnamomi* (Gui Zhi), 2. 5 g of *Fructus Evodiae* (Dan Wu Yu), 10 g of *Cervi Cornu Degelatinatum* (Lu Jiao Shuang), 10 g of *Radix Achyranthis Bidentatae* (Niu Xi), 10 g of *Rhizoma Cyperi* (Xiang Fu), 10 g of *Fructus Ligustri Lucidi* (Nu Zhen Zi) and 5 g of *Folium Artemistae Argyi* (Ai Ye).

各10克，川芎10克，白芍10克，桂枝3克，淡吴萸2.5克，鹿角霜10克，怀牛膝10克，香附10克，女贞10克，艾叶5克。

Modification　For severe cold, *Aconiti Radix Lateralis Tosta* (Pao Fu Zi) is added. For severe asthenia, *Radix Ginseng* (Ren Shen) is added. For clear urine and loose sloppy stool, *Fructus Psoraleae* (Bu Gu Zhi) and *Rhizoma Atractylodis Macrocephalae* (Bai Zhu) are added. For phlegm and dampness, *Rhizoma Atractylodis* (Cang Zhu) and *Semen Coicis* (Yi Yi Ren) are added.

加减　若寒甚者，加炮附子；虚甚者，加人参；若小便清，大便溏薄者，加补骨脂、白术；兼痰湿者，加苍术、薏苡仁。

2. 2. 3　Blood cold syndrome

2. 2. 3　血寒证

Main manifestations　Delayed menstruation with blackish, scanty menses and blood clot, abdominal cold and pain, aversion to cold, cold limbs, pale facial complexion, profuse clear urine, dark-red tongue with white fur and deep-tense or deep-slow pulse.

主要证候　经行错后，量少，色暗有块。小腹冷痛，畏寒肢冷，面色苍白，小便清长。舌暗红，苔白，脉沉紧或沉迟。

Therapeutic methods　Warming meridians to disperse cold, moving the blood to regulate menstruation.

治法　温经散寒，行血调经。

Formulas and herbs　*Channel-Warming Decoction* (Wen Jing Tang): 10 g of *Radix Ginseng* (Ren Shen), 12 g of *Radix Angelicae Sinensis* (Dang Gui), 6 g of *Rhizoma Ligustici Chuanxiong* (Chuan Xiong), 12 g of *Radix Paeoniae Alba* (Bai Shao), 3 g of *Cinnamomi Cortex Rasus* (Gui Xin), 9 g of *Rhizoma Zedoariae* (E Zhu), 12 g of *Cortex Moutan*

方药　代表方为温经汤；常用药如人参10克，当归12克，川芎6克，白芍12克，桂心3克，莪术9克，牡丹皮12克，甘草6克，牛膝9克。

Radicis (Mu Dan Pi), 6 g of *Radix Glycyrrhizae* (Gan Cao) and 9 g of *Radix Achyranthis Bidentatae* (Niu Xi, Huai Niu Xi).

Modification For scanty menses, *Caulis Spatholobi* (Ji Xue Teng) is added to activate the blood and regulate menstruation. For severe abdominal pain, *Pollen Typhae* (Pu Huang) and *Rhizoma Corydalis* (Yan Hu Suo) are added to activate the blood and relieve pain. For aching lumbus and knees, *Ramulus Loranthi* (Sang Ji Sheng), *Radix Dipsaci* (Xu Duan) and *Rhizoma Cibotii* (Gou Ji) are added to supplement kidney and strengthen lumber spine. For loose stool, *Rhizoma Atractylodis Macrocephalae* (Bai Zhu) and *Dioscoreae Rhizoma Frictum* (Chao Shan Yao) are added to fortify the spleen. For abdominal distention, *Rhizoma Cyperi* (Xiang Fu) and *Radix Linderae* (Wu Yao) are added to move qi and eliminate distention.

加减 若经血量少者,加鸡血藤以活血调经;若腹痛较甚者,加蒲黄、延胡索以活血止痛;若腰膝酸痛者,加桑寄生、续断、狗脊以补肾壮腰脊;便溏者加炒白术、炒山药以健脾;小腹胀满者加香附、乌药以行气除胀。

2.2.4 Qi stagnation syndrome

Main manifestations Delayed menstruation with scantyand dark-red menses and blood clot, abdominal distention or breast and hypochondriac distention and pain, mental depression with occasional sighs, normal or dark tongue with white fur and taut pulse.

Therapeutic methods Resolving depression and moving qi, harmonizing blood and regulating menstruation.

Formulas and herbs ① *Supplemented Lindera Decoction* (Jia Wei Wu Yao Tang): 9 g of *Radix Linderae* (Wu Yao), 3 g of *Fructus Amomi* (Sha Ren), 10 g of *Radix Aucklandiae* (Mu Xiang), 10 g of *Rhizoma Corydalis* (Yan Hu Suo), 12 g of *Rhizoma Cyperi* (Xiang Fu), 6 g

2.2.4 气滞证

主要证候 经行延后,量少,色暗红有块。小腹胀满,或胸胁乳房胀痛不适,精神抑郁,时欲太息。舌质正常或略暗,苔白,脉弦。

治法 开郁行气,和血调经。

方药 代表方:①加味乌药汤;常用药如乌药 9 克,砂仁 3 克,木香 10 克,延胡索 10 克,香附 12 克,甘草 6 克,槟榔 6 克。②七制香附丸;常用药如香附 15 克,当归 9

of *Radix Glycyrrhizae* (Gan Cao) and 6 g of *Semen Arecae* (Bing Lang). ② *Seven Fold Processed Cyperus Pill* (Qi Zhi Xiang Fu Wan): 15 g of *Rhizoma Cyperi* (Xiang Fu), 9 g of *Radix Angelicae Sinensis* (Dang Gui), 15 g of *Rhizoma Zedoariae* (E Zhu), 9 g of *Cortex Moutan Radicis* (Mu Dan Pi), 3 g of *Folium Artemistae Argyi* (Ai Ye), 9 g of *Radix Linderae* (Wu Yao), 12 g of *Rhizoma Ligustici Chuanxiong* (Chuan Xiong), 15 g of *Rhizoma Corydalis* (Yan Hu Suo), 9 g of *Rhizoma Sparganii Stoloniferi* (San Leng), 15 g of *Radix Bupleuri* (Chai Hu), 6 g of *Flos Carthami* (Hong Hua) and 5 g of *Fructus Mume* (Wu Mei).

克,莪术 15 克,牡丹皮 9 克,艾叶 3 克,乌药 9 克,川芎 12 克,延胡索 15 克,三棱 9 克,柴胡 15 克,红花 6 克,乌梅 5 克。

Modification For severe breast and hypochondriac distention and pain, *Radix Bupleuri* (Chai Hu), *Radix Curcumae* (Yu Jin) and *Fructus Meliae Toosendan* (Chuan Lian Zi) are added to course the liver and relieve pain. For scanty menses, *Caulis Spatholobi* (Ji Xue Teng) and *Radix Salviae Miltiorrhizae* (Dan Shen) are added to activate the blood and dredge the meridians. For abdominal cold and pain, *Folium Artemistae Argyi* (Ai Ye) and *Cortex Cinnamomi* (Rou Gui) are added to warm menstruation. For severe abdominal pain with blood clot in menses, *Pollen Typhae* (Pu Huang), *Radix Notoginseng* (San Qi) and *Herba Leonuri* (Yi Mu Cao) are added to activate the blood and dissolve stasis.

加减 若胸胁乳房胀痛较重者,加柴胡、郁金、川楝子以疏肝止痛;月经量少者加鸡血藤、丹参以活血通经;小腹冷痛者,加艾叶、肉桂以温经;经血有块,腹痛较重者,加蒲黄、三七、益母草以活血化瘀。

2.3 Other therapeutic methods

2.3.1 Chinese patent drugs

(1) *Channel-Regulating Leonurus* (Motherwort) Pill (Tiao Jing Yi Mu Wan): 2-4 g each time and twice a day, applicable to the treatment of blood stasis syndrome.

(2) *Mugwort and Cyperus Palace-Warming Pill*

2.3 其他疗法

2.3.1 中成药

(1) 调经益母丸:每次 2~4片,每日 2 次,适用于血瘀证。

(2) 艾附暖宫丸:每次 6

(Ai Fu Nuan Gong Wan): 6 g each time and twice or three times a day, applicable to the treatment of asthenia and cold syndrome.

克,每日 2～3 次,适用于虚寒证。

(3) *Compound Formula Leonurus (Motherwort) Oral Liquid* (Fu Fang Yi Mu Kou Fu Ye): 20 ml each time and twice a day, applicable to the treatment of blood stasis syndrome.

(3) 复方益母口服液:每次 20 毫升,每日 2 次,适用于血瘀证。

(4) *Ginseng and Young Deerhorn Bai Feng Pill* (Shen Rong Bai Feng Wan): For Water Honey Pill, 6 g each time and once a day; for Honey Pill, 1 pill each time and once a day.

(4) 参茸白凤丸:水蜜丸每次 6 克,大蜜丸每次 1 丸,每日 1 次,适用于气虚血瘀证。

2.3.2 Empirical and folk recipes

2.3.2 单验方

(1) 6 g of *Rhizoma Zingiberis Recens* (Sheng Jiang), 6 g of *Folium Artemistae Argyi* (Ai Ye) and 15 g of brown sugar are decocted. The decoction is taken orally twice a day, applicable to the treatment of blood cold syndrome.

(1) 生姜 6 克,艾叶 6 克,红糖 15 克,煎煮为饮,每日 2 次,适用于血寒证。

(2) 10 g of *Radix Salviae Miltiorrhizae* (Dan Shen), 10 g of *Rhizoma Cyperi* (Xiang Fu), 6 g of *Folium Artemistae Argyi* (Ai Ye), 6 g of *Radix Glycyrrhizae* (Gan Cao) and 15 g of *Herba Leonuri* (Yi Mu Cao) are decocted for oral taking applicable to the treatment of qi stagnation syndrome.

(2) 丹参 10 克,香附 10 克,艾叶 6 克,甘草 6 克,益母草 15 克,煎煮为饮,适用于气滞证。

3 Irregularity of menstrual cycle

3 月经先后无定期

Menstruation 1-2 weeks earlier or later, irregularity of menstrual cycle, is often caused by mental depression, stagnation of liver qi; or by frequent asthenia of the kidney, lack of proper care after prolonged illness, multiparity and over sex, consumption of kidney qi. Prolonged duration of the illness may lead to metrorrhagia and metrostaxis.

月经周期时或提前时或延后 1～2 周,连续出现 3 个周期以上,称为月经先后无定期。本病主要由于情志不畅,肝气郁滞,或素体肾虚,久病失养,多产房劳,肾气亏损所致。若病延日久,也可转为崩漏病。

3.1 Key points of diagnosis

(1) Irregular periods, menstruation occurs 1-2 weeks earlier or later, for three continuous cycles.

(2) Menstruation is not prolonged and menses is not profuse. Cares should be taken to differentiate it from metrorrhagia and metrotaxis.

3.2 Syndrome differentiation and treatment

The pathogenesis of irregularity of menstrual cycle is due to the liver failing to course freely and kidney failing to store, leading to irregular storage and drainage in uterus. Therapeutic principle is mainly coursing the liver and supplementing the kidney to harmonize the Thoroughfare and Conception Vessels. As soon as the storage and drainage is normalized in uterus, menstruation will come on time.

3.2.1 Liver stagnation syndrome

Main manifestations Early or delayed menstruation in profuse or scanty menorrhea, dark-red menses with blood clot, accompanied by emotional depression, breast and hypochondriac distention, discomfort in the epigastric region, preference for sighing, belching, poor appetite, normal or slight dark tongue with thin and white or thin and yellowish fur as well as taut pulse.

Therapeutic methods Coursing the liver and resolving stagnation, harmonizing the blood and regulating menstruation.

Formulas and herbs *Free Wanderer Powder* (Xiao Yao San): 6 g of *Radix Bupleuri* (Chai Hu), 10 g of *Radix Angelicae Sinensis* (Dang Gui), 10 g of *Rhizoma Atractylodis Macrocephalae* (Bai Zhu), 10 g of *Radix Paeoniae Alba* (Bai Shao), 10 g of *Poriae* (Fu Ling), 5 g of *Herba Menthae* (Bo He)

3.1 诊断要点

(1) 月经周期不定，时或提前、时或延后 1～2 周，连续 3 个月经周期以上者。

(2) 本病经期不长，经量不多，应注意与崩漏区别。

3.2 辨证论治

月经先后无定期的主要病机是肝失疏泄或肾失封藏，以致胞宫藏泻失常。治疗原则以疏肝补肾为主，使冲任调和，胞宫藏泻有度，则月经按期来潮。

3.2.1 肝郁证

主要证候　月经或提前，或错后，经量或多或少，色暗红有块。伴情志抑郁，胸胁乳房胀满，脘闷不舒，时叹息，嗳气食少。舌质正常或略暗，舌苔薄白，或薄黄，脉弦。

治法　疏肝解郁，和血调经。

方药　代表方为逍遥散；常用药如柴胡 6 克，当归 10 克，白术 10 克，白芍 10 克，茯苓 10 克，薄荷（后下）5 克，荆芥 6 克，甘草 3 克。

(to be decocted later), 6 g of *Herba Schizonepetae* (Jing Jie) and 3 g of *Radix Glycyrrhizae* (Gan Cao).

Shanghai doctor WANG Huiping's experience prescription, *Depression-Diffusing and Menstruation-Freeing Decoction* (Xuan Yu Tong Jing Tang): 12 g of *Radix Angelicae Sinensis* (Dang Gui), 12 g of *Radix Paeoniae Alba* (Bai Shao), 7 g of *Rhizoma Ligustici Chuanxiong* (Chuan Xiong), 12 g of *Radix Salviae Miltiorrhizae* (Dan Shen), 10 g of *Radix Bupleuri* (Chai Hu), 12 g of *Curcumae Radix & Australis* (Guang Yu Jin), 15 g of *Cyperi Rhizoma Praeparatum* (Zhi Xiang Fu), 12 g of *Rhizoma Dioscoreae* (Shan Yao) and 5 g of *Radix Glycyrrhizae* (Gan Cao).

上海医家王辉萍经验方(宣郁通经汤):当归 12 克,白芍 12 克,川芎 7 克,丹参 12 克,柴胡 10 克,广郁金 12 克,制香附 15 克,山药 12 克,甘草 5 克。

Modification For blood stasis and blood clot in menses due to liver stagnation, *Radix Salviae Miltiorrhizae* (Dan Shen), *Pollen Typhae* (Pu Huang) and *Rhizoma Ligustici Chuanxiong* (Chuan Xiong) are added to activate blood and move qi. For profuse menses, bitter mouth and dry throat due to heat transformed from liver stagnation, *Cortex Moutan Radicis* (Mu Dan Pi) and *Fructus Gardeniae* (Zhi Zi) are added to clear away liver heat. For stuffy sensation in the chest and epigastric region and poor appetite, *Pericarpium Citri Tangerinae* (Chen Pi), *Cortex Magnoliae Officinalis* (Hou Po) and *Massa Fermentata Medicinalis* (Shen Qu) are added to move qi and disperse stuffy sensation. For abdominal distension and pain, *Rhizoma Cyperi* (Xiang Fu) and *Radix Aucklandiae* (Mu Xiang) are added to move qi and relieve pain. For aching lumbs and knees, *Cortex Eucommiae* (Du Zhong) and *Ramulus Loranthi* (Sang Ji Sheng) are added to supplement the kidney and strengthen the lumbs and knees.

加减 若肝郁血滞,经血有块者,加丹参、蒲黄、川芎以活血行气;肝郁化热,经量多,口苦咽干者,加牡丹皮、栀子以清肝热;胸脘痞闷,纳呆者,加陈皮、厚朴、神曲以行气消痞;小腹胀痛者加香附、木香以行气止痛;腰膝酸痛者,加杜仲、桑寄生补肾壮腰膝。

3. 2. 2 Kidney asthenia syndrome

Main manifestations Early or delayed menstruation with scanty, light-colored, clear and thin menses, somber facial complexion, dizziness, tinnitus, aching lumbs and knees, abdominal empty sagging sensation, frequent urination, pale tongue with thin fur, and deep-weak pulse.

Therapeutic methods Supplementing the kidney and boosting qi, securing Thoroughfare Vessel and regulating menstruation.

Formulas and herbs *Yin-Securing Brew* (Gu Yin Jian): 10 g of *Radix Ginseng* (Ren Shen), 12 g of *Radix Rehmanniae Praeparata* (Shu Di Huang), 12 g of *Rhizoma Dioscoreae* (Shan Yao), 12 g of *Fructus Corni* (Shan Zhu Yu), 9 g of *Radix Polygalae* (Yuan Zhi), 6 g of *Radix Glycyrrhizae Praeparata* (Zhi Gan Cao), 6 g of *Fructus Schisandrae* (Wu Wei Zi) and 12 g of *Semen Cuscutae* (Tu Si Zi).

Shanghai doctor CAI Xiaosun's experience prescription, *Supplemented Eight-Gem Decoction* (Jia Wei Ba Zhen Tang): 10 g of *Angelicae Sinensis Radix Fricta* (Chao Dang Gui), 10 g of *Radix Rehmanniae Cruda* (Sheng Di Huang), 10 g of *Radix Rehmanniae Praeparata* (Shu Di Huang), 6 g of *Rhizoma Ligustici Chuanxiong* (Chuan Xiong), 10 g of *Radix Paeoniae Alba* (Bai Shao), 12 g of *Codonopsis Radix & Lu'anensis Fricta* (Chao Lu Dang), 10 g of *Atractylodis Macrocephalae Rhizoma Frictum* (Chao Bai Zhu), 12 g of *Poriae* (Fu Ling), 3 g of *Radix Glycyrrhizae Praeparata* (Zhi Gan Cao), 10 g of *Cyperi Rhizoma Praeparatum* (Zhi Xiang Fu), 10 g of *Herba Leonuri* (Yi Mu Cao) and 7 pieces of *Fructus Ziziphi Jujubae* (Da Zao).

Modification For profuse menses, *Ecliptae Herba* (Han Lian Cao), *Rosae Laevigatae Fructus* (Jin Ying Zi) and *Pyrolae Herba* (Lu Xian Cao) are

3. 2. 2 肾虚证

主要证候 经行或先或后，量少，色淡，质清稀。伴面色晦暗，头晕耳鸣，腰膝酸痛，小腹空坠，小便频数。舌淡，苔薄，脉沉细弱。

治法 补肾益气，固冲调经。

方药 代表方为固阴煎；常用药如人参 10 克，熟地黄 12 克，山药 12 克，山茱萸 12 克，远志 9 克，炙甘草 6 克，五味子 6 克，菟丝子 12 克。

上海医家蔡小荪经验方（加味八珍汤）：炒当归 10 克，生熟地各 10 克，川芎 6 克，白芍 10 克，炒潞党 12 克，炒白术 10 克，云茯苓 12 克，炙甘草 3 克，制香附 10 克，益母草 10 克，大枣 7 枚。

加减 若兼经血量多者加旱莲草、金樱子、鹿衔草以益肾固摄；腰痛如折者，加续

added to boost the kidney and promote the containing ability. For severe low back pain, *Radix Dipsaci* (Xu Duan) and *Ramulus Loranthi* (Sang Ji Sheng) are added to supplement the kidney and strengthen the lumbus. For abdominal cold and pain, *Cortex Cinnamomi* (Rou Gui) and *Fructus Foeniculi* (Xiao Hui Xiang) are added to warm the meridians and relieve pain. For physical cold and cold limbs, *Aconiti Radix Lateralis Tosta* (Pao Fu Zi) and *Ramulus Cinnamomi* (Gui Zhi) are added to free yang. For frequent urination, *Fructus Alpiniae Oxyphyllae* (Yi Zhi Ren) and *Ootheca Mantidis* (Sang Piao Xiao) are added to secure astringency. For loose stool and diarrhea, *Fructus Psoraleae* (Bu Gu Zhi) and *Fructus Evodiae* (Wu Zhu Yu) are added to warm and supplement the spleen and kidney. For vexation and sleeplessness, *Semen Zizyphi Spinosae* (Suan Zao Ren) and *Cortex Alibiziae* (He Huan Pi) are added to quiet the heart and spirit and resolve depression.

断、桑寄生以增强补肾强腰之效；小腹冷痛者，加肉桂、小茴香以温经止痛；形寒肢冷者，加炮附片、桂枝以通阳；小便频数者，加益智仁、桑螵蛸以固涩；大便溏泻者，加补骨脂、吴茱萸以温补脾肾；心烦不眠者，加酸枣仁、合欢皮以宁心安神解郁。

3.3 Other therapeutic methods

3.3.1 Chinese patent drugs

(1) *Free Wanderer Pill* (Xiao Yao Wan): 8 pills each time and 3 times a day, applicable to the treatment of qi stagnation syndrome.

(2) *Stagnancy-Relieving Pills* (Yue Ju Wan): 5 g each time and 3 times a day, applicable to the treatment of phlegm stagnation syndrome.

(3) *Nyu Jin Pill* (Nü Jin Wan): For water honey pill, 5 g each time, for honey pill, 1 pill each time and twice a day, applicable to the treatment of qi-blood vacuity, qi stagnation and blood stasis syndrome.

3.3 其他疗法

3.3.1 中成药

（1）逍遥丸：每次 8 丸，每日 3 次，适用于气滞之证。

（2）越鞠丸：每次 5 克，每日 3 次，适用于痰滞之证。

（3）女金丸：水蜜丸每次 5 克，大蜜丸每次 1 丸，每日 2 次，用于气血两虚、气滞血瘀之证。

3.3.2 Empirical and folk recipes

(1) Slices of 30 g of *Rhizoma Cyperi* (Xiang Fu) and 15 g of *Radix Angelicae Sinensis* (Dang Gui) are steeped in rice wine. After three days the wine is ready. Drink twice a day and 15 ml each time, applicable to the treatment of liver stagnation syndrome.

(2) 15 g of *Fructus Lycii* (Gou Qi Zi), 20 g of *Fresh Folium Citri Reticulatae* (Xian Ju Ye), 10 g of *Caulis Perillae* (Zi Su Geng) and 15 g of brown sugar are steeped in boiling water for 15 - 20 minutes. The decoction is taken orally as tea, applicable to the treatment of kidney asthenia and liver stagnation syndrome.

3.3.2 单验方

（1）香附 30 克，当归 15 克，黄酒 250 克，前两药切片泡酒，3 日后可饮用，每日 2 次，每次 15 毫升，适用于肝郁证。

（2）枸杞子 15 克，鲜橘叶 20 克，紫苏梗 10 克，红糖 15 克，置保温杯中，加开水泡 15～20 分钟，频作茶饮，适用于肾虚肝郁证。

4 Profuse menorrhea

Profuse menorrhea means that the quantity of menses increases noticeably, more than 80 ml, while menstrual cycle and period are basically normal. Early or delayed menstruation may happen but it is in a certain cycle. Abnormal menstruation may cause secondary anemia.

4 月经过多

月经量明显增多，超过 80 毫升，周期、经期基本正常，称为月经过多。可伴有月经提前或推后，但尚有一定的周期；经期的异常，可引起继发性贫血。

4.1 Key points for diagnosis

(1) Menorrhea increases noticeably but stops after a certain period of time.

(2) Profuse menorrhea usually appears together with early menstruation or delayed menstruation.

(3) Profuse menorrhea in fulminant downflow or incessant menorrhea, or metrorrhagia and metrostaxis if on irregular menstrual cycle.

4.1 诊断要点

（1）月经量明显增多，但在一定时间内能自行停止。

（2）本病常与月经先期、月经后期同时出现。

（3）经量过多，暴下如注或经血日久不止，或有周期紊乱者，则为崩漏。

4.2 Syndrome differentiation and treatment

The main pathogenesis of profuse menorrhea is storage and drainage failing in the uterus due to insecurity of the Thoroughfare and Conception Ves-

4.2 辨证论治

月经过多的主要病机是冲任不固，胞宫藏泻失职。治疗原则是益气清热，固冲

sels. Therapeutic methods are boosting qi and clearing heat, securing Thoroughfare Vessel and containing the blood. Qi asthenia, blood heat or blood stasis should be identified according to menstruation, general symptom, tongue and pulse. Therapeutic methods should be different for the menstrual time and normal time. Treatment should focuses on strengthening the Thoroughfare Vessel and stopping bleeding to reduce menstrual flow during menstruation and on regulating qi and blood and and strengthening the body according to the cause of disease and pathogenesis in normal times. Asthenia and sthenia are differentiated by their color and texture. Profuse menses in thin texture with light color are the characteristics of qi asthenia. Profuse menses in thick texture with bright red color are the characteristics of blood heat. Drugs of warm and dry nature should be avoided lest blood be disturbed. Methods to stop bleeding should be adopted according to pattern identification. For qi asthenia, boost qi and contain the blood. For blood heat, clear away heat and cool the blood. For blood stasis, resolve stasis and stop bleeding in order to achieve static and dynamic equilibrium, moderate storage and drainage in uterus.

摄血。要根据月经情况及全身症状与舌脉辨别气虚、血热或血瘀。其治法则需区分经期与平时。经期重在固冲止血,减少月经量;非经期则主要针对病因病机,调理气血以治本。辨证仍以经色质来别虚实,月经量多质薄、经色偏淡属气虚;量多质稠、经色鲜红属血热。临证用药,以少用温燥之品为宜,以免动血。止血之法,应根据辨证,气虚者宜益气摄血;血热者宜清热凉血;血瘀者宜化瘀止血。以达到动静平衡,胞宫藏泻有度。

4.2.1 Qi asthenia syndrome

Main manifestations Profuse, clear and thin menses with light red color, lusterless facial complexion, low spirit and lack of strength, shortness of breath and lazy to speak, insidious abdominal pain, slight red tongue with thin white fur, and thin and weak pulse.

Therapeutic methods Supplementing qi and strengthening the Thoroughfare Vessel, controlling

4.2.1 气虚证

主要证候 经行量多,经色淡红,经质清稀。面色无华,神疲乏力,气短懒言,小腹绵绵作痛。舌淡红,苔薄白,脉细弱。

治法 补气固冲,摄血调经。

blood and regulating menstruation.

Formulas and herbs *Original-Lifting Brew* (Ju Yuan Jian): 12 g of *Radix Ginseng* (Ren Shen), 12 g of *Radix Astragali Praeparata* (Zhi Huang Qi), 6 g of *Radix Glycyrrhizae Praeparata* (Zhi Gan Cao), 6 g of *Rhizoma Cimicifugae Frictum* (Chao Sheng Ma) and 9 g of *Rhizoma Atractylodis Macrocephalae Frictum* (Chao Bai Zhu).

方药 代表方为举元煎;常用药如人参12克,炙黄芪12克,炙甘草6克,炒升麻6克,炒白术9克。

Modification For profuse menorrhea during menstrual course, *Colla Corii Asini* (E Jiao), *Artemisiae Argyi Folium Carbonisatum* (Ai Ye Tan), *Os Sepiellae seu Sepiae* (Hai Piao Xiao) and *Ostreae Concha Cruda* (Sheng Mu Li) are added to astringe and stanch bleeding. For blood stasis and prolonged menstruation with blood clot in menses, *Herba Leonuri* (Yi Mu Cao) and *Typhae Pollen Frictus* (Chao Pu Huang) are added to dispel stasis and stanch bleeding. For palpitations and insomnia due to spirit deprived of nourishment, *Ziziphi Spinosi Semen Frictum* (Chao Zao Ren) and *Concha Margaritifera Usta* (Zhen Zhu Mu) are added to nourish the heart and quiet the spirit. For kidney qi vacuity and aching lumbs and knees, *Cortex Eucommiae* (Du Zhong), *Fructus Psoraleae* (Bu Gu Zhi) and *Halloysitum Rubrum* (Chi Shi Zhi) are added to secure the kidney and stanch bleeding.

加减 若值经期者,可选加阿胶、艾叶炭、乌贼骨、生牡蛎以收涩止血;若兼血瘀,伴经期延长,经血有块者,加益母草、炒蒲黄以祛瘀止血;若兼心神失养见心悸不眠者,加炒枣仁、珍珠母以养心安神;若兼肾气虚,腰膝酸痛者,加杜仲、补骨脂、赤石脂以固肾止血。

4.2.2 Blood heat syndrome

Main manifestations Profuse menorrhea with bright red or dark red color and thick and sticky menses, dysphoria, thirst, generalized heat sensation with red face, constipation, yellow or reddish urine with scorching heat sensation, red or crimson tongue with yellow fur, and slippery and rapid pulse.

4.2.2 血热证

主要证候 经行量多,经色鲜红或深红,有光泽,质稠黏。伴心烦口渴,身热面赤,大便干结,小便黄赤,或有灼热感。舌红绛,苔黄,脉滑数。

Therapeutic methods Clearing away heat, cooling blood and nourishing yin, dispelling stasis and stopping bleeding.

治法 清热凉血养阴，祛瘀止血。

Formulas and herbs *Yin-Protecting Decoction* (Bao Yin Jian): 9 g of *Radix Rehmanniae Cruda* (Sheng Di Huang), 9 g of *Radix Rehmanniae Praeparata* (Shu Di Huang), 6 g of *Radix Scutellariae* (Huang Qin), 9 g of *Radix Paeoniae Alba* (Bai Shao), 12 g of *Rhizoma Dioscoreae* (Shan Yao), 12 g of *Radix Dipsaci* (Xu Duan) and 6 g of *Radix Glycyrrhizae* (Can Cao).

方药 代表方为保阴煎；常用药如生地黄 9 克，熟地黄 9 克，黄芩 6 克，白芍 9 克，山药 12 克，续断 12 克，甘草 6 克。

Shanghai doctor TANG Jifu's experience prescription, *Radix Codonopsis Pilosulae/Rubiae RadixMenses-Securing Granules* (Shen Qian Gu Jing Chong Ji): 9 g of *Rhizoma Cimicifugae* (Sheng Ma), 12 g of *Radix Codonopsis Pilosulae* (Dang Shen), 9 g of *Rhizoma Atractylodis Macrocephalae* (Bai Zhu), 12 g of *Radix Rehmanniae Cruda* (Sheng Di Huang), 9 g of *Radix Paeoniae Alba* (Bai Shao), 12 g of *Fructus Ligustri Lucidi* (Nü Zhen Zi), 12 g of *Ecliptae Herba* (Han Lian Cao), 12 g of *Typhae Pollen* (Pu Huang), 12 g of *Sophorae Flos Immaturus* (Huai Mi), 12 g of *Herba seu Radix Cirsii Japonici* (Da Ji), 12 g of *Herba Cephalanoploris* (Xiao Ji), 12 g of *Fructus Crataegi* (Shan Zha) and 12 g of *Rubiae Radix* (Qian Cao).

上海医家唐吉父经验方（参茜固经冲剂）：升麻 9 克，党参 12 克，白术 9 克，生地黄 12 克，白芍 9 克，女贞子 12 克，旱莲草 12 克，蒲黄 12 克，槐米 12 克，大小蓟各 12 克，山楂 12 克，茜草 12 克。

Shanghai doctor TANG Xiyuan's experience prescription, *Cortex Mori Radicis and Folium Mori Four Agents Decoction* (Er Sang Si Wu Tang): 12 g of *Cortex Mori Radicis* (Sang Bai Pi), 9 g of *Folium Mori* (Sang Ye), 10 g of *Angelicae Sinensis Radix Frictum* (Chao Dang Gui), 10 g of *Radix Paeoniae Rubra Frictum* (Chao Chi Shao), 10 g of *Radix Rehmanniae Cruda* (Sheng Di Huang), 9 g of *Cortex Moutan Radicis* (Mu Dan Pi), 6 g of *Radix Scutellariae Frictum* (Chao Huang Qin), 12 g of *Rhizoma Imperatae* (Bai Mao Gen), 9 g of *Radix Cyathulae* (Chuan Niu Xi) and 5 g of *Radix Glycyrrhizae* (Gan Cao).

上海医家唐锡元经验方（二桑四物汤）：桑白皮 12 克，桑叶 9 克，炒当归 10 克，炒赤芍 9 克，生地黄 10 克，牡丹皮 9 克，炒黄芩 6 克，白茅根 12 克，川牛膝 9 克，甘草 5 克。

Modification If exogenous pathogenic heat

加减 若兼有感受热邪

transforms into fire and changes into toxin with the symptoms of fever, aversion to cold and lower abdominal hardness and pain aggravated by pressure, *Herba Patriniae* (Bai Jiang Cao), *Caulis Sargentodoxae* (Da Xue Teng), *Herba Taraxaci* (Pu Gong Ying) and *Typhae Pollen* (Pu Huang) are added. The prescription can be used together with *Pulse-Engendering Powder* (Sheng Mai San)to treat qi and yin vacuity due to prolonged illness with the symptoms of shortness of breath, palpitations, vexing heat in the five body parts, tinnitus, insomnia and dizziness.

而化火成毒，症见发热恶寒，少腹硬痛拒按者，加败酱草、红藤、蒲公英、蒲黄；患病日久兼见气阴两虚证，气短心悸，五心烦热，耳鸣失眠，头晕者，可与生脉散合用。

4.3 Other therapeutic methods

4.3.1 Chinese patent drugs

(1) *Gong Xue Ning Capsule* (Gong Xue Ning Jiao Nang): 2 capsules each time and three times a day, applicable to the treatment of frenetic blood heat syndrome.

(2) *Chinese Angelica Blood-Nourish Pill* (Dang Gui Yang Xue Wan): 9 g each time and three times a day, applicable to the treatment of qi and blood vacuity syndrome.

(3) *Compound Formula Colla Corii Asini Syrup* (Fu Fang E Jiao Jiang): 20 ml each time and three times a day, applicable to the treatment of qi and blood vacuity syndrome.

4.3.2 Empirical and folk recipes

(1) 60 g of *Sanguisorbae Radix* (Di Yu) is ground into powder. Each time 6 g of powder is decocted in sweet wine for oral administration. Such a recipe is applicable to the treatment of blood heat syndrome.

(2) 60 g of *Radix Ginseng* (Ren Shen) and 500 g of *Radix Astragali* (Huang Qi) are decocted

4.3 其他疗法

4.3.1 中成药

（1）宫血宁胶囊：每次 2 粒，每日 3 次，适用于血热妄行之证。

（2）当归养血丸：每次 9 克，每日 3 次，适用于气血两虚之证。

（3）复方阿胶浆：每次 20 毫升，每日 3 次，适用于气血两虚之证。

4.3.2 单验方

（1）地榆 60 克，甜酒适量，地榆研末，每次 6 克，甜酒煎服，适用于血热之证。

（2）人参 60 克，黄芪 500 克，饴糖 500 克，前两味药煎

for three times. After the removal of residue, 500 g of *Mattose* (Yi Tang) is added into the decoction. Each time 10 g of extract is taken, twice a day. This recipe is applicable to the treatment of qi asthenia syndrome.

熬 3 次，去渣后入饴糖，出膏，每次 10 克，每日 2 次，适用于气虚之证。

5 Scanty menstruation

Scanty menstruation means that, normal cycle, obviously reduced menorrhea, less than 30 ml, or the menstrual cycle in less than two days or just a little menses.

The cause of scanty menstruation is similar to that of delayed menstruation and is either asthenia or sthenia. Asthenia syndrome is due to constitutional blood asthenia or kidney asthenia, leading to deficiency of essence and blood, asthenia of nutrient blood and insufficiency of blood in the uterus. Sthenia syndrome is due to stagnation of exogenous cold in the meridians and collaterals; or due to qi stagnation and unsmooth circulation of blood that blocks the Thoroughfare and Conception Vessels and the uterus, inhibiting the occurrence of menorrhea; or due to internal retention of phlegm and dampness that hinders blood, and leading to scanty menorrhea.

5 月经过少

月经周期正常，经量明显减少，不足 30 毫升，或行经时间不足 2 日，甚或点滴即净，称为月经过少。

本病的发病机理基本上与月经后期类同，分虚实两证：虚者因素体血虚或肾虚，以致精血不足，营血亏虚，血海不充而月经过少；实者可由感寒，寒凝经脉，或气滞经不畅，致冲任胞宫瘀阻，经行不畅；或痰湿内阻，血不畅行而月经过少。

5.1 Key points for diagnosis

(1) Menstrual cycle is basically normal, but the amount of menses is scanty or just a few drops.

(2) Cares should be taken to exclude scanty menses due to administration of contraceptives in women of childbearing age.

(3) Menstruation in early pregnancy should be differentiated from the problem mentioned above.

5.1 诊断要点

(1) 月经周期基本正常，经量很少，甚或点滴即净。

(2) 注意排除育龄女性因服用避孕药而致经量过少。

(3) 注意早孕而有激经者应与本病区别。

5.2 Syndrome differentiation and treatment

The cause of scanty menstruation is either asthenia or sthenia. Asthenia includes kidney asthenia and blood asthenia. Sthenia includes blood stasis and phlegm dampness. Usually light-colored and clear menses without abdominal distention and pain is of asthenia syndrome. Purplish and blackish dark menses with blood clot and abdominal pain aggravated by pressure signifies blood stasis. Light-reddish menses sticky like phlegm suggests phlegm dampness. For asthenia, supplement the kidney, nourish the blood and regulate menstruation. For sthenia, dredge the meridians and collateral, dispel stasis and dissolve phlegm to free blood movement. The treatment of this syndrome should concentrate on replenishing and supplementing essence and blood. Since asthenia syndrome appears more frequently than sthenia, care must be taken when using purgative and strong herbs lest qi and blood are impaired and menstruation becomes difficult to restore. Scanty menstruation accompanied by delayed menstruation may turn into amenorrhea.

5.2 辨证论治

月经过少的病机有虚实两端。虚者有肾虚和血虚；实者有血瘀和痰湿。一般以色淡、质清、腹无胀痛为虚；色紫暗夹有血块，腹痛拒按者，为血瘀；色淡红、质黏如痰者为痰湿。虚者补肾养血调经；实者疏通经脉，祛瘀化痰，以畅血行。本病治法当重在填补精血。因虚多实少，慎不可恣投攻破之品，以免重伤气血，使经血难复。月经过少而常伴后期者，可发展为闭经。

5.2.1 Blood asthenia syndrome

Main manifestations Scanty menses with light color and thin texture, sallow complexion, dizziness, palpitation, shortness of breath, insidious abdominal pain during menstruation, slight red tongue with thin fur, and thin and weak pulse.

Therapeutic methods Nourishing blood and regulating menstruation.

Formulas and herbs *Blood-Enriching Decoction* (Zi Xue Tang) composed of 12 g of *Radix Codonopsis Pilosulae* (Dang Shen), 12 g of *Rhizoma Dioscoreae* (Shan Yao), 12 g of *Poriae* (Fu Ling),

5.2.1 血虚证

主要证候 经血量少，经色淡红，质稀薄。伴面色萎黄，头晕眼花，心悸气短，经行小腹绵绵作痛。舌淡红，苔薄，脉细弱。

治法 养血调经。

方药 代表方为滋血汤；常用药如党参 12 克，山药 12 克，茯苓 12 克，熟地黄 12 克，当归 12 克，白芍 9 克，

12 g of *Radix Rehmanniae Praeparata* (Shu Di Huang), 12 g of *Radix Angelicae Sinensis* (Dang Gui), 9 g of *Radix Paeoniae Alba* (Bai Shao), 6 g of *Rhizoma Ligustici Chuanxiong* (Chuan Xiong) and 12 g of *Radix Astragali* (Huang Qi).

川芎6克，黄芪12克。

Modification For asthenia heat, *Cortex Lycii Radicis* (Di Gu Pi) and *Radix Scrophulariae* (Xuan Shen) are added. For insomnia and palpitation due to blood asthenia, 15 g of *Caulis Polygoni Multiflori* (Ye Jiao Teng) and *Fructus Schisandrae* (Wu Wei Zi) are added. If it is accompanied by liver stagnation with hypochondriac distention or breast distention and pain, *Radix Bupleuri* (Chai Hu), *Rhizoma Cyperi* (Xiang Fu) and *Fructus Meliae Toosendan* (Chuan Lian Zi) are added.

加减 若虚热者，加地骨皮、玄参；血虚而失眠、心悸者，加夜交藤、五味子；兼肝郁有胁胀或乳胀作痛者，加柴胡、香附、川楝子。

5.2.2 Kidney-deficiency syndrome

5.2.2 肾虚证

Main symptoms Scanty and pale menses, withered complexion, dizziness and tinnitus, flaccid, weak, cold and painful waist and knees, cold in the lower abdomen, profuse urine at night, slight dark tongue with thin and white fur, deep and thin pulse and weak cubit pulse.

主要证候 经行量少，经色淡暗，伴面容憔悴，头晕耳鸣，腰骶酸软冷痛，小腹凉，夜尿多。舌淡暗，苔薄白，脉沉细，尺脉无力。

Therapeutic methods Supplementing the kidney and replenishing essence, nourishing blood and regulating menstruation.

治法 补肾填精，养血调经。

Formulas and herbs *Kidney-Returning Pill* (Gui Shen Wan) composed of 10 g of *Cortex Eucommiae* (Du Zhong), 10 g of *Semen Cuscutae* (Tu Si Zi), 10 g of *Radix Rehmanniae Praeparata* (Shu Di Huang), 10 g of *Radix Angelicae Sinensis* (Dang Gui), 15 g of *Rhizoma Dioscoreae* (Shan Yao), 10 g of *Poriae* (Fu Ling), 10 g of *Fructus Corni* (Shan Zhu Yu) and 10 g of *Fructus Lycii* (Gou Qi Zi).

方药 代表方为归肾丸；常用药如杜仲10克，菟丝子10克，熟地黄10克，当归10克，山药15克，茯苓10克，山茱萸10克，枸杞子10克。

Shanghai doctor WANG Huiping's experience prescrip-

上海医家王辉萍经验方（定

tion, *Modified Menses-Stabilizing Decoction* (Ding Jing Tang): 20 g of *Semen Cuscutae* (Tu Si Zi), 12 g of *Radix Rehmanniae Praeparata* (Shu Di Huang), 12 g of *Radix Angelicae Sinensis* (Dang Gui), 10 g of *Radix Paeoniae Alba* (Bai Shao), 12 g of *Radix Bupleuri* (Chai Hu), 15 g of *Epimedium davidii* (Xian Ling Pi), 15 g of *Radix Morindae Officinalis* (Ba Ji Tian), 12 g of *Fructus Corni* (Shan Zhu Yu), 12 g of *Cortex Moutan Radicis* (Mu Dan Pi) and 10 g of *Radix Aucklandiae* (Guang Mu Xiang).

经汤)加减:菟丝子 20 克,熟地 12 克,当归 12 克,白芍 10 克,柴胡 12 克,仙灵脾 15 克,巴戟天 15 克,山茱萸 12 克,牡丹皮 12 克,广木香 10 克。

Modification For cold abdomen, frequent nocturia and lack of warmth in the extremities, *Epimedium davidii* (Yin Yang Huo), *Radix Morindae Officinalis* (Ba Ji Tian), *Cortex Cinnamomi* (Rou Gui, Shanghai Gui, Guan Gui) and *Fructus Alpiniae Oxyphyllae* (Yi Zhi Ren) are added to warm and supplement kidney yang; For vexing heat in the five body parts and red tongue, *Fructus Ligustri Lucidi* (Nü Zhen Zi), *Radix Scrophulariae* (Xuan Shen) and *Testudinis Carapax et Plastrum cum Liquido Fricti* (Zhi Gui Ban) are added to enrich and nourish kidney yin. For dry throat and mouth, tidal heat sensation and sweating, *Radix Trichosanthis* (Tian Hua Fen), *Rhizoma Anemarrhenae* (Zhi Mu) and *Herba Dendrobii* (Shi Hu) are added to nourish yin and clear away heat.

加减　若小腹凉,夜尿多,手足不温者,加入淫羊藿、巴戟天、肉桂、益智仁以温补肾阳;若五心烦热,舌红者,加女贞子、玄参、炙龟板以滋养肾阴;若咽干口燥,潮热汗出者,加天花粉、知母、石斛以养阴清热。

5.2.3 Blood stasis syndrome

Main manifestations Scanty and dark-red menses with blood clot, abdominal distention and pain alleviated after menstruation, pain and distention in the chest and rib-side, lumbosacral pain, dark purple tongue with stasis macules or petechiae, deep and choppy or deep and stringlike pulse.

Therapeutic methods Activating blood to resolve blood stasis and nourishing blood to regulate

5.2.3 血瘀证

主要证候　经血量少,色暗红,或挟有小血块。小腹胀痛不适,经行后痛减,或伴胸胁胀痛,腰骶疼痛。舌紫暗,有瘀斑或瘀点,脉沉涩或沉弦。

治法　活血化瘀,养血调经。

menstruation.

Formulas and herbs *Peach Pit, Safflower and Four Agents Decoction* (Tao Hong Si Wu Tang) composed of 10 g of *Semen Persicae* (Tao Ren), 6 g of *Flos Carthami* (Hong Hua), 10 g *Radix Angelicae Sinensis* (Dang Gui), 5 g of *Rhizoma Ligustici Chuanxiong* (Chuan Xiong), 10 g of *Radix Paeoniae Alba* (Bai Shao), 10 g of *Radix Rehmanniae Praeparata* (Shu Di Huang), 12 g of *Herba Lycopi* (Ze Lan), 10 g of *Faeces Trogopterorum* (Wu Ling Zhi), 12 g of *Radix Salviae Miltiorrhizae* (Dan Shen) and 3 g of *Radix Glycyrrhizae* (Gan Cao).

方药 代表方为桃红四物汤；常用药如桃仁10克，红花6克，当归10克，川芎5克，白芍10克，熟地黄10克，泽兰12克，五灵脂10克，丹参12克，甘草3克。

Modification For distension in the chest and hypochodrium, *Fructus Aurantii* (Zhi Qiao), *Rhizoma Cyperi* (Xiang Fu) and *Fructus Meliae Toosendan* (Chuan Lian Zi) are added to move qi and relieve pain. For abdominal cold and pain, *Cortex Cinnamomi* (Rou Gui) and *Rhizoma Zingiberis Praeparata* (Pao Jiang) are added to warm the meridians and dredge the collaterals. For dry throat, bitter taste in the mouth and generalized heat, *Radix Scutellariae* (Huang Qin) and *Cortex Moutan Radicis* (Mu Dan Pi) are added to cool and activate the blood. For fatigued spirit and lack of strength, *Radix Astragali* (Huang Qi), *Radix Ginseng* (Ren Shen) and *Rhizoma Atractylodis Macrocephalae* (Bai Zhu) are added to fortify the spleen and boost qi.

加减 若胸胁小腹胀满者，加枳壳、香附、川楝子以行气止痛；小腹冷痛者，加肉桂、炮姜以温经通络；若咽干口苦身热者，加黄芩、牡丹皮以凉血活血；若神疲乏力者，加黄芪、人参、白术以健脾益气。

5.2.4 Phlegm-dampness syndrome

Main manifestations Scanty, slight red and sticky menses with grume, fat body, fullness and oppression in the chest and epigastric region, fatigue and lack of strength, profuse vaginal discharge, enlarged tongue with whitish greasy fur, and tooth marks on the margins of the tongue, taut

5.2.4 痰湿证

主要证候 经血量少，色淡红，质黏稠或夹杂黏液。形体肥胖，胸脘满闷，倦怠乏力，或带下量多。舌体胖大，边有齿痕，苔白腻，脉弦滑。

and slippery pulse.

Therapeutic methods Drying up dampness, resolving phlegm, activating blood and regulating menstruation.

治法　燥湿化痰，活血调经。

Formulas and herbs *Atractylodes and Cyperus Phlegm-Abducting Pill* (Cang Fu Dao Tan Wan) composed of 10 g of *Rhizoma Atractylodis* (Cang Zhu), 10 g of *Rhizoma Cyperi* (Xiang Fu), 12 g of *Poriae* (Fu Ling), 10 g of *Pinelliae Rhizoma Praeparatum* (Fa Ban Xia), 10 g of *Pericarpium Citri Tangerinae* (Chen Pi), 3 g of *Radix Glycyrrhizae* (Gan Cao), 10 g of *Arisaema cum Bile* (Dan Nan Xing), 10 g of *Fructus Aurantii* (Zhi Qiao), 12 g of *Massa Fermentata Medicinalis* (Shen Qu) and 3 slices of *Rhizoma Zingiberis Recens* (Sheng Jiang).

方药　代表方为苍附导痰丸；常用药如苍术10克，香附10克，茯苓12克，法半夏10克，陈皮10克，甘草3克，胆南星10克，枳壳10克，神曲12克，生姜3片。

Modification For delayed scanty menses or gradual amenorrhea, *Herba Lycopi* (Ze Lan) and *Radix Cyathulae* (Chuan Niu Xi) are added to nourish and activate blood to regulate menstruation. For profuse phlegm and fat body, *Rhizoma Acori Graminei* (Shi Chang Pu) and *Radix Polygalae* (Zhi Yuan Zhi) are added to resolve phlegm and activate the collaterals.

加减　若月经量少落后或渐闭经者，酌加泽兰、川牛膝以养血活血通经；若痰多，形体肥胖者，加石菖蒲、炙远志以化痰活络。

5.3 Other therapeutic methods

5.3 其他疗法

5.3.1 Chinese patent drugs

5.3.1 中成药

(1) *Black Chicken and White Phoenix Pill* (Wu Ji Bai Feng Wan): 10 g each time and three times a day, applicable to blood deficiency syndrome.

（1）乌鸡白凤丸：每次10克，每日3次，适用于阴血虚证。

(2) *An Kun Zan Yu Pill* (An Kun Zan Yu Wan): 1 pill each time and twice a day, applicable to dual depletion of qi and blood and insufficiency in the liver and kidney.

（2）安坤赞育丸：每次1丸，每日2次，适用于气血两亏，肝肾不足之证。

(3) *Four Agents Mixture* (Si Wu He Ji): 10-15 ml each time and three times a day, applicable to

（3）四物合剂：每次10～15毫升，每日3次，适用于血

blood deficiency syndrome.

虚证。

(4) *Placenta Major Bollus* (He Che Da Zao Wan): For big honey pill, 6 g or 1 pill each time and twice a day; for small honey pill, 9 g each time and twice a day, applicable to dual depletion of lung and kidney.

(4) 河车大造丸：大蜜丸每次 6 克，小蜜丸每次 9 克，大蜜丸每次 1 丸，每日 2 次，适用于肺肾两亏之证。

(5) *Donkey Glue Blood-Supplementing Granules* (Lu Jiao Bu Xue Ke Li): 20 g each time and 4 times a day, applicable to bodily vacuity and blood depletion syndrome.

(5) 阿胶补血颗粒：每次 20 克，每日 4 次，适用于体虚血亏之证。

(6) *Blood-Activating and Menstruation-Regulating Tablet* (Huo Xue Tiao Jing Pian): 5 tablets each time and three times a day, applicable to blood stasis syndrome.

(6) 活血调经片：每次 5 片，每日 3 次，适用于血瘀证。

5.3.2 Empirical and folk recipes

5.3.2 单验方

(1) 15 pieces of Chinese roses, proportional amount of rice wine. Charred Chinese roses are taken with rice wine, applicable to qi stagnation and blood stasis syndrome.

(1) 月季花 15 朵，黄酒适量，月季花烧炭，温黄酒送下，适用于气滞血瘀证。

(2) 250 g of pig trotters and 20 g of *Radix Achyranthis Bidentatae* (Niu Xi) are cooked with 20-50 g of rice wine, applicable to kidney deficiency syndrome.

(2) 猪蹄 250 克，牛膝 20 克，炖煮过程中加入米酒 20～50 克，适用于肾虚证。

Intermenstrual bleeding

经间期出血

Intermenstrual bleeding refers to periodic uterine bleeding or red and white vaginal discharge during ovulation or red leukorrhea. The characteristic of intermenstrual bleeding is that it happens during ovulation with scanty uterine bleeding and lasts about 1-2 days and generally stops automatically.

两次月经中间，即氤氲乐育之时，出现周期性的阴道出血，或者赤白带，称为“经间期出血”。其特点是阴道流血发生在经间期，即氤氲之时，且量甚少，一般一二日即自止。

This disease, pertaining to functional uterine

本病多发生于 20～30

bleeding in Western medicine and known as intermenstrual bleeding in TCM, usually occurs in the women aging from 20 to 30.

The occurrence of the disease is closely related to the decrease, increase and conversion of qi, blood, yin and yang during menstrual cycle. The main pathogenesis is yin vacuity, dampness and heat or blood stasis motivating yang qi, uncoordinated conversion in yin and yang, injury of yin-collaterals, weakness of the Thoroughfare and Conception Vessels, and blood spillage out of vessels, resulting in intermenstrual bleeding. If yin and blood are nourished yang qi is stored and yin and yang are balanced, the bleeding stops.

岁的女性，多属于西医学功能失调性子宫出血，中医学称之为经间期出血。

本病的发生与月经周期中的气血阴阳消长转化有密切关系。主要病因病机是阴虚、湿热或血瘀引动阳气，使阴阳转化不协调，损伤阴络，冲任不固，血溢脉外，遂发生经间期出血。当滋阴养血，使阳气潜藏，阴阳平衡，出血乃止。

1　Key points for diagnosis

1.1　Medical history

It is more common in young women, with medical history of irregular menstruation, or abortion and miscarriage.

1.2　Symptoms

Scanty uterine bleeding occurs repeatedly between two menstruations during 10-16 days in the menstrual cycle, lasts about 2-3 days and generally stops automatically. It may be accompanied by backache, one-side lower abdominal distention and pain, breast distention and pain, or increased vaginal discharge with transparent and sticky substance like egg white, or red and white vaginal discharge.

1.3　Examination

①Gynecological examination, cervical mucus is transparent and filiform with bloodshot in it. ② Other examination, basal body temperature is measured. There is bleeding when the high and low tem-

1　诊断要点

1.1　病史

多见于青年女子，可有月经不调史，或堕胎、小产史。

1.2　症状

在两次月经中间，一般是周期的第 10～16 日出现少量阴道流血，持续 2～3 日或数日则自止，反复发生。可伴腰酸，一侧少腹胀痛，乳房胀痛，或带下增多，质黏透明如蛋清样，或赤白带下。

1.3　检查

①妇科检查，宫颈黏液透明，呈拉丝状，夹有血丝。②其他检查，测量基础体温，在高、低温相交替时出血，一

perature alternate. Usually the bleeding stops after the basal body temperature rises. Sometimes bleeding continues during the high basal body temperature too. Serum estrogen and progesterone levels are usually lower.

般在基础体温升高后则出血停止，亦有高温相时继续出血；血清雌、孕激素水平通常偏低。

2 Syndrome differentiation and treatment

Asthenia and sthenia should be differentiated in the light of the amount, color and quality of bleeding as well as general symptoms, tongue and pulse. The syndrome of kidney yin deficiency is marked by minor, bright red bleeding with sticky texture. The syndrome of damp-heat is usually marked by slightly increased bleeding with red and white color and thick texture. The syndrome of blood stasis is marked by increased or scanty dark-red or purplish black bleeding. Treatment principles are mainly balancing the yin and yang, promoting the smooth transformation of yin and yang. According to the relationship of mutual dependance between yin and yang, pay attention to seeking yin in yang, supplementing yin without forgetting yang. The treatment time is focused on late menstrual periods. It can be treated by nourishing the kidney and enriching blood, clearing away heat, eliminating dampness and dissolving stasis. In bleeding, some herbs should be used to secure the Thoroughfare Vessel and stanch bleeding.

2 辨证论治

本病的辨证要点是根据出血的量、色、质，结合全身症状与舌脉辨虚实。若出血量少，色鲜红，质黏者，多为肾阴虚证；若出血量稍多，赤白相兼，质稠者，多为湿热证；若出血量时多时少，色暗红，或紫黑如酱，则为血瘀证。治疗原则以平衡阴阳为主，促进阴阳的顺利转化。根据阴阳互根的关系，要注意阳中求阴，补阴不忘阳。治疗时机重在经后期。一般以滋肾养血为主，热者清之，湿者除之，瘀者化之。出血时适当配伍一些固冲止血药。

2.1 Syndrome of kidney yin deficiency

Main manifestations Scanty intermenstrual bleeding with bright red color and sticky texture, dizziness, tinnitus, restless sleep, vexing heat in the five hearts, weakness of the waist and knees, constipation, red tongue with scanty coating, thin and

2.1 肾阴虚证

主要证候 两次月经中间阴道少量出血，色鲜红，质黏，头晕耳鸣，夜寐不宁，五心烦热，腰膝酸软，大便秘结。舌红，苔少，脉细数。

rapid pulse.

Therapeutic methods Enriching the kidney and nourishing yin, securing the Thoroughfare Vessel and stanching bleeding.

治法 滋肾养阴,固冲止血。

Formulas and herbs *Rehmannia and Lycium Root Bark Decoction* (Liang Di Tang) combined with *Double Supreme Pills* (Er Zhi Wan), composed of 12 g of *Fructus Ligustri Lucidi* (Nü Zhen Zi), 15 g of *Herba Ecliptae* (Mo Han Lian), 15 g of *Radix Rehmanniae Cruda* (Sheng Di Huang), 12 g of *Cortex Lycii Radicis* (Di Gu Pi), 12 g of *Radix Scrophulariae* (Xuan Shen), 12 g of *Radix Paeoniae Alba* (Bai Shao), 10 g of *Colla Corii Asini* (E Jiao) and 9 g of *Ophiopogonis Radix* (Mai Dong).

方药 代表方为两地汤合二至丸;常用药如女贞子12克,墨旱莲15克,生地黄15克,地骨皮12克,玄参12克,白芍12克,阿胶10克,麦冬9克。

Modification For scanty menses, *Processed Radix Polygoni Multiflori* (Zhi He Shou Wu) and *Fructus Lycii* (Gou Qi Zi) are added to nourish the blood and regulate menstruation. For vexing heat in the five body parts, *Radix Cynanchi Atrati* (Bai Wei), *Processed Plastrum Testudinis* (Zhi Gui Ban) and *Radix Stellariae* (Yin Chai Hu) are added to nourish yin and clear away heat.

加减 若经行量少加制何首乌、枸杞子以养血调经,五心烦热选加白薇、炙龟板、银柴胡以滋阴清热。

2.2 Damp-heat syndrome

2.2 湿热证

Main manifestations Scanty intermenstrual bleeding with dark red color and sticky and slimy texture, profuse yellowish leukorrhea, abdominal pain, fatigued spirit and lack of strength, fullness and oppression in chest and rib-side, bitterness in the mouth and poor appetite, yellow urine and sloppy stool, red tongue with yellow and greasy fur, and slippery rapid pulse.

主要证候 两次月经中间阴道少量出血,色深红,质黏腻,平时带下量多,色黄,小腹作痛,神疲乏力,胸胁满闷,口苦纳呆,溺黄便溏。舌红,苔黄腻,脉滑数。

Therapeutic methods Clearing away heat and removing dampness.

治法 清热利湿。

Formulas and herbs *Liver-Clearing and Strangury-*

方药 代表方为清肝止

Stopping Decoction (Qing Gan Zhi Lin Tang) composed of 10 g of *Radix Angelicae Sinensis* (Dang Gui), 10 g of *Radix Paeoniae Rubra* (Chi Shao), 10 g of *Radix Paeoniae Alba* (Bai Shao), 10 g of *Radix Rehmanniae Cruda* (Sheng Di Huang), 10 g of *Cortex Moutan Radicis Carbonisata* (Mu Dan Pi Tan), 20 g of *Semen Coicis* (Yi Yi Ren), 10 g of *Spica Schizonepetae Tenuifolia* (Jing Jie Sui), 10 g of *Fried Rhizoma Atractylodis* (Chao Cang Zhu), 6 g of *Cortex Phellodendri* (Huang Bo), 10 g of *Caumen Biotae Carbonisata* (Ce Bai Tan), 12 g of *Herba Cephalanoploris* (Xiao Ji) and 9 g of *Poriae* (Fu Ling).

淋汤;常用药如当归10克,赤芍10克,白芍10克,生地黄10克,牡丹皮炭10克,薏苡仁20克,荆芥穗10克,炒苍术10克,黄柏6克,侧柏炭10克,小蓟12克,茯苓9克。

Modification For profuse thick yellow vaginal discharge, *Herba Portulacae* (Ma Chi Xian) and *Toonae Radicis Cortex* (Chun Gen Pi) are added to clear away heat and dissolve dampness. For heat vexation and thirst, *Fructus Gardeniae* (Zhi Zi) and *Rhizoma Phragmitis* (Lu Gen) are added. For abdominal distention and pain, *Fructus Meliae Toosendan* (Chuan Lian Zi) and *Rhizoma Corydalis* (Yan Hu Suo) are added. For oppression in the chest and sliminess in the mouth, *Herba Agastachis* (Huo Xiang) and *Herba Eupatorii* (Pei Lan) are added. For scanty and reddish stranguria, *Caulis Akebiae* (Mu Tong), *Herba Plantaginis* (Che Qian Cao) and *Radix Glycyrrhizae* (Gan Cao) are added.

加减 若带下多而黄稠者,加马齿苋、椿根皮以清热化湿;烦热口渴者,加栀子、芦根;小腹胀痛者,加川楝子、延胡索;胸闷口腻者,加藿香、佩兰;小便短赤淋痛者,加木通、车前草、甘草。

2.3 Blood stasis syndrome

Main manifestations Scanty or profuse intermenstrual bleeding, in purple black color, distending pain or stabbing pain in lower abdomen, emotional depression, oppression and dysphoria, grayish tongue or with stasis macule, thready and

2.3 血瘀证

主要证候 经间期出血量时多时少,色暗红,或紫黑如酱,少腹胀痛或刺痛;情志抑郁,胸闷烦躁。舌暗或有瘀斑,脉细弦。

taut pulse.

Therapeutic methods Resolving stasis and stopping bleeding.

Formulas and herbs *Stasis-Expelling and Blood-Stanching Decoction* (Zhu Yu Zhi Xue Tang) composed of 10 g of *Radix Rehmanniae Cruda* (Sheng Di Huang), 5 g of *Radix et Rhizoma Rhei* (Da Huang) (to be decocted later), 12 g of *Radix Paeoniae Rubra* (Chi Shao), 12 g of *Cortex Moutan Radicis* (Mu Dan Pi), 10 g of *Angelicae Sinensis Radicis Extremitas* (Dang Gui Wei), 10 g of *Fructus Aurantii* (Zhi Qiao), 10 g of *Semen Persicae* (Tao Ren) and 10 g of *Testudinis Carapax et Plastrum cum Liquido Fricti* (Zhi Gui Ban).

Modification For profuse bleeding, *Radix Paeoniae Rubra* (Chi Shao) and *Angelicae Sinensis Radicis Extremitas* (Dang Gui Wei) are deleted, while combined with *Great Guffaw Powder* (Shi Xiao San) to dispel stasis and stanch bleeding. For severe abdominal pain, *Rhizoma Corydalis* (Yan Hu Suo) and *Rhizoma Cyperi* (Xiang Fu) are added to move qi and relieve pain. For damp heat and yellow vaginal discharge, *Semen Coicis* (Yi Yi Ren), *Caulis Sargentodoxae* (Da Xue Teng) and *Herba Patriniae* (Bai Jiang Cao) are added to clear away heat and remove dampness For spleen vacuity, poor appetite and sloppy stool, *Radix Rehmanniae Cruda* (Sheng Di Huang), *Semen Persicae* (Tao Ren) and *Radix et Rhizoma Rhei* (Da Huang) are deleted, while *Rhizoma Atractylodis Macrocephalae* (Bai Zhu), *Pericarpium Citri Tangerinae* (Chen Pi) and *Fructus Amomi* (Sha Ren) are added to fortify the spleen and harmonize the stomach. For kidney vacuity, aching lumbus and knees, *Radix Dipsaci* (Xu

治法 化瘀止血。

方药 代表方为逐瘀止血汤;常用药如生地黄 10 克,大黄(后下)5 克,赤芍 12 克,牡丹皮 12 克,当归尾 10 克,枳壳 10 克,桃仁 10 克,炙龟板 10 克。

加减 若出血偏多者,宜去赤芍、当归尾,合失笑散以祛瘀止血;若少腹痛甚者,加延胡索、香附以行气止痛;若兼湿热,带下黄者,加薏苡仁、红藤、败酱草以清利湿热;若兼脾虚,纳呆便溏者,去生地黄、桃仁、大黄,加白术、陈皮、砂仁以健脾和胃;若兼肾虚,腰膝酸软者,加续断、桑寄生、菟丝子以补益肾气。

Duan), *Ramulus Loranthi* (Sang Ji Sheng) and *Semen Cuscutae* (Tu Si Zi) are added to supplement kidney qi.

3 Other therapeutic methods

3.1 Chinese patent drugs

(1) *Black Chicken and White Phoenix Pill* (Wu Ji Bai Feng Wan): 1 pill each time and twice a day, applicable to the syndrome of kidney-yin deficiency.

(2) *Gong Xue Ning Capsule* (Gong Xue Ning Jiao Nang): 1-2 capsules each time and three times a day, applicable to the syndrome of blood stasis or yin deficiency and fire exuberance.

3.2 Empirical and folk recipes

(1) 60 g of fresh *Rhizoma Nelumbinis* (Ou) and 60 g of *Cacumen Platycladi* (Ce Bai Ye) are pounded. The juice is taken orally with wine, applicable to bleeding of damp-heat syndrome.

(2) 250 g of *Tuber Asparagi* (Tian Men Dong), 250 g of *Radix Ophiopogonis* (Mai Men Dong) and 250 g of *Os Sepiae* (Wu Zei Gu) are decocted. After the removal of residue, the decoction is concentrated into paste with honey and is taken 10-15 ml each time and twice a day, applicable to the syndrome of kidney-yin deficiency.

3 其他疗法

3.1 中成药

（1）乌鸡白凤丸：每次1丸，每日2次，适用于肾阴亏虚证。

（2）宫血宁胶囊：每次1～2粒，每日3次，适用于血瘀证或阴虚火旺证。

3.2 单验方

（1）鲜藕60克，侧柏叶60克，打碎取汁，陈酒分送服，适用于湿热证出血。

（2）天冬250克，麦冬250克，乌贼骨250克，浓煎去渣，炼蜜成膏，每服10～15毫升，每日2次，适用于肾阴亏虚证。

Metrorrhagia and metrostaxis

Metrorrhagia and metrostaxis refer to sudden profuse discharge or dripping menses, the former is called flooding or menstrual flooding, the latter is called mestrual leakage. They often transform into each other, so they are called metrorrhagia and

崩 漏

崩漏是指经血非时暴下不止或淋漓不尽，前者称“崩中”或“经崩”，后者称“漏下”或“经漏”。由于崩与漏二者常相互转化，故概称崩漏。

metrostaxis. It is a menstrual disease due to severe disorder of menstrual cycle, period and amount.

The main pathogenesis of this disease is consumptive damage in blood and qi, injury of organs, abnormal amassment and overflow in the sea of blood, the Thoroughfare and Conception Vessels failing to restrain menstrual blood, resulting in sudden discharge of menstrual blood.

1 Key points for diagnosis

1.1 Medical history

Detailed medical history should be required. Pregnancy and puerperal-related diseases, systemic and organic diseases should be excluded. Such as: ① early menstruation, menstruation at irregular intervals, prolonged menstruation, profuse menstruation and other medical history; ② age, pregnancy history, current contraceptive use, hormone drug use history; ③ history of liver disease, blood disease, hypertension and thyroid gland, adrenal, pituitary diseases.

1.2 Manifestations

Irregular menstrual cycle and frenetic menstruation, profuse and sudden menses or scanty and dripping menses. Bleeding can be manifested in many forms, such as a sudden menstruation after a few months' cessation and then constant dripping; or scanty menstruation and dripping for a few months followed by sudden and profuse menstruation; or intermittent bleeding alternatively in profuse amount or in scanty amount. Secondary anemia, or even hemorrhagic shock often occurs.

1.3 Examination

The purpose is to exclude organic diseases of

其是月经周期、经期、经量严重紊乱的月经病。

本病主要发病机理是劳伤血气，脏腑损伤，血海蓄溢失常，冲任二脉不能约制经血，以致经血非时而下。

1 诊断要点

1.1 病史

详细询问病史，需排除与妊娠和产褥有关的病变、全身性和器质性疾患。如：①既往多有月经先期、先后无定期、经期延长、月经过多等病史；②年龄、孕产史、目前采取的避孕措施、激素类药物的使用史；③肝病、血液病、高血压以及甲状腺、肾上腺、脑垂体病史。

1.2 症状

主要是月经不按周期妄行，出血量多如山之崩，或量少淋漓漏下不止。出血情况可有多种表现形式，如停经数月而后骤然暴下，继而淋漓不断；或淋漓量少累月不止，突然又暴下量多如注；或流血时断时续、血量时多时少。常常继发贫血，甚至发生失血性休克。

1.3 检查

目的是排除生殖器官器

the reproductive organs, various diseases related to pregnancy and puerperium, and determine the severity and the presence of malignant lesions.

质性病变、与妊娠和产褥有关的各种病变,判断病情轻重及有无恶性病变。

1.3.1 Gynecological examination

Bleeding is from the uterine cavity. There are no organic disease of the genital organs and no signs of pregnancy.

1.3.1 妇科检查

出血来自子宫腔。生殖器官无器质性病变。无妊娠迹象。

1.3.2 Auxiliary examination

① B ultrasound: Evaluate uterine size and endometrial thickness, exclude pregnancy, genital tumors or neoplasms; ② blood test: blood routine examination, platelet count, clotting time, and coagulation tests, etc. in order to understand the degree of anemia and exclude blood diseases; ③ ovarian function and hormone determination: basal body temperature in a single-phase type. Serum estrogen, progesterone and pituitary hormones should be measured. Pregnancy test should be done if with sexual life; ④ diagnostic curettage: Bleeding can be stopped and the diagnosis can be confirmed. As to patients of the reproductive age and during menopausal period, the curettage can be done a few days before the hemorrhage, or within 6 hours of the bleeding. As for the patient with bleeding, dripping or irregular bleeding, diagnostic scraping of endometria may be sent for biopsy at any time to confirm the presence of ovulation and exclude endometrial malignancy. But for unmarried patients, curettage can only be taken after failed drug treatment or in suspision of organic disease and by their parents' informed consent.

1.3.2 辅助检查

① B超检查:了解子宫大小及内膜厚度,排除妊娠、生殖器肿瘤或赘生物等;②血液检查:如血常规、血小板计数、出凝血时间和凝血功能检查等以了解贫血程度并排除血液病;③卵巢功能及激素测定:基础体温呈单相型;血清雌、孕激素及垂体激素测定等。有性生活史者,应做妊娠试验;④诊断性刮宫:可止血并明确诊断。对育龄期和绝经过渡期患者可在出血前数天、或出血6小时之内诊刮;对大出血、或淋漓不净或不规则出血者,可随时诊刮取子宫内膜送病理检查,以明确有无排卵及排除子宫内膜恶性病变。但对未婚患者,仅在药物治疗失败或疑有器质性病变,并征得本人或其家长知情同意后方可诊刮。

2 Syndrome differentiation and treatment

The syndrome should firstly be differentiated

2 辨证论治

崩漏辨证首先要根据出

according to the quantity, color and texture of bleeding to decide whether it is of asthenia or sthenia, of cold or heat. Sudden discharge of profuse menstrual blood and then dripping with light color and thin texture is of asthenia. Sudden discharge of profuse menstrual blood with bright or dark red color and thick and sticky texture is of repletion heat. Dripping and spotting discharge of menstrual blood with purplish red color and thick texture is of vacuity heat. Irregular menstrual cycle, period and amount with dark color and clot is of stasis and stagnation. Sudden discharge of profuse menstrual blood is of qi vacuity or blood heat. Continuous dribbling is of vacuity heat or blood stasis. In accordance with CAI Xiaosun's theory, metrorrhagia and metrostaxis is either in yang or yin nature. Early menstruation with thick texture is of yang nature. Metrorrhagia and metrostaxis and spotting for a long time with light color and thin texture is of yin nature.

血的量、色、质辨明血证的属性,以分清寒、热、虚、实。一般经血非时崩下,量多势急,继而淋漓不止,色淡,质稀多属虚;经血非时暴下,血色鲜红或深红,质地稠黏多属实热;淋漓漏下,血色紫红,质稠多属虚热;经来无期,时来时止,时多时少,或久漏不止,色暗挟血块,多属瘀滞。出血急骤多属气虚或血热,淋漓不断多属虚热或血瘀。蔡小苏将崩分为阳崩和阴崩,经来先期,质较浓或稠,属阳崩;久崩久漏,色较淡而稀薄,属阴崩。

Usually, metrorrhagia and metrostaxis are more numerous in asthenia pattern than in sthenia pattern. Even in heat nature, it is mostly asthenia heat. But, it is sthenia heat at the early stage of disease, and it can be transformed to asthenia heat, if blood is lost and yin is damaged.

一般而言,崩漏虚证多而实证少,热证多而寒证少。即便是热亦是虚热为多,但发病初期可为实热,失血伤阴即转为虚热。

Metrorrhagia and metrostaxis should be treated based upon the principle "to deal with the symptoms in emergency, and to treat the causative reason in the remission stage", by the voluntary application of the three methods to block the flow, to check the source, and to promote the restoration.

治疗崩漏,尚需本着"急则治其标,缓则治其本"的原则,灵活掌握塞流、澄源、复旧三法。

To block the flow: i.e. a method to stop bleeding. In the moment of sudden bleeding, it is neces-

塞流:即是止血之法。暴崩之际,急当止血防脱,一

sary to stop bleeding for avoiding prostration, usually by the qi-boosting and blood-checking method. If bleeding cannot be stopped, blood transfusion must be given promptly. If bleeding is alleviated, treatment should be decided for dealing with the pathogenesis by pattern identification.

般用益气摄血法。血势不减者，宜输血救急，血势渐缓，则谨守病机，辨证论治。

To check the source: When bleeding is alleviated, treatment is given in light of syndrome differentiation, in order to avoid using the cold-cool or war-tonic agents without exception and to avoid mingling deficiency and excess by only promoting astringency.

澄源：一般用止血法后，待血势稍缓便须根据不同病证辨证论治，切忌不问原由，概投寒凉或温补之剂，或专事止涩，致犯虚虚实实之戒。

To promote the restoration: Restoration means nourishing the kidney, regulating the liver or strengthening the spleen; Since menstrual disease is usually related to the kidney, the treatment should concentrate on nourishing the kidney, strengthening the Thoroughfare Vessel and regulating menstruation.

复旧：即固本善后，治法或补肾，或调肝，或扶脾。然月经病之本在肾，故总宜益肾固冲调经。

In the clinical treatment, these three therapeutic methods should be used in combination. It is necessary to check out the source in blocking the flow and to consolidate the constitution in checking out the source. It is appropriate to promote the raising and uplifting ability for astringency, instead of the method to circulate blood with spicy and warm herbs, and to nourish blood and regulate qi in treating bleeding, without stressing on astringency. For example, the treatment for the patients during adolescence should focus on nourishing kidney qi and invigorating the Thoroughfare and Conception Vessels. The treatment for the patients of childbearing age should concentrate on soothing the liver, nourishing the liver and regulating the thoroughfare and

治崩漏三法不可截然分割，塞流需澄源，澄源当固本。治崩宜升提固涩，不宜辛温行血；治漏宜养血理气，不可偏于固涩。青春期患者，重在补肾气，益冲任；育龄期患者重在舒肝养肝，调冲任；围绝经期患者重在滋肾调肝，扶脾固冲任。

conception vessels. The treatment for the patients during perimenopausal period should emphasize nourishing the kidney, regulating the liver, strengthening the spleen and reinforcing the Thoroughfare and Conception Vessels.

2.1 Syndrome of failure of consolidation due to kidney asthenia

Main manifestations Menstrual blood not at the due time, or profuse and fulminant blood flow, dripping bleeding, dark red or bright red color, accompanied by dizziness, tinnitus, aching sensation and weakness in the loins, grayish complexion, deep and thready or fast pulse.

Therapeutic methods Nourishing the kidney to boost qi, nourishing blood to strengthen the Thoroughfare Vessel.

Formulas and herbs *Vital Gate Pills* (You Gui Wan) combined with *Kidney Pills* (Zuo Gui Wan), composed of 10 g of *Radix Rehmanniae Praeparata* (Shu Di Huang), 10 g of *Fructus Corni* (Shan Zhu Yu), 10 g of *Fructus Lycii* (Gou Qi Zi), 12 g of *Semen Cuscutae* (Tu Si Zi), 10 g of *Colla Cornus Cervi* (Lu Jiao Jiao)(to be melted), 15 g of *Fructus Ligustri Lucidi* (Nü Zhen Zi), 15 g of *Herba Ecliptae* (Mo Han Lian), 12 g of *Ramulus Loranthi* (Sang Ji Sheng), 10 g of *Colla Corii Asini* (E Jiao)(to be melted) and 10 g of *Cortex Eucommiae* (Du Zhong).

Modification For palpitation and shortness of breath, *Radix Codonopsis Pilosulae* (Dang Shen) and *Radix Astragali* (Huang Qi) are added. For dysphoria and insomnia, Semen *Zizyphi Spinosae* (Suan Zao Ren) and *Ramulus Uncariae cum Uncis* (Gou Teng) are added. For aversion to cold and

2.1 肾虚不固证

主要证候 经血非时而下，或量多如注，淋漓不断，色暗红或鲜红，头晕耳鸣，腰酸乏力，面色晦暗，脉沉细或数。

治法 补肾益气，养血固冲。

方药 代表方为右归丸合左归丸；常用药如熟地黄10克，山茱萸10克，枸杞子10克，菟丝子12克，鹿角胶（烊化）10克，女贞子15克，墨旱莲15克，桑寄生12克，阿胶（烊化）10克，杜仲10克。

加减 若心悸气短者，加党参、黄芪；心烦失寐者，加酸枣仁、钩藤；畏寒肢冷者，加炮附片、覆盆子；小便频数者，加桑螵蛸、益智仁。

cold limbs, *Aconite Radix Lateralis Tosta* (Pao Fu Zi) and *Fructus Rubi* (Fu Pen Zi) are added. For frequent urination, *Ootheca Mantidis* (Sang Piao Xiao) and *Fructus Alpiniae Oxyphyllae* (Yi Zhi Ren) are added.

Shanghai doctor LUO Yijun's experience prescription: 20 g of *Radix Astragali Praeparata* (Zhi Huang Qi), 15 g of *Radix Codonopsis Pilosulae* (Dang Shen), 12 g of *Burnt Radix Paeoniae Alba* (Jiao Bai Shao), 12 g of *Burnt Rhizoma Atractylodis Macrocephalae* (Jiao Bai Zhu), 9 g of *Colla Corii Asini* (E Jiao) (to be melted), 15 g of *Herba Agrimoniae* (Xian He Cao), 15 g of *Mastodi Ossis Fossilia Calcinata* (Duan Long Gu) (to be decocted first), 30 g of *Ostreae Concha Calcinata* (Duan Mu Li) (to be decocted first), 10 g of *Trachycarpi Petiolus Vetus Carbonisatus* (Chen Zong Tan), 5 g of *Burnt Folium Artemistae Argyi* (Jiao Ai Ye), 15 g of *Fructus Ligustri Lucidi* (Nü Zhen Zi), 6 g of *Fructus Citri Saroodactylis Sectus* (Fo Shou Pian), 15 g of *Processed Radix Polygoni Multiflori* (Zhi He Shou Wu), 6 g of *Processed Rhizoma Cimicifugae* (Zhi Sheng Ma) and 20 g of *Fructus Ziziphi Jujubae* (Da Zao).

上海医家骆益君经验方加减：炙黄芪20克，党参15克，焦白芍12克，焦白术12克，阿胶（烊化）9克，仙鹤草15克，煅龙骨（先煎）15克，煅牡蛎（先煎）30克，陈棕炭10克，焦艾叶5克，女贞子15克，佛手片6克，制首乌15克，炙升麻6克，红枣20克。

2.2 Syndrome of asthenia spleen failing to command blood

2.2 脾虚失统证

Main manifestations Menstrual blood not at the due time, or profuse and fulminant blood flow, or dripping bleeding with thin texture, bright-pale complexion or sallow complexion, edema of limbs, lassitude, cold limbs, lack of qi and no desire to speak, anorexia and loose stool, empty prolapsing sensation in the lower abdomen, light and bulgy tongue or tooth-printed tongue with thin and white fur, thready and weak pulse.

主要证候 经血非时而下，或量多如注，或淋漓不断，色淡红，质稀薄，面色㿠白或萎黄不泽，面浮肢肿、倦怠乏力，四肢不温，少气懒言，纳少便溏，小腹空坠，舌质淡胖或有齿印，苔薄白，脉细弱。

Therapeutic methods Nourishing qi to elevate yang, strengthening the spleen to control blood.

治法 益气升阳，健脾摄血。

Formulas and herbs ① *Root-Securing and*

方药 代表方：①固本

Flood-Stanching Decoction (Gu Ben Zhi Beng Tang), composed of 15 g of *Radix Codonopsis Pilosulae* (Dang Shen), 10 g of *Radix Astragali* (Huang Qi), 10 g of *Rhizoma Atractylodis Macrocephalae* (Bai Zhu), 6 g of *Processed Rhizoma Cimicifugae* (Zhi Sheng Ma), 12 g of *Rhizoma Dioscoreae* (Shan Yao), 10 g of *Roasting Radix Aucklandiae* (Wei Mu Xiang), 6 g of *Zingiberis Rhizoma Praeparatum* (Pao Jiang Tan), 12 g of *Radix Dipsaci* (Xu Duan) and 5 g of *Radix Glycyrrhizae Praeparata* (Zhi Gan Cao). ② *Original-Lifting Brew* (Ju Yuan Jian), composed of 10 g of *Radix Ginseng* (Ren Shen), 10 g of *Radix Astragali Praeparata* (Zhi Huang Qi), 3 g of *Radix Glycyrrhizae Praeparata* (Zhi Gan Cao), 5 g of *Rhizoma Cimicifugae* (Sheng Ma) and 6 g of *Rhizoma Atractylodis Macrocephalae* (Bai Zhu).

止崩汤；常用药如党参 15 克，黄芪 10 克，白术 10 克，炙升麻 6 克，山药 12 克，煨木香 10 克，炮姜炭 6 克，续断 12 克，炙甘草 5 克。②举元煎；常用药如人参 10 克，炙黄芪 10 克，炙甘草 3 克，升麻 5 克，白术 6 克。

Modification For profuse bleeding, *Fructus Corni* (Shan Zhu Yu), *Herba Agrimoniae* (Xian He Cao) and *Crinis Carbonisatus* (Xue Yu Tan) are added to preserve yin, secure blood and stanch bleeding. For bleeding with blood clot, *Faeces Trogopterorum* (Wu Ling Zhi) is added. For dripping bleeding, *Herba Leonuri* (Yi Mu Cao) and *Radix Rubiae* (Qian Cao) are added. For prolonged bleeding, dizziness, lack of strength and insomnia, *Processed Radix Polygoni Multiflori* (Zhi He Shou Wu), *Ramulus Loranthi* (Sang Ji Sheng) and *Fructus Schisandrae* (Wu Wei Zi) are added to nourish the heart and quiet the spirit. For yang bleeding, 9 g of *Aconiti Radix Lateralis Tosta* (Pao Fu Pian), 3 g of *Rhizoma Zingiberis Praeparata* (Pao Jiang) and 15-30 g of *Rehmanniae Radix Praeparatum* (Sheng Di Tan) are added.

加减　若崩中量多者，加山茱萸、仙鹤草、血余炭以敛阴涩血止血；血块多者，加炒五灵脂；淋漓不净者，加益母草、茜草；久崩不止，症见头昏、乏力、心悸、失眠者，酌加制首乌、桑寄生、五味子以养心安神；阳崩者可加炮附片 9 克，炮姜 3 克，重用生地炭 15～30 克。

Shanghai doctor SHEN Zhongli's experience prescrip-

上海医家沈仲理经验方加

tion: 30 g of *Radix Codonopsis Pilosulae* (Dang Shen), 50 g of *Radix Astragali* (Huang Qi), 15 g of *Rhizoma Atractylodis Macrocephalae* (Bai Zhu), 15 g of *Rhizoma Cimicifugae* (Sheng Ma), 30 g of *Mastodi Ossis Fossilia Calcinata* (Duan Long Gu), 20 g of *Herba Agrimoniae* (Xian He Cao), 10 g of *Rhois Chinensis Surculus* (Wu Bei Zi), 10 g of *Trachycarpi Petiolus Vetus Carbonisatus* (Chen Zong Tan), 6 g of *Zingiberis Rhizoma Praeparatum* (Pao Jiang Tan), 20 g of *Maydis Stigma* (Yu Mi Xu), 6 g of *Artemisiae Argyi Folium Carbonisatum* (Ai Ye Tan) and 12 g of *Radix Glycyrrhizae Praeparata* (Zhi Gan Cao).

减：党参30克，黄芪50克，白术15克，升麻15克，煅龙骨30克，仙鹤草20克，五倍子10克，陈棕炭10克，炮姜炭6克，玉米须20克，艾叶炭6克，炙甘草12克。

Shanghai doctor CAI Xiaosun's experience prescription, *Qi-Boosting Uprising Prescription* (Yi Qi Sheng Ti Fang): 15 g of *Radix Codonopsis Pilosulae* (Dang Shen), 20 g of *Astragali Radix Cruda* (Sheng Huang Qi), 10 g of *Rhizoma Atractylodis Macrocephalae Frictum* (Chao Bai Zhu), 10 g of *Angelicae Sinensis Radix Frictum* (Chao Dang Gui), 10 g of *Radix Rehmanniae Praeparata* (Shu Di Huang), 3 g of *Fructus Amomi* (Sha Ren), 12 g of *Radix Paeoniae Alba* (Bai Shao), 5 g of *Rhizoma Cimicifugae* (Sheng Ma), 5 g of *Radix Bupleuri* (Chai Hu), 20 g of *Herba Agrimoniae* (Xian He Cao) and 20 g of *Eclipta* (Han Lian Cao).

上海医家蔡小荪经验方（益气升提方）加减：党参15克，生黄芪20克，炒白术10克，炒当归10克，熟地黄10克，砂仁3克，白芍12克，升麻5克，柴胡5克，仙鹤草20克，旱莲草20克。

2.3 Syndrome of abnormal flow of blood due to blood heat

2.3 血热妄行证

Main manifestations Menstrual blood not at the due time, dripping or profuse bleeding, dark red or bright red color and thick texture, or with blood clots, red lips and eyes, dysphoria and thirst, constipation, yellowish urine, red tongue with yellow fur, slippery and rapid pulse.

主要证候 经血非时暴下，或淋漓不净又时而增多，血色深红或鲜红，质稠，或有血块；唇红目赤，烦热口渴，或大便干结，小便黄，舌红，苔黄，脉滑数。

Therapeutic methods Clearing away heat and cooling blood, stanching blood and regulating menstruation.

治法 清热凉血，止血调经。

Formulas and herbs *Heat-Clearing and Menses-Securing Granules* (Qing Re Gu Jing Tang) com-

方药 代表方为清热固经汤；常用药如黄芩10克，

posed of 10 g of *Radix Scutellariae* (Huang Qin), 6 g of *Gardeniae Fructus Frictus* (Chao Zhi Zi), 10 g of *Radix Rehmanniae Cruda* (Sheng Di Huang), 12 g of *Cortex Lycii Radicis* (Di Gu Pi), 15 g of *Sanguisorbae Radix*(Di Yu), 10 g of *Cortex Moutan Radicis* (Mu Dan Pi), 10 g of *Testudinis Carapax et Plastrum cum Liquido Fricti* (Zhi Gui Ban), 10 g of *Colla Corii Asini* (E Jiao), 10 g of *Trachycarpi Petiolus Vetus Carbonisatus* (Chen Zong Tan), 10 g of *Nelumbinis Rhizomatis Nodus Carbonisatus* (Ou Jie Tan) and 5 g of *Glycyrrhizae Radix* (Gan Cao).

Modification For blood clot in menses, *Typhae Pollen Frictus* (Chao Pu Huang) and *Trogopteri Faeces Frictum* (Chao Wu Ling Zhi) are added. For vexation, tidal heat sensation with flushed cheeks, heat in the palms and soles, red and dry tongue, thready and rapid pulse, *Yin-Protecting Decoction* (Bao Yin Jian), *Ophiopogonis Radix* (Mai Dong), *Adenophorae seu Glehniae Radix* (Sha Shen) and *Herba Artemisiae Chinghao* (Qing Hao) are added. For pain and distention in the chest and rib-side, vexation and irascibility, sigh and string like pulse due to exuberant fire in the liver meridian, *Moutan and Gardenia Free Wanderer Powder* (Dan Zhi Xiao Yao San) is added instead of *Zingiberis Rhizoma Tostum* (Wei Jiang), with *Herba Leonuri* (Yi Mu Cao), *Typhae Pollen Frictus* (Chao Pu Huang), *Crinis Carbonisatus* (Xue Yu Tan) and *Cyperi Rhizoma Frictum* (Chao Xiang Fu) added to stanch and activate blood and regulate qi.

Shanghai doctor CHEN Danian's experience prescription, *Black Catta Pollen Powder* (Hei Pu Huang San): 30 g of *Pollen Typhae* (Pu Huang), 10 g of *Trachycarpi Petiolus*

炒栀子6克，生地黄10克，地骨皮12克，地榆15克，牡丹皮10克，炙龟板10克，阿胶10克，陈棕炭10克，藕节炭10克，甘草5克。

加减　若血块多者，加炒蒲黄、炒五灵脂；若以心烦，潮热颧红，手足心热，舌红而干，脉细数为主症者，用保阴煎加麦冬、沙参、青蒿；若症见胸胁胀痛，心烦易怒，时欲叹息，脉弦等，为肝经火炽，宜疏肝清热佐以止血，用丹栀逍遥散去煨姜，加益母草、炒蒲黄、血余炭、醋炒香附以止血活血调气。

上海医家陈大年经验方（黑蒲黄散）加减：蒲黄30克，棕皮10克，川芎9克，牡丹皮9克，香附

Vetus (Zong Pi), 9 g of *Rhizoma Ligustici Chuanxiong* (Chuan Xiong), 9 g of *Cortex Moutan Radicis* (Mu Dan Pi), 12 g of *Rhizoma Cyperi* (Xiang Fu), 12 g of *Radix Paeoniae Alba* (Bai Shao), 9 g of *Colla Corii Asini* (E Jiao), 15 g of *Radix Angelicae Sinensis* (Dang Gui), 15 g of *Radix Sanguisorbae* (Di Yu), 15 g of *Radix Rehmanniae Praeparata* (Shu Di Huang), 9 g of *Herba Schizonepetae* (Jing Jie) and 12 g of *Crinis Carbonisatus* (Xue Yu Tan).

12克，白芍12克，阿胶9克，当归15克，地榆15克，熟地黄15克，荆芥9克，血余炭12克。

2.4 Syndrome of retention of blood stasis

Main manifestations Menstrual blood not at the due time, occasional bleeding or dripping bleeding, in purple and black color and blood clot, or abdominal pain, dark purplish tongue with thin and white fur, unsmooth or thready and taut pulse.

Therapeutic methods Activating blood to dissolve stasis, stanching bleeding to regulate menstruation.

Formulas and herbs *Great Guffaw Powder* (Jia Wei Shi Xiao San), composed of 10 g of *Typhae Pollen Frictus* (Chao Pu Huang), 10 g of *Trogopteri Faeces Frictum* (Chao Wu Ling Zhi), 6 g of *Rhei Radix et Rhizoma Carbonisatum* (Da Huang Tan), 12 g of *Stir-Fried Chinese Angelica* (Chao Dang Gui), 12 g of *Radix Paeoniae Rubra* (Chi Shao), 12 g of *Radix Paeoniae Alba* (Bai Shao), 30 g of *Madder Carbonisatum* (Qian Cao Tan), 10 g of *Fructus Crataegi* (Shan Zha), 30 g of *Herba Leonuri* (Yi Mu Cao), 30 g of *Pyrolae Herba* (Lu Xian Cao) and 30 g of *Verbenae Herba* (Ma Bian Cao).

Modification For excessive blood clots in the menstrual blood, *Rhizome Dryopteris Gassirhizomae* (Guan Zhong Tan) is added. For severe abdominal distention and pain, *Rhizoma Cyperi* (Xiang Fu) and *Rhizoma Corydalis* (Yan Hu Suo) are added.

2.4 瘀血阻滞证

主要证候 经血非时而下，时下时止，或淋漓不净，色紫黑有块；或有小腹疼痛，舌质紫暗，苔薄白，脉涩或细弦。

治法 活血化瘀，止血调经。

方药 代表方为加味失笑散；常用药如炒蒲黄10克，炒五灵脂10克，大黄炭6克，炒当归12克，赤白芍各12克，茜草炭30克，山楂10克，益母草30克，鹿衔草30克，马鞭草30克。

加减 若瘀块较多者，加贯众炭；小腹胀痛显著者，加香附、延胡索；小腹觉冷者，加艾叶炭、补骨脂。

For cold sensation in the lower abdomen, *Artemisiae Argyi Folium Carbonisatum* (Ai Ye Tan) and *Fructus Psoraleae* (Bu Gu Zhi) are added.

Shanghai doctor CAI Xiaosun's experience prescription, *Stasis-Dissolving and Bleeding-Stopping Prescription* (Hua Yu Ding Beng Fang): 10 g of *Radix Angelicae Sinensis* (Dang Gui), 10 g of *Radix Rehmanniae Cruda* (Sheng Di Huang), 10 g of *Radix Salviae Miltiorrhizae* (Dan Shen), 10 g of *Radix Paeoniae Alba* (Bai Shao), 10 g of *Rhizoma Cyperi* (Xiang Fu), 30 g of *Typhae Pollen Crudum* (Sheng Pu Huang) (to be wrapped for decocting), 20 g of *Ophicalcitum* (Hua Xin Shi), 10 g of *Rhei Radix et Rhizoma Carbonisati* (Shu Jun Tan), 2 g of *Notoginseng Radix Pulverata* (San Qi Mo)(to be taken separately) and 12 g of *Rousing Spirit Elixir* (Zhen Ling Dan)(to be wrapped for decocting).

上海医家蔡小荪经验方(化瘀定崩方):当归 10 克,生地黄 10 克,丹参 10 克,白芍 10 克,香附 10 克,生蒲黄(包煎)30 克,花蕊石 20 克,熟军炭 10 克,三七末(吞)2 克,震灵丹(包煎)12 克。

3 Other therapeutic methods

3 其他疗法

3.1 Chinese patent drugs

3.1 中成药

(1) *Heat-Clearing and Menses-Securing Pill* (Qing Re Gu Jing Wan): 6 g each time and twice a day, applicable to the treatment of yin vacuity and blood heat syndrome.

(1) 清热固经丸:每次服 6 克,每日 2 次,适用于阴虚血热证。

(2) *Ginseng and Angelica Splenic Pill* (Ren Shen Gui Pi Wan): 6 g each time and twice a day, applicable to the treatment of dual vacuity of the heart and spleen syndrome.

(2) 人参归脾丸:每次 6 克,每日 2 次,适用于心脾两虚,气血不足证。

(3) *Bleeding-Stopping Capsule* (Duan Xue Liu Jiao Nang): 3-6 capsules each time and three times a day, applicable to the treatment of blood heat syndrome.

(3) 断血流胶囊:每次服 3~6 粒,每日 3 次,适用于血热证。

(4) *Rotating Jerusalem Sage Capsule* (Du Yi Wei Jiao Nang): 3 capsules each time and three times a day, applicable to the treatment of obstruction of collaterals by blood stasis.

(4) 独一味胶囊:每次服 3 粒,每日 3 次,适用于血瘀闭阻经络证。

3.2 Empirical and folk recipes

(1) Shanghai doctor ZHU Nanshan's experience prescription, *General Chopping the Commissioner Decoction* (Jiang Jun Zhan Guan Tang): 3 g of *Radix et Rhizoma Rhei Carbonisatum* (Shu Da Huang Tan), 18 g of *Radix Morindae Officinalis* (Ba Ji Tian), 18 g of *Herba Agrimoniae* (Xian He Cao), 9 g of *Poria cum Ligno Hospite* (Fu Shen), 9 g of *Stir-fried Pollen Typhae* (Pu Huang) and *Colla Corii Asini* (E Jiao), 4.5 g of *Radix Astragali* (Huang Qi), 18 g of *Stir-Fried Chinese Angelica* (Chao Dang Gui), 4.5 g of *Burnt Rhizoma Atractylodis Macrocephalae* (Jiao Bai Zhu), 6 g of *Radix Rehmanniae Cruda* (Sheng Di Huang), 6 g of *Radix Rehmanniae Praeparata* (Shu Di Huang), 9 g of *Burnt Fructus Oryzae Germinatus* (Jiao Gu Ya). 0.9 g of *Croci Stigma* (Zang Hong Hua) and 0.9 g of *Notoginseng Radix Pulverata* (San Qi Mo) are added for oral taking with black tea to dispel stasis, engender the new and stanch bleeding, applicable to the treatment of blood stasis, syndrome of severe metrorrhagia and metrostaxis.

(2) 30 g of *Fructificatio Auriculariae Auriculae* (Hei Mu Er) and 30 *Fructus Ziziphi Jujubae* (Da Zao) are decocted for oral taking for several days. This treatment is applicable to blood heat syndrome.

(3) 250 g of fresh *Radix Boehmeriae Niveae* (Xian Zhu Ma Gen) is washed and ground to extract juice, and mixed up with 30 g of sugar for oral taking, once a day for several days. This treatment is applicable to the treatment of yin asthenia and blood heat syndrome.

3.2 单验方

（1）上海医家朱南山经验方（将军斩关汤）：熟大黄炭3克，巴戟天18克，仙鹤草18克，茯神9克，蒲黄炒阿胶9克，黄芪4.5克，炒当归9克，焦白术4.5克，生熟地各6克，焦谷芽9克，另用藏红花0.9克，三七末0.9克，红茶汁送服。祛瘀生新止血，用于重症崩漏之血瘀证。

（2）黑木耳30克，红枣30枚，煎汤食服，每日1次，连服数日，适用于血热证。

（3）鲜苎麻根250克，砂糖30克，将苎麻根洗净捣绒取汁，砂糖冲服，每日1次，连服数日，适用于阴虚血热证。

Dysmenorrhea

Dysmenorrhea or abdominal pain during menstruation refers to periodic lower abdominal pain or lumbosacral pain before, after or during menstruation, affecting normal work and life. Mild abdominal or lumbosacral distention, pain and discomfort before or during menstruation, without affecting normal work and life, is a common physiological phenomenon, not a disease.

No apparent abnormities are found in pelvic organs in gynecologic examination. Pains because of endometriosis, adenomyosis, pelvic inflammation, cervical stenosis and so on are called secondary dysmenorrheal.

Pathogenesis of dysmenorrhea during this period is mainly due to the impact of pathogenic factors, which leads to qi and blood stagnation in the Thoroughfare and Conception Vessels, uterus, or malnutrition in the Thoroughfare and Conception Vessels and uterus. The positions of the disease are in Thoroughfare and Conception Vessels and uterus, changes are in qi and blood, manifested as pain syndrome. It occurs with the onset of the menstrual cycle, because it is associated with the changes of qi and blood during menstruation. During, before or after menstruation, because of overflow in the sea of blood, due to exuberance, qi and blood are preponderant and excessive, inducing sudden deficiency. When qi and blood change suddenly in the Thoroughfare Vessel and Conception Vessel and uterus, the pathogenic factors take the chance to attack, leading to dysmenorrhea.

痛　经

妇女正值经期或经行前后出现周期性下腹部疼痛，或伴腰骶酸痛，影响正常工作及生活，称为“痛经”，亦称“经行腹痛”。若经前或经期仅有小腹或腰部轻微的胀痛不适，不影响日常工作和生活者，则属经期常见生理现象，不作病论。

妇科检查未发现盆腔器官有明显异常，西医学子宫内膜异位症、子宫腺肌病、盆腔炎性疾病、宫颈狭窄等出现的痛经，称为继发性痛经。

痛经发病机理主要是在这个期间受到致病因素的影响，导致冲任、胞宫气血阻滞，“不通则痛”；或冲任胞宫失于濡养，“不荣而痛”。其病位在冲任、胞宫，变化在气血，表现为痛证。其所以随月经周期而发作，是与经期冲任气血变化有关。在经期或经期前后，由于血海由满盈而溢泻，气血盛实而骤虚，冲任、胞宫气血变化急骤，致病因素乘时而作，导致痛经。

1 Key points for diagnosis

1.1 Medical history

Periodic abdominal pain during menstruation, accompanied by regular seizure in the menstrual cycle, or infertility, pelvic inflammation or surgery of uterine cavity.

1.2 Manifestations

Abdominal pain mostly occurs 1-2 days before menstruation or during the first and the second days of menstrual period, manifested by paroxysmal spasmodic pain or distending pain in the lower abdomen, pain radiating to the lumbosacral region, anus, vagina. In severe cases, pale complexion, cold sweating, cold hands and feet or even syncope may occur. Generally, the pain is mild or severe, but with no muscle tension or rebound tenderness. In some cases, pain may persist until the end of menstruation.

1.3 Examinations

1.3.1 Gynecological examination

Patients with no positive signs are functional dysmenorrhea. Extreme flexion of the uterus or cervical stenosis existsin some patients. Adhesion, masses, nodules, thickening in adnexal area or even increase in uterus body may be caused by pelvic inflammaton, endometriosis, adenomyosis or other diseases.

1.3.2 Auxiliary examination

B ultrasound, laparoscopy, hysteroscopy, hysterosalpingography are helpful to identify the cause of dysmenorrhea.

1 诊断要点

1.1 病史

经行小腹疼痛，伴随月经周期规律性发作，或有不孕、盆腔炎、宫腔手术史。

1.2 症状

腹痛多发生于行经第1～2日或经期前1～2日，可呈阵发性痉挛性或胀痛下坠感，疼痛可引及全腹或腰骶部，或外阴、肛门坠痛，严重者可出现面色苍白、出冷汗、手足发凉等晕厥现象。疼痛程度虽有轻有重，但一般无腹肌紧张或反跳痛。偶有经行腹痛延续至经净或于经净后1～2日始发病。

1.3 检查

1.3.1 妇科检查

无阳性体征者属功能性痛经，部分患者可见子宫体极度屈曲或宫颈口狭窄；如盆腔内有粘连、包块、结节、附件区增厚或子宫体均匀增大者，可能是盆腔炎症、子宫内膜异位症、子宫腺肌病等病所致。

1.3.2 辅助检查

B超、腹腔镜、宫腔镜检查，子宫输卵管造影有助于明确痛经的原因。

2 Syndrome differentiation and treatment

In differentiation of dysmenorrheal, first it is necessary to identify its nature of deficiency, excess, cold or heat. In accordance with the time, nature, location and degree of pain, in combination of the menstrual cycle, amount, color and quality, and accompanying symptoms, pulse situation, and body condition, its cold, heat, deficiency or excess must be investigated by reference to the relavant factors of the morbidity. Generally, pain happening before, at the beginning of or during menstruation belongs to excessive pattern. Pain happening at the end of or after menstruation belongs to deficient pattern, or deficiency mixed with blood stasis. Severe pain, pain aggravated by pressure, dragging pain, colic pain, burning pain, and pricking pain belong to excessive pattern. Insidious pain, dropping pain and pain relieved by pressure mostly belong to deficiency. Pain more severe than distention, pain relieved after discharge of blood clots, or pricking pain, continuous pain are due to blood stasis, while distention more severe than pain and intermittent pain are due to qi stagnation. Colic pain and pain alleviated with warmth belong to cold. Burning pain worsened with warmth is due to heat. Pain in the sides of the abdomen is mostly related to liver, while pain involving the loins is mostly related to kidney.

The basic therapeutic principle for treating dysmenorrhea is regulating qi and blood in the thoroughfare and conception vessels and uterus, including regulating qi, activating blood, dissipating cold, clearing away heat, correcting asthenia and getting

2 辨证论治

痛经辨证首先当识别痛证的虚实寒热。根据疼痛发生的时间、性质、部位以及痛的程度,结合月经期、量、色、质及兼证、舌脉,并根据素体情况,参考发病相关因素等审其寒热虚实。一般痛在经前、经期之初、中多属实;痛在月经将净或经后多属虚或虚中挟瘀。疼痛剧烈、拒按、掣痛、绞痛、灼痛、刺痛多属实;隐隐作痛、坠痛、喜按揉多属虚。痛甚于胀,血块排出疼痛则减轻或刺痛、持续作痛者多为血瘀;胀甚于痛,时痛时止者多为气滞。绞痛、冷痛得热痛减多属寒;灼痛得热痛增多为热。痛在两侧少腹病多在肝,痛在腰际病多在肾。

痛经的治疗原则,以调理冲任、胞宫气血为主。根据不同的证候,或行气,或活血,或散寒,或清热,或补虚,或泻实。治法分两步:月经

rid of sthenia according to the syndromes. The treatment focuses either on the principal symptoms by regulating blood to stop pain during menstruation or on the cause based on syndrome differentiation at the ordinary time.

期调血止痛以治标，平时辨证求因而治本。

2.1 Syndrome of qi stagnation and blood stasis

Main manifestations Abdominal pain or prolapsing pain aggravated by pressure before menstruation or during menstruation, scanty menstruation, unsmooth menorrhea, purplish and black color menses with blood clot, alleviation after the removal of blood clot, distention and pain in breasts, oppression in the chest, purplish tongue or with ecchymosis, and taut pulse.

Therapeutic methods Soothing the liver to regulate qi and resolving stasis to stop pain.

Formulas and herbs *Sanguine Mansion Stasis-Expelling Decoction* (Xue Fu Zhu Yu Tang), composed of 10 g of *Radix Angelicae Sinensis* (Dang Gui), 6 g of *Rhizoma Ligustici Chuanxiong* (Chuan Xiong), 10 g of *Radix Paeoniae Rubra* (Chi Shao), 10 g of *Semen Persicae* (Tao Ren), 10 g of *Flos Carthami* (Hong Hua), 10 g of *Radix Cyathulae* (Chuan Niu Xi), 10 g of *Rhizoma Cyperi* (Xiang Fu), 6 g of *Pericarpium Citri Reticulatae Viride* (Qing Pi), 10 g of *Fructus Aurantii* (Zhi Qiao), 6 g of *Radix Aucklandiae* (Mu Xiang), 10 g of *Rhizoma Corydalis* (Yan Hu Suo), 10 g of *Faeces Trogopterorum* (Wu Ling Zhi) and 3 g of *Radix Glycyrrhizae* (Gan Cao).

Modification For abdominal pain with cold sensation or sloppy stool, *Rhizoma Cyperi* (Xiang Fu) is deleted, while *Radix Aucklandiae* (Mu Xiang), *Fructus Foeniculi* (Xiao Hui Xiang),

2.1 气滞血瘀证

主要证候 经前或经期小腹胀痛拒按，经血量少，经行不畅，血色紫暗有块，块下痛暂减，乳房胀痛，胸闷不舒，舌质紫暗或有瘀点，脉弦。

治法 疏肝理气，化瘀止痛。

方药 代表方为血府逐瘀汤；常用药如当归10克，川芎6克，赤芍10克，桃仁10克，红花10克，川牛膝10克，香附10克，青皮6克，枳壳10克，木香6克，延胡索10克，五灵脂10克，甘草3克。

加减 若小腹疼痛伴有冷感，或伴有便溏者，去香附，加木香、小茴香、吴茱萸、肉桂；膜样痛经者，加花蕊

Fructus Evodiae (Wu Zhu Yu) and *Cortex Cinnamomi* (Rou Gui) are added. For membraniform dysmenorrhea, *Ophicalcitum* (Hua Rui Shi), *Myrrha* (Mo Yao) and *Great Guffaw Powder* (Shi Xiao San) are added.

石、没药、失笑散。

Shanghai doctor ZHU Nansun's experience prescription, *Supplemented Mo Jie Decoction* (Jia Wei Mo Jie Tang): 20 g of *Typhae Pollen Crudum* (Sheng Pu Huang), 12 g of *Rhizoma Sparganii Stoloniferi* (San Leng), 12 g of *Rhizoma Zedoariae* (E Zhu), 3 g of *Olibanum Praeparatum* (Zhi Ru Xiang), 3 g of *Myrrha Praeparata* (Zhi Mo Yao), 12 g of *Fructus Crataegi Cruda* (Sheng Shan Zha), 6 g of *Pericarpium Citri Reticulate Viride* (Qing Pi) and 2 g of *Daemonoropis Resina Pulverata* (Xue Jie Fen)(orally taken with water).

上海医家朱南孙经验方(加味膜竭汤)加减:生蒲黄20克,三棱12克,莪术12克,炙孔香3克,炙没药3克,生山楂12克,青皮6克,血竭粉2克(冲服)。

Shanghai doctor CAI Xiaosun's experience prescription, *Stasis-Dissolving and Pain-Relieving Prescription* (Hua Yu Ding Tong Fang): 10 g of *Chinese Angelica* (Chao Dang Gui), 12 g of *Radix Salviae Miltiorrhizae* (Dan Shen), 10 g of *Radix Cyathulae* (Chuan Niu Xi), 10 g of *Cyperi Rhizoma Praeparatum* (Zhi Xiang Fu), 6 g of *Rhizoma Ligustici Chuanxiong* (Chuan Xiong), 10 g of *Radix Paeoniae Rubra* (Chi Shao), 6 g of *Myrrha Praeparata* (Zhi Mo Yao), 12 g of *Rhizoma Corydalis* (Yan Hu Suo), 12 g of *Typhae Pollen Crudum* (Sheng Pu Huang), 10 g of *Faeces Trogopterorum* (Wu Ling Zhi) and 3 g of *Resina Draconis* (Xue Jie).

上海医家蔡小荪经验方(化瘀定痛方):炒当归10克,丹参12克,川牛膝10克,制香附10克,川芎6克,赤芍10克,制没药6克,延胡索12克,生蒲黄12克,五灵脂10克,血竭3克。

2.2 Syndrome of coagulation of cold dampness

2.2 寒湿凝滞证

Main manifestations Unpressable lower abdominal cold pain before or during menstruation, alleviation of pain with warmth, scanty menorrhea with purplish color menses and clot or like juice of black soybean, cold sensation in the body and aversion to cold, loose stool, slight purplish tongue with white and moist or white and greasy fur, deep and tense pulse.

主要证候 经前或经期小腹冷痛,按之痛甚,得热则舒,经行量少,色紫暗有块,或如黑豆汁,形寒畏冷,大便溏薄,舌淡紫,苔白润或白腻,脉沉紧。

Therapeutic methods Warming meridians to

治法 温经散寒,利湿

disperse cold and draining dampness to eliminate stagnation.

逐瘀。

Formulas and herbs *Lesser Abdomen Stasis-Expelling Decoction* (Shao Fu Zhu Yu Tang) composed of 6 g of *Cortex Cinnamomi* (Rou Gui) (to be decocted later), 6 g of *Fructus Foeniculi* (Xiao Hui Xiang), 6 g of *Rhizoma Zingiberis Praeparata* (Pao Jiang), 10 g of *Rhizoma Corydalis* (Yan Hu Suo), 10 g of *Faeces Trogopterorum* (Wu Ling Zhi), 6 g of *Myrrha* (Mo Yao), 10 g of *Radix Angelicae Sinensis* (Dang Gui), 5 g of *Rhizoma Ligustici Chuanxiong* (Chuan Xiong), 10 g of *Pollen Typhae* (Pu Huang), 10 g of *Radix Paeoniae Rubra* (Chi Shao) and 10 g of *Rhizoma Atractylodis* (Cang Zhu).

方药 代表方为少腹逐瘀汤；常用药如肉桂（后下）6克，小茴香6克，炮姜6克，延胡索10克，五灵脂10克，没药6克，当归10克，川芎5克，蒲黄10克，赤芍10克，苍术10克。

Modification For severe infection of cold, *Fructus Evodiae* (Wu Zhu Yu), *Ramulus Cinnamomi* (Gui Zhi) and *Aconiti Radix Lateralis Lateralis Tosta* (Pao Fu Zi) are added. For severe blood stasis, *Semen Persicae* (Tao Ren) and *Flos Carthami* (Hong Hua) are added. For severe pain and vomiting, *Fructus Evodiae* (Wu Zhu Yu) is added. For severe pain, aversion to cold and cold limbs, *Ramulus Cinnamomi* (Gui Zhi) is added. For intractable dysmenorrhea, *Scorpio* (Quan Xie) and *Scolopendra subspinipes* (Wu Gong) are added to free the meridians and relieve pain, or *Scorpio* (Quan Xie) and *Rhizoma Typhonii* (Bai Fu Zi) are added to dispel wind and relieve spasm, disperse cold and relieve pain.

加减 受寒重者，酌加吴茱萸、桂枝、炮附片；血瘀重者，加桃仁、红花；痛甚呕吐者，加吴茱萸；痛甚，畏寒四肢冷者，加桂枝；顽固性痛经者，加用全蝎、蜈蚣搜剔通络止痛，或全蝎配白附子，祛风止痉、散寒止痛。

Shanghai doctor SHEN Zhongli's experience prescription, *Channels-Warming and Cold-Dispersing Decoction* (Wen Jing San Han Tang): 12 g of *Radix Angelicae Sinensis* (Dang Gui), 6 g of *Rhizoma Ligustici Chuanxiong* (Chuan Xiong), 12 g of *Radix Paeoniae Rubra* (Chi Shao), 15 g of *Amethyst*

上海医家沈仲理经验方（温经散寒汤）加减：当归12克，川芎6克，赤芍12克，紫石英15克，葫芦巴12克，五灵脂12克，金铃子9克，延胡索10克，制香附12克，

(Zi Shi Ying), 12 g of *Trigonellae Semen* (Hu Lu Ba), 12 g of *Faeces Trogopterorum* (Wu Ling Zhi), 9 g of *Toosendan Fructus* (Jin Ling Zi), 10 g of *Rhizoma Corydalis* (Yan Hu Suo), 12 g of *Cyperi Rhizoma Praeparatum* (Zhi Xiang Fu), 6 g of *Fructus Foeniculi* (Xiao Hui Xiang) and 6 g of *Folium Artemistae Argyi* (Ai Ye).

小茴香6克,艾叶6克。

2.3 Syndrome of qi and blood asthenia

Main manifestations　Insidious pain or prolapsing sensation in the lower abdomen during or after menstruation, alleviated by pressure, scanty menses with light color and thin texture, lusterless facial complexion, dizziness, palpitation, lassitude, light-colored tongue as well as thready and weak pulse.

Therapeutic methods　Nourishing qi and blood, regulating menstruation and relieving pain.

Formulas and herbs　*Eight Jewel Decoction* (Ba Zhen Tang), composed of 12 g of *Radix Codonopsis Pilosulae* (Dang Shen), 12 g of *Rhizoma Atractylodis Macrocephalae* (Bai Zhu), 10 g of *Poriae* (Fu Ling), 10 g of *Radix Angelicae Sinensis* (Dang Gui), 10 g of *Radix Paeoniae Alba* (Bai Shao), 10 g of *Radix Rehmanniae Praeparata* (Shu Di Huang), 5 g of *Radix Glycyrrhizae Praeparata* (Zhi Gan Cao), 10 g of *Radix Astragali* (Huang Qi) and 6 g of *Radix Aucklandiae* (Mu Xiang).

Modification　For rib-side pain, breast distention and abdominal distention and pain due to blood asthenia and liver qi stagnation, *Fructus Meliae Toosendan* (Chuan Lian Zi), *Radix Bupleuri* (Chai Hu), *Fructus Foeniculi* (Xiao Hui Xiang) and *Radix Linderae* (Wu Yao) are added to move qi and relieve pain. For aching lumbus and knees, *Semen Cuscutae* (Tu Si Zi), *Radix Dipsaci* (Xu Duan) and *Ramulus Loranthi* (Sang Ji Sheng) are added to

2.3　气血虚弱证

主要证候　经期或经后小腹隐隐作痛,喜按或小腹及阴部空坠不适,月经量少,色淡,质清稀,面色无华,头晕心悸,神疲乏力。舌淡,脉细无力。

治法　益气养血,调经止痛。

方药　代表方为八珍汤;常用药如党参12克,白术12克,茯苓10克,当归10克,白芍10克,熟地黄10克,炙甘草5克,黄芪10克,木香6克。

加减　若症见胁痛,乳胀,小腹胀痛者,乃血虚肝郁,加川楝子、柴胡、小茴香、乌药以行气止痛;若伴腰腿酸软者,加菟丝子、续断、桑寄生补肾强腰脊;经量过多者,加阿胶、艾叶炭。

supplement the kidney and strengthen lumbar spine. For profuse menstruation, *Colla Corii Asini* (E Jiao) and *Artemisiae Argyi Folium Carbonisatum* (Ai Ye Tan) are added.

2.4 Syndrome of liver and kidney asthenia

Main manifestations Continuous abdominal pain during or after menstruation, scanty menses with light color and thin texture, aching sensation in the loins and knees, dizziness and tinnitus, slight red tongue with thin fur, deep and thready pulse.

Therapeutic methods Boosting the kidney and nourishing the liver, relieving emergency and relieving pain.

Formulas and herbs *Liver-Regulating Decoction* (Tiao Gan Tang) composed of 10 g of *Radix Angelicae Sinensis* (Dang Gui), 10 g of *Radix Paeoniae Alba* (Bai Shao), 6 g of *Fructus Corni* (Shan Zhu Yu), 10 g of *Radix Morindae Officinalis* (Ba Ji Tian), 10 g of *Colla Corii Asini* (E Jiao), 10 g of *Rhizoma Dioscoreae* (Shan Yao) and 3 g of *Radix Glycyrrhizae* (Gan Cao).

Modification For severe pain in the loins, *Radix Dipsaci* (Xu Duan) and *Cortex Eucommiae* (Du Zhong) are added to supplement the kidney and strengthen the loins. For abdominal or hypochondriac distension and pain due to liver qi stagnation, *Fructus Meliae Toosendan* (Chuan Lian Zi), *Rhizoma Corydalis* (Yan Hu Suo), *Semen Citri Reticulatae* (Ju He) and *Radix Curcumae* (Yu Jin) are added to soothe the liver, move qi and relieve pain.

3 Other therapeutic methods

3.1 Chinese patent drugs

(1) *Dysmenorrhea Pill* (Fu Nu Tong Jing

2.4 肝肾亏损证

主要证候 经期或经后小腹绵绵作痛，经行量少，色暗淡，质稀薄，腰膝酸软，头晕耳鸣，舌淡红，苔薄，脉沉细。

治法 益肾养肝，缓急止痛。

方药 代表方为调肝汤；常用药如当归10克，白芍10克，山茱萸6克，巴戟天10克，阿胶10克，山药10克，甘草3克。

加减 若腰酸甚者，加续断、杜仲以补肾壮腰。兼少腹或两胁胀痛者，乃挟肝郁所致，加川楝子、延胡索、橘核、郁金以疏肝行气止痛。

3 其他疗法

3.1 中成药

（1）妇女痛经丸：每次

Wan): 50 pills each time and twice a day, applicable to the treatment of syndrome of qi stagnation and blood stasis.

50粒,每日2次,适用于气血凝滞证。

(2) *Mugwort and Cyperus Uterus-Warming Pill* (Ai Fu Nuan Gong Wan): For small honey pill, 9 g each time. For big honey pill, 1 pill each time and twice to three times a day, applicable to the treatment of blood stasis, qi stagnation and vacuity cold syndrome of the Lower Energizer.

(2) 艾附暖宫丸:小蜜丸每次9克,大蜜丸每次1丸,每日2～3次,适用于血虚气滞、下焦虚寒证。

(3) *Dysmenorrhea Granules* (Yue Yue Shu Tong Jing Bao Ke Li): 1 bag each time and twice a day, applicable to the treatment of congealing cold, qi stagnation and blood stasis syndrome.

(3) 月月舒(痛经宝颗粒):每次1袋,每日2次,适用于寒凝气滞血瘀证。

(4) *Corydalis Pain-Relieving Granules* (Yuan Hu Zhi Tong Ke Li): 1 bag each time and three times a day, applicable to the treatment of qi stagnation and blood stasis syndrome.

(4) 元胡止痛颗粒:每次1袋,每日3次,适用于气滞血瘀证。

3.2 Empirical and folk recipes

3.2 单验方

(1) 30 g of *Herba Leonuri* (Yi Mu Cao) is decocted with proper amount of brown sugar for oral taking, three times a day, applicable to the treatment of dysmenorrhea due to blood stasis.

(1) 益母草30克,红糖适量,水煎服,每日3剂,适用于血瘀证痛经。

(2) 15 g of Rhizoma Zingiberis Recens (Sheng Jiang) is decocted with 3 scallion stalks and proper amount of brown sugar, applicable to the treatment of dysmenorrhea due to cold dampness.

(2) 生姜15克,葱白3根,红糖适量,水煎服;适用于寒湿痛经。

(3) Shanghai doctor CAI Xiaosun's experience prescription, *Stasis-Expelling and Membraniform Dysmenorrhea-Relieving Prescription* (Zhu Yu Hua Mo Fang): 10 g of *Angelicae Sinensis Radicis Extremitas* (Dang Gui Wei), 6 g of *Rhizoma Ligustici Chuanxiong* (Chuan Xiong), 10 g of *Achyranthis Radix* (Tu Niu Xi), 3 g of *Ramulus Cinnamomi* (Gui Zhi), 10 g of *Radix Paeoniae Rubra* (Chi

(3) 上海医家蔡小荪经验方(逐瘀化膜方):当归尾10克,川芎6克,土牛膝10克,桂枝3克,赤芍10克,延胡索12克,花蕊石15克,制香附10克,没药6克,桃仁10克,失笑散12克,适用于膜样痛经。

Shao), 12 g of *Rhizoma Corydalis* (Yan Hu Suo), 15 g of *Ophicalcitum* (Hua Rui Shi), 10 g of *Cyperi Rhizoma Praeparatum* (Zhi Xiang Fu), 6 g of *Myrrha* (Mo Yao), 10 g of *Semen Persicae* (Tao Ren) and 12 g of *Great Guffaw Powder* (Shi Xiao San), applicable to the treatment of membraniform dysmenorrhea.

(4) Shanghai doctor CHEN Xiaobao's experience prescription, *Eightfold Processed Cyperus Pill* (Ba Zhi Xiang Fu Wan): Eightfold processed *Rhizoma Cyperi* (Xiang Fu), *Radix Angelicae Sinensis* (Dang Gui), *Radix Rehmanniae Praeparata* (Shu Di Huang), *Radix Paeoniae Alba* (Bai Shao), *Rhizoma Ligustici Chuanxiong* (Chuan Xiong), *Flos Carthami* (Hong Hua), *Coptidis Rhizoma & Sichuanense* (Chuan Lian), *Rhizoma Pinelliae* (Ban Xia), *Gentianae Macrophyllae Radix* (Qin Jiu), *Cortex Moutan Radicis* (Mu Dan Pi) and *Pericarpium Citri Reticulatae Viride* (Qing Pi) are prepared into pills.

(4) 上海医家陈筱宝经验方(八制香附丸):以香附为君,经过八制,配合当归、熟地黄、白芍、川芎、红花、川连、半夏、秦艽、牡丹皮、青皮等药为丸。

Amenorrhea

Amenorrhea refers to no menstruation in female over 16 years old, or interruption of menstruation for over 6 months after the establishment of menstrual cycle, or no menstruation for over past six menstrual cycles. The former is primary amenorrhea, and the latter is secondary amenorrhea. Amenorrhea in pregnancy and breast-feeding is physiological phenomenon. Tis disease was termed "no period in females", "interrupted menstruation" and "blood depletion" in the medical classics of Chinese medicine.

Pathogenesis of amenorrhea is complex, but the

闭　经

女子年逾 16 周岁月经尚未来潮,或月经周期建立后又中断 6 个月以上,或月经停闭超过既往月经 3 个周期以上,称为闭经。前者为原发性闭经,后者为继发性闭经。妊娠期、哺乳期以及绝经后的无月经均属生理现象。中医古代医籍中称本病为"女子不月""经水断绝""血枯"等。

闭经的病因病机复杂,

cause is nothing more than asthenia or sthenia. Sthenia is caused by the obstruction of Thoroughfare Vessel, Conception Vessel and uterus, resulting in the inability of menses to move down. Asthenia is caused by congenital insufficiency of kidney qi, no blood nourishment in Thoroughfare and Conception Vessels and emptiness of the sea of blood, leading to amenorrhea.

但究其病因不外乎虚实两端。实者为冲任胞宫阻滞，经血不得下行；虚者多由先天肾气不足，冲任未充血海空虚，以致经闭。

1　Key points for diagnosis

1.1　General condition

(1) Non-occurrence of menarche after the age of 16 or non-physiological stoppage of menstruation for 3 cycles or 6 months, after the establishment of menstrual cycle.

(2) Careful examination is given to observe the general development, nutrition, mental state and development of the secondary sex character, in order to analyze the cause and nature of amenorrhea.

1.2　Gynecologicai examination

Examination is made to see whether the external and internal genitals are normal and whether there is mass in the pelvis.

1.3　Auxiliary examination

(1) Iodized oil roentgenography is performed to see whether there is abnormal development of the uterus, metrosynizesis and tuberculosis of endometrium.

(2) Diagnostic uterine curettage and pathological examination of endometrium are performed to examine the functional states of the ovary and to see whether there are tuberculosis of endometrium and severe damage of endometrium.

(3) When necessary CT or MRI can be used,

1　诊断要点

1.1　一般情况

(1) 年逾 16 岁月经尚未初潮，或月经周期建立以后非生理性停经 3 个周期或 6 个月以上。

(2) 注意观察患者一般发育、营养、精神及第二性征发育等状态，有助于分析判断闭经的原因与性质。

1.2　妇科检查

注意检查患者内外生殖器官的发育状况，有无畸形或缺如，有无盆腔肿块。

1.3　辅助检查

(1) 通过子宫碘油造影，了解有无子宫畸形、宫腔粘连及子宫内膜结核。

(2) 诊断性刮宫及子宫内膜病理检查，有助于了解卵巢功能状态、有无子宫内膜结核及子宫内膜严重损伤。

(3) 必要时可行 CT、

which is helpful for excluding pituitary tumor.

MRI 检查有助于排除垂体肿瘤。

(4) Uteroscopy and peritoneoscopy are helpful for detecting organic pathological change of the uterus and pelvis.

(4) 宫腔镜、腹腔镜检查可发现宫腔及盆腔器质性病变。

(5) Chomosome nuclear analysis can be made for the patients with primary amenorrhea.

(5) 对原发性闭经患者可进行染色体核型分析。

(6) Test of hormones in the blood: Obvious increase in FSH and decrease in estrogen (E_2) suggest hypo function of the ovary. Low FSH and LH values suggest hypofunction of the pituitary or hypothalamus. Increased LH, FSH and T values indicate amenorrhea due to polycystic ovary syndrome. Increase of PRL value indicates amenorrhea due to hyperprolactin hematopathy.

(6) 血中激素水平测定：促卵泡激素(FSH)明显升高、雌激素(E_2)水平低下，提示卵巢功能减退，FSH 及 LH 促黄体生成激素)值低下，提示垂体或下丘脑功能低下；LH/FSH 比值升高、T(睾酮)值升高，提示多囊卵巢综合征性闭经；泌乳素(PRL)值升高，提示高泌乳素血症性闭经。

(7) Cares should be taken to differentiate athis disease from physiological amenorrhea due to pregnancy, breastfeeding and menopause.

(7) 本病应与妊娠、哺乳期、绝经期的生理性闭经相鉴别。

2 Syndrome differentiation and treatment

2 辨证论治

Asthenia and sthenia must be differentiated in amenorrhea. No menstruation in females after the normal age of menarche or gradually scarce menstrual cycle to amenorrhea, accompanied by other asthenia symptoms, is of asthenia syndrome, while sudden amenorrhea accompanied by other sthenia symptoms is of sthenia syndrome.

闭经当分清虚实。一般而论，已逾正常女性初潮年龄而尚未行经，或月经逐渐稀发而停闭，伴有其他虚象的，多属虚证；如以往月经尚属正常而突然停闭，又伴其他实象的，则多是实证。

The therapeutical principles for amenorrhea are based upon asthenia, sthenia, cold or heat of the disease. Asthenia syndrome is treated by the tonifying and dredging method, by either nourishing the

闭经的治疗原则，是根据病证的虚实寒热，虚者补而通之，或补益肝肾，或调养气血；实者泻而通之，或活血

liver and kidney or regulating and nourishing qi and blood. The sthenia syndrome is treated by the reducing and dredging method, by either activating blood to resolve stasis, or regulating qi to remove stagnation, or dissolving phlegm to regulate menstruation. It is necessary not to abuse the representative herbal formula to promote menstruation by the attacking and breaking action, without differentiation between asthenia and sthenia. For instance, the sthenia syndrome must not be treated just by harsh tonification, for the pathogenic factor would be retained instead, blocking essence and blood. As for amenorrhea caused by other diseases, such as consumptive disease, blood disorder, parasitic infestation, the other diseases should be treated first. As soon as the disease is cured, menstruation can be regulated.

化瘀,或理气行滞,或化痰调经。切不可不分虚实,滥用攻破通经之代表方,如有实证,亦不可一味峻补,反而留邪,而阻滞精血。至于因他病而致经闭者,如虚痨、血痨、虫积等,又当先治他病,病愈则经可调。

2.1 Syndrome of insufficiency of the liver and kidney

2.1 肝肾不足证

Main manifestations Non-occurrence of menarche after the normal age, or delayed menarche, delayed menstruation, scanty menorrhea, gradual amenorrhea, dizziness, tinnitus, aching and flaccid sensation in the loins and knees, dry mouth, feverish sensation over the palms, soles and chest, tidal fever and sweating, dark complexion or flushed cheeks, slight red tongue with scanty fur, and thready and taut pulse.

主要证候 月经超龄未至,或初潮延迟,月经后期、量少,渐至经闭,头晕耳鸣,腰酸膝软,口干咽燥,五心烦热、潮热汗出,面色晦暗或两颧潮红,舌质淡红少苔,脉细弦。

Therapeutic methods Nourishing the liver and kidney, nourishing blood and regulating menstruation.

治法 补益肝肾,养血调经。

Formulas and herbs *Kidney-Returning Pill* (Gui Shen Wan), composed of 10 g of *Radix Rehmanniae Praeparata* (Shu Di Huang), 10 g of

方药 代表方为归肾丸;常用药如熟地黄 10 克,当归 10 克,山茱萸 10 克,枸

Radix Angelicae Sinensis (Dang Gui), 10 g of *Fructus Corni* (Shan Zhu Yu), 10 g of *Fructus Lycii* (Gou Qi Zi), 12 g of *Semen Cuscutae* (Tu Si Zi), 10 g of *Astragali Complanati Semen* (Tong Ji Li), 20 g of *Rhizoma Dioscoreae* (Shan Yao), 20 g of *Caulis Spatholobi* (Ji Xue Teng), 10 g of *Colla Corii Asini* (E Jiao), 10 g of *Radix Achyranthis Bidentatae* (Niu Xi) and 10 g of *Herba Lycopi* (Ze Lan).

杞子10克，菟丝子12克，潼蒺藜10克，山药20克，鸡血藤20克，阿胶10克，怀牛膝10克，泽兰10克。

Modification For unsolid stool, *Radix Rehmanniae Cruda* (Sheng Di Huang) is deleted while *Semen Cuscutae* (Tu Si Zi) is added. For coldness in abdomen and lumbar region, *Aconiti Radix Lateralis Tosta* (Pao Fu Zi) and *Folium Artemistae Argyi* (Ai Ye) are added. For obvious tidal heat sensation, *Cortex Lycii Radicis* (Di Gu Pi), *Trionycis Carapax cum Liquido Frictus* (Zhi Bie Jia) and *Radix Cynanchi Atrati* (Bai Wei) are added. For anorexia and loose stool, *Poriae* (Fu Ling) and *Rhizoma Atractylodis Macrocephalae* (Bai Zhu) are added.

加减 若大便不实者，可去生地黄，加菟丝子；腰腹冷者，加炮附片、艾叶；潮热明显者，加地骨皮、炙鳖甲、白薇；纳差便溏者，加茯苓、白术。

Shanghai doctor CAI Xiaosun's experience prescription, *Kidney-Nourishing and Network Vessels-Freeing Prescription* (Yu Shen Tong Luo Fang): 12 g of *Poria* (Yun Fu Ling), 10 g of *Radix Rehmanniae Cruda* (Sheng Di Huang), 10 g of *Radix Achyranthis Bidentatae* (Niu Xi), 10 g of *Liquidambaris Fructus* (Lu Lu Tong), 2.5 g of *Caryophylli Flos* (Gong Ding Xiang), 12 g of *Rhizoma Polygonati Praeparata* (Zhi Huang Jing), 10 g of *Ophiopogonis Radix* (Mai Dong), 12 g of *Epimedium davidii* (Yin Yang Huo), 10 g of *Photiniae Folium* (Shi Nan Ye) and 3 g of *Sliced Dalbergiae Lignum Pulveratum* (Jiang Xiang Pian).

上海医家蔡小荪经验方（育肾通络方）：云茯苓12克，生地黄10克，怀牛膝10克，路路通10克，公丁香2.5克，制黄精12克，麦冬10克，淫羊藿12克，石楠叶10克，降香片3克。

2.2 Syndrome of asthenia of qi and blood

2.2 气血虚弱证

Main manifestations Gradual development of

主要证候 月经由后

menorrhea from delayed menorrhea, scanty menorrhea and light-colored menorrhea into amenorrhea, bright-pale complexion or sallow complexion, lusterless hair or loss of hair, dizziness, blurred vision, palpitation, shortness of breath, no desire to speak, spiritual lassitude, anorexia, loose stool, light-colored lips and tongue as well as thready and weak pulse.

期、量少、色淡而渐至经闭，面色㿠白或萎黄，毛发不泽或脱落，头昏眼花，心悸怔忡，气短懒言，神疲肢倦，纳少便溏，唇舌色淡，脉细弱。

Therapeutic methods Supplementing qi, nourishing blood and regulating menstruation.

治法 补气养血调经。

Formulas and herbs *Ginseng Construction-Nourishing Decoction* (Ren Shen Yang Rong Tang) composed of 15 g of *Radix Ginseng* (Ren Shen), 10 g of *Radix Astragali* (Huang Qi), 10 g of *Stir-Fried Rhizoma Atractylodis Macrocephalae* (Chao Bai Zhu), 10 g of *Poriae* (Fu Ling), 6 g of *Radix Polygalae* (Yuan Zhi), 6 g of *Pericarpium Citri Tangerinae* (Chen Pi), 6 g of *Fructus Schisandrae* (Wu Wei Zi), 15 g of *Radix Angelicae Sinensis* (Dang Gui), 9 g of *Radix Paeoniae Alba* (Bai Shao), 12 g of *Radix Rehmanniae Praeparata* (Shu Di Huang), 3 g of *Cinnamomi Cortex Rasus* (Gui Xin) and 6 g of *Radix Glycyrrhizae Praeparata* (Zhi Gan Cao).

方药 代表方为人参养荣汤；常用药如人参15克，黄芪10克，炒白术10克，茯苓10克，远志6克，陈皮6克，五味子6克，当归15克，白芍9克，熟地黄12克，桂心3克，炙甘草6克。

Modification For peaceless sleep, *Caulis Polygoni Multiflori* (Ye Jiao Teng) and *Semen Zizyphi Spinosae* (Suan Zao Ren) are added. For aching lumbus, *Fructus Lycii* (Gou Qi Zi) and *Cortex Eucommiae* (Du Zhong) are added. For anorexia, *Radix Aucklandiae* (Mu Xiang) and *Fructus Oryzae Germinatus* (Gu Ya) are added.

加减 若夜寐欠安者，加夜交藤、酸枣仁；腰酸者，加狗脊、杜仲；纳差者，加木香、谷芽。

2.3 Syndrome of qi stagnation and blood stasis

2.3 气滞血瘀证

Main manifestations Amenorrhea, mental depression, irritability, susceptibility to rage, disten-

主要证候 月经闭止不行，精神抑郁，烦躁易怒，胸

ding fullness in the chest and hypochondria, distending pain or aggravated by pressure in the lower abdomen, purplish tongue or with ecchymosis, deep and unsmooth pulse.

胁胀满，小腹胀痛或拒按，舌紫暗，或有瘀点，脉沉涩。

Therapeutic methods Nourishing blood and promoting qi, resolving stasis and promoting menstruation.

治法 养血行气，化瘀通经。

Formulas and herbs *Sanguine Mansion Stasis-Expelling Decoction* (Xue Fu Zhu Yu Tang) compose of 10 g of *Radix Angelicae Sinensis* (Dang Gui), 5 g of *Rhizoma Ligustici Chuanxiong* (Chuan Xiong), 10 g of *Radix Paeoniae Rubra* (Chi Shao), 10 g of *Semen Persicae* (Tao Ren), 6 g of *Radix Bupleuri* (Chai Hu), 10 g of *Flos Carthami* (Hong Hua), 10 g of *Fructus Aurantii* (Zhi Qiao), 12 g of *Rhizoma Cyperi* (Xiang Fu), 10 g of *Radix Cyathulae* (Chuan Niu Xi) and 15 g of *Herba Lycopi* (Ze Lan).

方药 代表方为血府逐瘀汤；常用药如当归 10 克，川芎 5 克，赤芍 10 克，桃仁 10 克，柴胡 6 克，红花 10 克，枳壳 10 克，香附 12 克，川牛膝 10 克，泽兰 15 克。

Modification For abdominal pain aggravated by pressure, *Radix Cyathulae* (Chuan Niu Xi), *Rhizoma Zedoariae* (E Zhu) and *Flos Carthami* (Hong Hua) are added to break qi and disperse stasis. For breast distention and pain, *Pericarpium Citri Reticulatae Viride* (Qing Pi), *Pericarpium Citri Tangerinae* (Chen Pi) and *Fructus Crataegi* (Shan Zha) are added.

加减 如兼见腹部疼痛拒按者，可加川牛膝、莪术、红花等破气消瘀之品；乳房胀痛者，加青皮、陈皮、山楂。

Shanghai doctor CHEN Xiaobao's experience prescription, *Rhizoma Cyperi and Herba Leonuri Decoction* (Xiang Cao Tang): 12 g of *Rhizoma Cyperi* (Xiang Fu), 15 g of *Herba Leonuri* (Yi Mu Cao), 15 g of *Caulis Spatholobi* (Ji Xue Teng), 15 g of *Radix Angelicae Sinensis* (Dang Gui), 10 g of *Herba Lycopi* (Ze Lan), 6 g of *Rhizoma Ligustici Chuanxiong* (Chuan Xiong), 10 g of *Semen Biotae* (Bai Zi Ren) and 10 g of brown sugar.

上海医家陈筱宝经验方（香草汤）加减：香附 12 克，益母草 15 克，鸡血藤 15 克，当归 15 克，泽兰草 10 克，川芎 6 克，柏子仁 10 克，红糖 10 克。

2.4 Syndrome of phlegm-dampness obstruction

Main manifestations Amenorrhea, obesity, fullness and oppression in the chest and hypochondria, retching and nausea, and copious phlegm, low spirit, lassitude, puffy face and swollen feet, leukorrhagia, greasy tongue fur and slippery pulse.

Therapeutic methods Eliminating phlegm and dampness, regulating qi, activating blood and promoting menstruation.

Formulas and herbs *Atractylodes and Cyperus Phlegm-Abducting Decoction* (Cang Fu Dao Tan Tang) composed of 12 g of *Rhizoma Atractylodis* (Cang Zhu), 10 g of *Poriae* (Fu Ling), 10 g of *Rhizoma Pinelliae* (Ban Xia), 10 g of *Pericarpium Citri Tangerinae* (Chen Pi), 10 g of *Arisaema cum Bile* (Dan Nan Xing), 12 g of *Rhizoma Cyperi* (Xiang Fu), 10 g of *Radix Angelicae Sinensis* (Dang Gui), 5 g of *Rhizoma Ligustici Chuanxiong* (Chuan Xiong), 10 g of *Fructus Aurantii* (Zhi Qiao), 10 g of *Fructus Crataegi* (Shan Zha), 10 g of *Herba Lycopi* (Ze Lan) and 6 g of *Cortex Phellodendri* (Huang Bo).

Modification For chest distress, *Cortex Magnoliae Officinalis* (Hou Pu), *Fructus Trichosanthis* (Quan Gua Lou) and *Rhizoma Acori Graminei* (Shi Chang Pu) are added. For sticky and greasy taste in the mouth, *Herba Eupatorii* (Pei Lan) and *Fructus Oryzae Germinatus* (Gu Ya) are added. For edema, *Semen Coicis* (Yi Yi Ren) and *Rhizoma Alismatis* (Ze Xie) are added. For nausea and poor appetite, *Fructus Amomi* (Sha Ren) and *Rhizoma Atractylodis Macrocephalae* (Bai Zhu) are added.

Shanghai doctor CAI Xiaosu's experience prescription, *Fat-Transforming and Menstruation-Regulating Prescription*

2.4 痰湿阻滞证

主要证候 月经停闭，形体肥胖，胸胁满闷，呕恶痰多，神疲倦怠，或面浮足肿，或带下量多色白。苔腻，脉滑。

治法 豁痰除湿，调气活血通经。

方药 代表方为苍附导痰汤；常用药如苍术 12 克，茯苓 10 克，半夏 10 克，陈皮 10 克，胆南星 10 克，香附 12 克，当归 10 克，川芎 5 克，枳壳 10 克，山楂 10 克，泽兰 10 克，黄柏 6 克。

加减 胸闷者，加厚朴、全瓜蒌、石菖蒲；口中黏腻者，加佩兰、谷芽；浮肿者，加薏苡仁、泽泻；泛恶纳少者，加砂仁、白术。

上海医家蔡小荪经验方（化脂调经方）：全当归 10 克，川芎 6

(Hua Zhi Tiao Jing Prescription): 10 g of *Angelicae Sinensis Radix Integra* (Quan Dang Gui), 6 g of *Rhizoma Ligustici Chuanxiong* (Chuan Xiong), 5 g of *Rhizoma Atractylodis* (Cang Zhu), 10 g of *Cyperi Rhizoma Praeparatum* (Zhi Xiang Fu), 12 g of *Poriae* (Fu Ling), 6 g of *Rhizoma Arisaematis cum Bile* (Dan Nan Xing), 5 g of *Burnt Fructus Aurantii* (Jiao Zhi Qiao), 3 g of *Semen Sinapis Albae* (Bai Jie Zi), 5 g of *Pericarpium Citri Reticulatae Viride* (Qing Pi), 5 g of *Pericarpium Citri Tangerinae* (Chen Pi) and 15 g of *Fructus Crataegi Crudum* (Sheng Shan Zha).

克，苍术 5 克，制香附 10 克，云茯苓 12 克，胆南星 6 克，焦枳壳 5 克，白芥子 3 克，青皮、陈皮各 5 克，生山楂 15 克。

3 Other therapeutic methods

3.1 Chinese patent durgs

(1) *Eight-Gem Leonurus (Motherwort) Pill* (Ba Zhen Yi Mu Wan): 6 g each time and three times a day, applicable to the treatment of asthenia syndrome of qi and blood.

(2) *Sevenfold Processed Cyperus Pill* (Qi Zhi Xiang Fu Wan): 10 g each time and three times a day, applicable to the treatment of phlegm-dampness syndrome.

(3) *Rehmannia Pills with Six Ingredients* (Liu Wei Di Huang Wan) (Condensed Pill): 8 pills each time and three times a day, applicable to the treatment of deficiency syndrome of the liver and kidney.

3.2 Empirical and folk recipes

(1) 30-60 g of *Herba Leonuri* (Yi Mu Cao) is decocted with water and proper amount of brown sugar, one dose a day.

(2) 15 g of *Radix Angelicae Sinensis* (Dang Gui), 30 g of *Herba Leonuri* (Yi Mu Cao) and 15 g of *Radix Astragali* (Huang Qi) are decocted with water. The decoction, applicable to the treatment of amenorrhea of asthenia syndrome, is taken one

3 其他疗法

3.1 中成药

（1）八珍益母丸：每次服 6 克，每日 3 次，适用于气血虚弱证。

（2）七制香附丸：每次服 10 克，每日 3 次，适用于痰湿证。

（3）六味地黄丸（浓缩丸）：每次服 8 粒，每日 3 次，适用于肝肾不足证。

3.2 单验方

（1）益母草 30～60 g，红糖适量，水煎服，每日 1 剂。

（2）当归 15 克，益母草 30 克，黄芪 15 克，水煎服每日 1 剂，适用于虚证闭经。

dose a day.

(3) 30 g of *Radix Salviae Miltiorrhizae* (Dan Shen) and two eggs are decocted with water for 2 hours. Eat eggs and drink soup, one dose a day, applicable to the treatment of amenorrhea of blood asthenia syndrome, is taken one dose a day.

（3）丹参 30 克，鸡蛋 2 枚水煮 2 小时，食蛋饮汤，每日 1 剂，适用于血虚证闭经。

Polycystic ovary syndrome

多囊卵巢综合征

Polycystic ovary syndrome is endocrine syndrome of multiple-factor and polymorphic manifestations, clinically characterized by by irregular menstruation, sterility, obesity, pilosity, acne, bilateral cystic enlargement of ovary, androgen excess and persistent anovulation, and is a common disease of endocrine disturbance in women of childbearing age. Because of the diversity of its clinical manifestations, its discussion are seen in different texts on delayed menstruation, amenorrhea, uterine bleeding, sterility and other syndromes in TCM.

This disease is mainly caused by congenital weakness or early marriage, excessive sexual life and injury of kidney qi, or by obesity or excessive intake of greasy and rich food or intemperance of food, which leads to impairment of the spleen and stomach and endogenous dampness; or by retention of blood after delivery, depression or impairment of the liver due to rage, stagnation of liver qi and qi stagnation and blood stasis, or by fire developed from prolonged stagnation, which leads to disharmony between qi and blood. All of these factors may result in dysfunction of the viscera, disorder of qi and blood, obstruction of the meridians, accumu-

多囊卵巢综合征是是一种发病多因性，临床表现多态性的内分泌失调综合征。以月经紊乱、不孕、多毛、肥胖、痤疮、双侧卵巢持续增大，以及雄激素过多、持续无排卵为临床特征。这是生育年龄妇女常见的内分泌紊乱性疾病。由于其临床表现的多样性，中医论述散见于月经后期、闭经、崩漏、不孕等病证。

本病的主要病因可由禀赋薄弱或早婚房劳，肾气受损；素体肥胖或恣食膏粱厚味，或饮食失节，损伤脾胃，脾虚痰湿内生；经期产后余血末尽，抑郁或恼怒伤肝，肝气郁结，气滞血瘀，郁久化火气血失和。以上均可导致脏腑功能失常，气血失调，经络不畅，痰湿脂膜积聚，血海蓄溢失常而致本病。

lation of phlegm and dampness, and lipid accumulation, dysfunction of acumulation and overflow in the sea of blood, which lead to polycystic ovary syndrome.

1 Key points for diagnosis

1.1 Medical history

Sparce menstruation and scanty menorrhea after menarche, or even amenorrhea or irregular vaginal bleeding and infertility, overweight or pilosity before or after menarche.

1.2 Symptoms auxiliary examination

(1) Irregular menorrhea: It is mainly manifested by amenorrhea, mostly secondary amenorrhea. Sparce menstruation and scanty menses, intermittent amenorrhea or uterine bleeding in some patients.

(2) Sterility: It is mainly caused by menstrual disorder and anovulation, accompanied by insufficient luteal function. If pregnant, abortion happens easily.

(3) Pilosity: It occurs before and after the puberty, manifested by increased and thickened hair, with pubic hair masculinely distributed around the areola, below the belly button, on belly line, mouth and upper lip. Some patients are accompanied by greasy hair or acne.

(4) Obesity: It starts at puberty, but without specificity in physical posture and fat distribution.

(5) Acanthosis nigricans: Gray-brown pigmentation often appears in the labia, back of the neck, armpits, skin folds regions under the breasts and

1 诊断要点

1.1 病史

初潮后月经稀发或稀少，甚或闭经，或不规则阴道流血，不孕等，月经初潮前后即有多毛现象，或初潮前即有体重超重的趋势。

1.2 症状

（1）月经失调主要表现闭经，绝大多数为继发性闭经，闭经前常有月经稀发或过少；部分患者可表现为闭经与崩漏相间出现。

（2）不孕主要由月经失调和无排卵所致，且多伴有黄体功能不足，即使怀孕，也极易流产。

（3）多毛多发生在青春期前后，表现为毛发增多增粗，阴毛呈男性化分布，乳晕周围、脐下腹中线、口角上唇等部位有毛发。部分患者伴油脂性脱发或痤疮。

（4）肥胖多始于青春期前后，但其脂肪分布及体态并无特异性。

（5）黑棘皮症常在阴唇、颈背部、腋下、乳房下和腹股沟等皮肤皱褶部位出现灰褐

groin, symmetrically with thickened skin of soft texture.

1.3 Examinations

(1) B ultrasonic examination indicates polycystic change of ovary.

(2) Clinical and (or) biochemical indexes suggest the presence of hyperandrogenism.

(3) FSH value is normal or low, but LH value is elevated, serum LH/FSH is>2-3.

2 Syndrome differentiation and treatment

The internal cause of the disease is dysfunction of the liver, spleen and kidney. The external cause is phlegm-damp invasion. Both factors interact as both cause and effect on the organism to induce the disease. Therefore, syndromes with asthenia and sthenia mixed are more common clinically. Differentiation is mainly based on clinical symptoms, signs, tongue and pulse.

According to the characteristics of obesity, pilosity, ovarian enlargement and envelope thickening, the treatment is decided to tonify the kidney for dealing with the causative reason, and to strengthen the spleen to regulate qi and resolve phlegm, soothe the liver to relieve stagnation and reduce fire, activate blood to resolve stasis as well as regulate menstruation for dealing with the symptoms.

2.1 Kidney asthenia syndrome

Main manifestations Delayed menophania, in later period, small amount, light color, and thin nature, gradual amenorrhea, occasional uterine bleeding or prolonged menstruation, lusterless facial

色色素沉着，呈对称性，皮肤增厚，质地柔软。

1.3 检查

（1）B超检查提示卵巢呈多囊样改变。

（2）临床和(或)生化指标提示存在高雄激素血症。

（3）血清FSH值正常或偏低而LH值升高，LH/FSH>2～3。

2 辨证论治

本病内因为肝、脾、肾三脏功能失调，外因以痰湿之邪侵袭为主，且二者互为因果作用于机体而致病，故临床以虚实夹杂证多见。辨证主要根据临床症状、体征与舌脉。

根据体胖、多毛、卵巢增大、包膜增厚的特点，治疗以补肾治其本，健脾理气化痰，疏肝解郁泻火，活血化瘀调经治其标，标本同治。

2.1 肾虚证

主要证候　月经初潮迟至、后期、量少，色淡质稀，渐至停闭。偶有崩漏不止，或经期延长。面色无华，头晕

complexion, dizziness and tinnitus, aching and weak sensation in the loins and knees, lack of strength and fear of cold, sloppy stool, scanty vaginal discharge, dry and astringent sensation in vagina, sterility long after marriage, light-colored tongue with thin fur and deep-thready pulse.

耳鸣,腰膝酸软,乏力怕冷,大便溏薄。带下量少,阴中干涩,婚后日久不孕。舌质淡苔薄,脉沉细。

Therapeutic methods Nourishing the kidney to replenish essence, regulating and nourishing the Thoroughfare and Conception Vessels.

治法 补肾填精,调补冲任。

Formulas and herbs *Vital Gate Pills* (You Gui Wan), composed of 10 g of *Radix Rehmanniae Praeparata* (Shu Di Huang), 20 g of *Rhizoma Dioscoreae* (Shan Yao), 10 g of *Fructus Corni* (Shan Zhu Yu), 10 g of *Fructus Lycii* (Gou Qi Zi), 10 g of *Colla Cornus Cervi* (Lu Jiao Jiao), 12 g of *Semen Cuscutae* (Tu Si Zi), 10 g of *Cortex Eucommiae* (Du Zhong), 10 g of *Radix Angelicae Sinensis* (Dang Gui), 6 g of *Cortex Cinnamomi* (Rou Gui) and 6 g of *Aconiti Radix Lateralis Tosta* (Pao Fu Zi).

方药 代表方为右归丸;常用药如熟地黄 10 克,山药 20 克,山茱萸 10 克,枸杞子 10 克,鹿角胶 10 克,菟丝子 12 克,杜仲 10 克,当归 10 克,肉桂 6 克,炮附片 6 克。

Modification For absence of menstruation due to obstruction of meridians by phlegm-dampness, *Rhizoma Pinelliae* (Ban Xia), *Pericarpium Citri Tangerinae* (Chen Pi), *Bulbus Fritillariae Cirrhosae* (Chuan Bei Mu) and *Rhizoma Cyperi* (Xiang Fu) are added to rectify qi, dissolve phlegm and dredge the collaterals For abdominal stabbing pain and pain relieved after discharge of blood clot due to blood stasis, *Semen Persicae* (Tao Ren) and *Flos Carthami* (Hong Hua) are added to activate the blood and remove stagnation. For scanty menstruation, delayed menstruation or amenorrhea, *Herba Lycopi* (Ze Lan), *Radix Cyathulae* (Chuan Niu Xi) and *Caulis Spatholobi* (Ji Xue Teng) are added.

加减 月经不行或衍期,为痰湿阻滞脉络所致者,可加半夏、陈皮、川贝母、香附以理气化痰通络;兼见少腹刺痛不适,月经有血块而块出痛减者,为血滞,可酌加桃仁、红花以活血行滞;月经量少、错后或闭经者,加泽兰、川牛膝、鸡血藤。

2.2 Phlegm-dampness syndrome

Main manifestations Scanty menorrhea, delayed menstruation or even amenorrhea, obesity, pilosity, dizziness and oppression in the chest, copious phlegm in throat, lassitude of limbs, fatigue and lack of strength, profuse vaginal discharge, sterility long after marriage, enlarged tongue with light color and thick greasy fur, deep and slippery pulse.

Therapeutic methods Resolving phlegm and eliminating dampness, dredging the collaterals and regulating menstruation.

Formulas and herbs *Atractylodes and Cyperus Phlegm-Abducting Decoction* (Cang Fu Dao Tan Tang), composed of 10 g of *Rhizoma Atractylodis* (Cang Zhu), 10 g of *Rhizoma Cyperi* (Xiang Fu), 12 g of *Poriae* (Fu Ling), 10 g of *Rhizoma Pinelliae* (Ban Xia), 10 g of *Pericarpium Citri Tangerinae* (Chen Pi), 3 g of *Radix Glycyrrhizae* (Gan Cao), 10 g of *Arisaema cum Bile* (Dan Nan Xing), 10 g of *Fructus Aurantii* (Zhi Qiao), 10 g of *Massa Fermentata Medicinalis* (Shen Qu) and 3 slices of *Rhizoma Zingiberis Recens* (Sheng Jiang).

Modification For absence of menstruation blocked by phlegm, *Bulbus Fritillariae Thumbergii* (Zhe Bei Mu), *Sargassum* (Hai Zao) and *Rhizoma Acori Graminei* (Shi Chang Pu) are added to soften hardness, disperse accumulation, dissolve phlegm and open the orifices. For blood stagnation after phlegm dissolved, *Rhizoma Ligustici Chuanxiong* (Chuan Xiong) and *Radix Angelicae Sinensis* (Dang Gui) are added to activate the blood and dredge the collaterals. For spleen vacuity and phlegm dampness failing to be dissolved, *Rhizoma Atractylodis Macrocephalae* (Bai Zhu) and *Radix Codonopsis Pilosulae*

2.2 痰湿证

主要证候 月经后期、量少,甚则停闭。形体丰满肥胖,多毛,头晕胸闷,喉间多痰,四肢倦怠,疲乏无力。带下量多,婚久不孕。舌体胖大,色淡,苔厚腻,脉沉滑。

治法 化痰除湿,通络调经。

方药 代表方为苍附导痰汤;常用药如苍术 10 克,香附 10 克,茯苓 12 克,半夏 10 克,陈皮 10 克,甘草 3 克,胆南星 10 克,枳壳 10 克,神曲 10 克,生姜 3 片。

加减 若月经不行,为顽痰闭塞者,可加浙贝母、海藻、石菖蒲软坚散结,化痰开窍;若痰湿已化,血滞不行者,加川芎、当归活血通络;若脾虚痰湿不化者,加白术、党参以健脾祛湿;若胸膈满闷加郁金、薤白以行气解郁;若形体肥胖,多毛明显者,酌加山慈姑、夏枯草、皂角刺、石菖蒲以化痰活络。

(Dang Shen) are added to fortify the spleen and dispel dampness. For fullness and oppression in the chest and diaphragm, *Radix Curcumae* (Yu Jin) and *Bulbus Allii Macrostemi* (Xie Bai) are added to move qi and resolve depression. For obesity and pilosity, *Rhizoma Pleionis* (Shan Ci Gu), *Spica Prunellae* (Xia Ku Cao), *Spina Gleditsiae* (Zao Jiao Ci) and *Rhizoma Acori Graminei* (Shi Chang Pu) are added to dissolve phlegm and activate the collaterals.

2.3 Syndrome of liver qi stagnation transforming into fire

2.3 肝郁化火证

Main manifestations Scanty menorrhea or amenorrhea, or irregular menstruation, functional uterine and dripping bleeding, muscular physique, thick hair, acne on the face, distending pain in the chest, hypochondria and breasts, swelling in limbs and body; constipation and yellow urine, profuse vaginal discharge, genital itch, red tongue with thick yellow fur, deep taut or deep fast pulse.

主要证候 月经稀发、量少,甚则经闭不行,或月经紊乱,崩漏淋漓。形盛体壮,毛发浓密,面部痤疮,经前胸胁乳房胀痛,肢体肿胀;大便秘结,小便黄,带下量多,阴痒。舌红苔黄厚,脉沉弦或弦数。

Therapeutic methods Soothing the liver and rectifying qi, clearing away heat and regulating menstruation.

治法 舒肝理气,泻火调经。

Formulas and herbs *Moutan and Gardenia Free Wanderer Powder* (Dan Zhi Xiao Yao San) composed of 10 g of *Cortex Moutan Radicis* (Mu Dan Pi), 10 g of *Fructus Gardeniae* (Zhi Zi), 10 g of *Radix Angelicae Sinensis* (Dang Gui), 15 g of *Radix Paeoniae Alba* (Bai Shao), 6 g of *Radix Bupleuri* (Chai Hu), 10 g of *Rhizoma Atractylodis Macrocephalae* (Bai Zhu), 5 g of *Radix Glycyrrhizae Praeparata* (Zhi Gan Cao) and 10 g of *Radix Cyathulae* (Chuan Niu Xi).

方药 代表方为丹栀逍遥散;常用药如牡丹皮 10 克,栀子 10 克,当归 10 克,白芍 15 克,柴胡 6 克,白术 10 克,炙甘草 5 克,川牛膝 10 克。

Modification For obstruction of the Lower En-

加减 若湿热之邪阻滞

ergizer by damp-heat evil, which leads to constipation, *Radix et Rhizoma Rhei* (Da Huang) is added to clear and disinhibit stool. For constrained liver qi leading to lactorrhea, *Radix Curcumae* (Yu Jin) and *Hordei Fructus Germinatus Frictus* (Chao Mai Ya) are added to soothe the liver to terminate lactation. For fullness and pain in the chest and hypochondria, *Radix Curcumae* (Yu Jin) and *Semen Vaccariae* (Wang Bu Liu Xing) are added to activate blood and rectify qi. For amenorrhea, *Fructus Crataegi* (Shan Zha) and *Radix Salviae Miltiorrhizae* (Dan Shen) are added to activate blood and free menstruation. For severe constipation, proper amount of *Radix et Rhizoma Rhei* (Da Huang) is added for clearing away heat and reducing fire to promote defecation.

下焦,大便秘结者,加大黄清通便;若肝气不舒,溢乳者,加郁金、炒麦芽以疏肝回乳;胸胁满痛者,加郁金、王不留行以活血理气;月经不行者,加山楂、丹参以活血通经;若大便秘结明显者,加大黄适量清热泻火通便。

2.4 Syndrome of qi stagnation and blood stasis

Main manifestations Delayed menstruation with scanty menorrhea and blood clot or even amenorrhea and sterility, mental depression, vexation and irascibility, unpressable abdominal pain with distention and fullness, pain and distention in the chest, rib-side and breasts, dark-red tongue with ecchymosis and stasis macule, deep, taut and hesitent pulse.

Therapeutic methods Moving qi and activating blood, dispelling stasis and freeing menstruation.

Formulas and herbs *Infradiaphragmatic Stasis-Expelling Decoction* (Ge Xia Zhu Yu Tang), composed of 15 g of *Radix Angelicae Sinensis* (Dang Gui), 6 g of *Rhizoma Ligustici Chuanxiong* (Chuan Xiong), 10 g of *Radix Paeoniae Rubra* (Chi Shao), 10 g of *Semen Persicae* (Tao Ren), 6 g of *Flos Carthami* (Hong Hua), 10 g of *Fructus Aurantii*

2.4 气滞血瘀证

主要证候 月经后期量少,经行有块,甚则经闭不孕。精神抑郁,心烦易怒,小腹胀满拒按,或胸胁满痛,乳房胀痛。舌体暗红有瘀点、瘀斑,脉沉弦涩。

治法 行气活血,祛瘀通经。

方药 代表方为膈下逐瘀汤;常用药如当归 15 克,川芎 6 克,赤芍 10 克,桃仁 10 克,红花 6 克,枳壳 10 克,延胡索 10 克,五灵脂 10 克,牡丹皮 10 克,白芍 10 克,香附 12 克,甘草 6 克。

(Zhi Qiao), 10 g of *Rhizoma Corydalis* (Yan Hu Suo, Yuan Hu), 10 g of *Faeces Trogopterorum* (Wu Ling Zhi), 10 g of *Cortex Moutan Radicis* (Mu Dan Pi), 10 g of *Radix Paeoniae Alba* (Bai Shao), 12 g of *Rhizoma Cyperi* (Xiang Fu) and 6 g of *Radix Glycyrrhizae* (Gan Cao).

Modification For distending pain in chest, breast and lower abdomen, vexation and irascibility, *Pericarpium Citri Reticulatae Viride* (Qing Pi), *Radix Aucklandiae* (Mu Xiang) and *Radix Bupleuri* (Chai Hu) are added to soothe the liver, resolve depression, move qi and relieve pain. For mass in the abdomen, *Rhizoma Sparganii Stoloniferi* (San Leng), *Rhizoma Zedoariae* (E Zhu) and *Liquidambaris Fructus* (Lu Lu Tong) are added for activating blood, resolving stasis and dissipating abdominal mass.

加减 若经前胸胁、乳房、少腹胀痛，心烦易怒者，加青皮、木香、柴胡以疏肝解郁，行气止痛；若腹中包块久不消散者，加三棱、莪术、路路通以活血化瘀消癥。

3 Other therapeutic methods

3.1 Chinese patent drugs

(1) *Vital Gate Pills* (You Gui Wan): 1 pill each time and three times a day, applicable to the treatment of kidney asthenia syndrome.

(2) *Sevenfold Processed Cyperus Pill* (Qi Zhi Xiang Fu Wan): 6 g each time and three times a day, applicable to the treatment of phlegm-dampness syndrome.

(3) *Free Wanderer Pill* (Xiao Yao Wan): 10 g each time and three times a day, applicable to the treatment of liver qi stagnation syndrome.

(4) *Rhubarb and Ground Beetle Pill* (Da Huang Zhe Chong Wan): Take 1 pill each time, and twice or three times a day, with boiled water or ginger decoction, applicable to the treatment of blood stasis

3 其他疗法

3.1 中成药

(1) 右归丸：每次 1 丸，每日 3 次，适用于肾虚型。

(2) 七制香附丸：每次 6 克，每日 3 次，适用于痰湿证。

(3) 逍遥丸：每次 10 克，每日 3 次，适用于肝郁证。

(4) 大黄䗪虫丸：每次 1 丸，每日 2～3 次，温开水或姜水送下，适用于血瘀证。

syndrome.

3.2 Empirical and folk recipes

(1) *Cyst-Dissolving Decoction* (Hua Nang Tang) composed of 30 g of *Semen Benincasae* (Dong Gua Ren), 30 g of *Spica Prunellae* (Ju He), 20 g of *Bulbus Fritillariae Thumbergii* (Zhe Bei Mu), 10 g of *Semen Persicae* (Tao Ren), 10 g of *Cortex Moutan Radicis* (Mu Dan Pi), 10 g of *Radix Paeoniae Rubra* (Chi Shao), 10 g of *Herba Polygoni Aviculari*a (Bian Xu) and 10 g of *Ramulus Mori* (Sang Zhi). These herbs are decocted in water and the decoction is orally taken one dose a day. One menstrual cycle is a course of treatment. This treatment is applicable to the dampness-heat syndrome.

(2) *Semen Coicis, Fructus Crataegi and Herba Leonuri Decoction* (Yi Ren Shan Zha Yi Mu Cao Tang), composed of 30 g of *Semen Coicis* (Yi Yi Ren), 15 g of *Fructus Crataegi* (Shan Zha), 30 g of *Herba Leonuri* (Yi Mu Cao) and 20 g of *Semen Lablab Album* (Chao Bai Bian Dou). These ingredients are cooked into porridge for treating phlegm-dampness syndrome.

3.2 单验方

(1) 化囊汤：冬瓜仁30克，夏枯草30克，橘核30克，浙贝母20克，桃仁10克，牡丹皮10克，赤芍10克，萹蓄10克，桑枝10克，水煎服，每日1次，1个周期为1个疗程，适用于湿热证。

(2) 苡仁山楂益母草汤：薏苡仁30克，山楂15克，益母草30克，炒白扁豆20克，煮粥常食用，适用于痰湿证。

Premenstrual syndrome

The premenstrual syndrome refers to cyclical physical, mental and behavioral changes and other symptoms during luteal phase.

The occurrence of the disease is closely related to the menstrual cycle. It occurs before or during menstruation, eases after menstruation and reoccursduring the next menstrual period.

The syndrome is usually caused by emotional

经前期综合征

经前期综合征是妇女反复在黄体期周期性出现以躯体、精神和行为改变等症状为特征的综合征。

本病的发生与月经周期关系密切，具有经前、经期发病，经净自然缓解，下次月经期重现的特点。

本病的发生与情志因素

factors and dysfunction of viscera, especially the dysfunction of the liver. It is related to the heart, spleen and kidney.

及脏腑功能失调有关，其中尤以肝的功能失调为主要原因，与心、脾、肾等脏密切相关。

According to the clinical symptoms, this syndrome pertains to the conceptions of "abnormal emotional changes during menstruation", "distending pain in breasts during menstruation", "headache during menstruation", "fever during menstruation", "body pain during menstruation", "edema during menstruation", "diarrhea during menstruation", and "dizziness during menstruation" in TCM, generally known as "symptoms before and after menstruation".

根据本病的临床症状，可分属于中医学的"经行情志异常""经行乳房胀痛""经行头痛""经行发热""经行身痛""经行浮肿""经行泄泻""经行眩晕"等范畴，总称为"经行前后诸证"。

1 Key points for diagnosis

1 诊断要点

1.1 Clinical manifestation

1.1 临床表现

Before or during the menstruation, there are regular mental stress, depression, anxiety, irritability, insomnia, headache, vertigo, distending pain in chest, hypochondria and breasts, fever, edema, diarrhea and oral ulceration. Fewer patients with severe symptoms can be similar to those with mental disorders.

在经前或经期周期性出现精神紧张、抑郁忧虑、烦躁失眠、头痛眩晕、胸胁乳房胀痛、发热、浮肿、泄泻、口腔溃疡等症状，极少数症状严重者可类似精神病患者。

1.2 Auxiliary examination

1.2 辅助检查

The basal body temperature appears bi-directionally and no organic changes are found in examination. The breasts are normal or have nodules with tenderness. Estrogenis increased. Progesterone is low. The ratio between estrogen and progestogen is increased. In a few cases lactin is elevated.

基础体温多呈双相型曲线，妇科检查无器质性改变；乳房检查可正常或有触痛性结节；性激素测定可有雌激素水平升高，孕酮偏低，雌/孕激素比值增高，少数病例可有泌乳素增高。

1.3 Differential diagnosis

1.3 鉴别诊断

This syndrome should be differentiated from

本病应与其他功能性或

other functional or organic diseases, such as neurosis, schizophrenia, periodic psychosis, cardiac renal, and gastrointestinal diseases as well as breast tumor.

2 Syndrome differentiation and treatment

This syndrome is clinically divided into asthenia and sthenia types. The asthenia type is marked by kidney asthenia and spleen asthenia. The sthenia syndrome is marked by qi stagnation. The viscera involved are the liver, the spleen and the kidney, usually manifested by simultaneous involvement in the two viscera or three viscera are involved, or simultaneous incidence of qi and blood. Since clinical symptoms are complicated, treatment methodsshould be taken in light of causes. Treatment should be focused on supplementing the kidney, fortifying the spleen, coursing the liver, rectifying qi, activating the blood and dispelling stasis, in order to balance the function of viscera and achieve the mutual aid between yin and yang, qi and blood. There should be two steps for treatment: dealing with the causative factor based on syndrome differentiation at ordinary times, modifying prescriptions according to the symptoms to control symptoms on the basis of syndrome differentiation before and during menstruation.

2.1 Syndrome of liver qi stagnation

Main manifestations Distending, full and painful sensation in breasts before or during menstruation, aggravated by touching the clothes, depression, frequent sighing, abdominal distending pain, inhibited menstruation with dark-red color, oppression in the chest, rib-side distention, thin and white

器质性疾病鉴别。如与神经官能症，精神分裂症，周期性精神病，心、肾疾病，肠胃道疾病，乳房肿瘤等病相鉴别。

2 辨证论治

本病在临床上分为虚、实两大类。虚证以肾虚、脾虚多见；实证则以气滞多见。涉及的脏腑以肝、脾、肾功能失调为主，常表现为两脏或三脏同时发病或气血同病。由于本病临床症状复杂多样，须审因论治。治疗重在补肾、健脾、疏肝理气、活血祛瘀，使脏腑功能平衡，阴阳气血互济。治疗应分两步，平时辨证施治以治本，经前、经期辨证基础上随证加减以控制症状。

2.1 肝郁气滞证

主要证候　经前或经行乳房胀满疼痛，甚则痛不可触衣，精神抑郁，时欲叹息，小腹胀痛，经行不畅，血色暗红，胸闷胁胀。苔薄白，脉弦。

tongue fur and taut pulse.

Therapeutic methods Soothing the liver to regulate qi and activating blood to dredge collaterals.

治法 疏肝理气，活血通络。

Formulas and herbs *Free Wanderer Powder* (Xiao Yao San) composed of 6 g of *Radix Bupleuri* (Chai Hu), 12 g of *Radix Paeoniae Alba* (Bai Shao), 12 g of *Radix Angelicae Sinensis* (Dang Gui), 10 g of *Rhizoma Cyperi* (Xiang Fu), 6 g of *Pericarpium Citri Reticulatae Viride* (Qing Pi), 6 g of *Pericarpium Citri Tangerinae* (Chen Pi), 10 g of *Radix Curcumae* (Yu Jin), 10 g of *Luffae Fructus Retinervus* (Si Gua Luo), 10 g of *Radix Salviae Miltiorrhizae* (Dan Shen) and 3 g of *Glycyrrhizae Radix* (Gan Cao).

方药 代表方为逍遥散；常用药如柴胡 6 克，白芍 12 克，当归 12 克，香附 10 克，青陈皮各 6 克，郁金 10 克，丝瓜络 10 克，丹参 10 克，甘草 3 克。

Modification For distending pain in the breasts, aggravated by touching the clothes, *Liquidambaris Fructus* (Lu Lu Tong) and *Radix Paeoniae Rubra* (Chi Shao) are added. For mass in breasts, *Semen Citri Reticulatae* (Ju He), *Semen Vaccariae* (Wang Bu Liu Xing) and *Spica Prunellae* (Xia Ku Cao) are added. For restless sleep at night, *Dens Draconis* (Qing Long Chi), *Caulis Polygoni Multiflori* (Ye Jiao Teng) and *Cortex Alibiziae* (He Huan Pi) are added.

加减 若乳房胀痛不能触衣者，加路路通、赤芍；乳房有块者，加橘核、王不留行、夏枯草；夜寐欠安者，加青龙齿、夜交藤、合欢皮。

Shanghai doctor LUO Yijun's experience prescription: 6 g of *Radix Bupleuri* (Chai Hu), 12 g of *Radix Curcumae* (Yu Jin), 12 g of *Rhizoma Cyperi* (Xiang Fu), 10 g of *Folium Citri Reticulatae* (Ju Ye), 10 g of *Semen Citri Reticulatae* (Ju He), 30 g of *Spica Prunellae* (Xia Ku Cao), 10 g of *Chinese Angelica* (Chao Dang Gui), 30 g of *Radix Salviae Miltiorrhizae* (Dan Shen), 9 g of *Rhizoma Ligustici Chuanxiong* (Chao Chuan Xiong) and 30 g of *Radix Puerariae* (Ge Gen).

上海医家骆益君经验方：柴胡 6 克，郁金 12 克，香附 12 克，橘叶核各 10 克，夏枯草 30 克，炒当归 10 克，丹参 30 克，炒川芎 9 克，葛根 30 克。

2.2 Syndrome of yin asthenia and liver hyperactivity

Main manifestations Dizziness and headache during menstruation or before and after menstruation, restlessness, occasional tidal fever, feverish sensation over palms, soles and chest, irritating sensation in the eyes, tinnitus, dry mouth and throat, aching sensation in the loins and spine, red tongue, thready and rapid pulse.

Therapeutic methods Enriching the kidney and calming the liver, coursing the Thoroughfare Vessel and harmonizing collaterals.

Formulas and herbs *Lycium, Chrysanthemun and Rehmannia Pills* (Qi Ju Di Huang Wan), composed of 10 g of *Fructus Lycii* (Gou Qi Zi), 10 g of *Flos Chrysanthemi* (Ju Hua), 20 g of *Rhizoma Dioscoreae* (Shan Yao), 10 g of *Radix Rehmanniae Praeparata* (Shu Di Huang), 10 g of *Cortex Moutan Radicis* (Mu Dan Pi), 10 g of *Poriae* (Fu Ling), 10 g of *Fructus Corni* (Shan Zhu Yu), 10 g of *Radix Angelicae Sinensis* (Dang Gui), 10 g of *Radix Paeoniae Alba* (Bai Shao), 15 g of *Ramulus Uncariae cum Uncis* (Gou Teng) (to be decocted later), 10 g of *Fructus Tribuli* (Bai Ji Li) and 3 g of *Glycyrrhizae Radix* (Gan Cao).

Modification For loose stool, *Rhizoma Atractylodis Macrocephalae* (Bai Zhu) and *Radix Aucklaneliae* (Wei Mu Xiang) are added. For insomnia, *Semen Zizyphi Spinosae* (Suan Zao Ren) and *Caulis Polygoni Multiflori* (Ye Jiao Teng) are added. For pain in the limbs, *Caulis Spatholobi* (Ji Xue Teng) and *Radix Angelicae Pubescentis* (Du Huo) are added.

2.2 阴虚肝旺证

主要证候 经期或月经前后眩晕头痛，烦躁不安，时有潮热，五心烦热，目涩耳鸣，咽干口燥，腰脊酸楚，舌质偏红，脉细数。

治法 滋肾平肝，疏冲和络。

方药 代表方为杞菊地黄丸；常用药如枸杞子 10 克，菊花 10 克，山药 20 克，熟地黄 10 克，牡丹皮 10 克，茯苓 10 克，山茱萸 10 克，当归 10 克，白芍 10 克，钩藤(后下)15 克，白蒺藜 10 克，甘草 3 克。

加减 若大便溏薄者，加白术、煨木香；失眠者，加酸枣仁、夜交藤；肢体疼痛者，加鸡血藤、独活。

2.3 Syndrome of spleen and kidney asthenia

Main manifestations During, or before or after

2.3 脾肾两虚证

主要证候 经期或经行

menstruation, facial dropsy, edema of limbs, loose stool, even diarrhea, anorexia, epigastric distention, aching and weak sensation in the loins and knees, lassitude, dizziness, nausea, aversion to cold, and cold limbs, whitish and slippery tongue fur as well as deep and weak pulse.

前后,面浮肢肿,大便不实,甚则泄泻,纳少脘胀,腰膝酸软,身倦乏力,头晕呕恶,畏寒肢冷,舌苔白滑,脉沉弱。

Therapeutic methods Warming and invigorating kidney yang, strengthening the spleen and resolving dampness.

治法 温补肾阳,健脾化湿。

Formulas and herbs *Fortifying and Securing Decoction* (Jian Gu Tang), composed of 15 g of *Radix Codonopsis Pilosulae* (Dang Shen), 10 g of *Rhizoma Atractylodis Macrocephalae* (Bai Zhu), 10 g of *Poriae* (Fu Ling), 12 g of *Rhizoma Dioscoreae* (Shan Yao), 20 g of *Semen Coicis* (Yi Yi Ren), 10 g of *Radix Morindae Officinalis* (Ba Ji Tian), 10 g of *Fructus Psoraleae* (Bu Gu Zhi), 6 g of *Pericarpium Citri Tangerinae* (Chen Pi), 5 g of *Rhizoma Zingiberis Praeparata* (Pao Jiang), 10 g of *Radix Aucklandiae* (Mu Xiang) and 5 g of *Radix Glycyrrhizae Praeparata* (Zhi Gan Cao).

方药 代表方为健固汤;常用药如党参 15 克,白术 10 克,茯苓 10 克,山药 12 克,薏苡仁 20 克,巴戟天 10 克,补骨脂 10 克,陈皮 6 克,炮姜 5 克,木香 10 克,炙甘草 5 克。

Modification For nausea, *Rhizoma Pinelliae* (Ban Xia) and *Fructus Amomi* (Sha Ren) are added. For poor appetite, *Fructus Crataegi* (Shan Zha) and *Fructus Oryzae Germinatus* (Gu Ya) are added. For morning diarrhea, *Semen Myristicae* (Rou Dou Kou) and *Fructus Alpiniae Oxyphyllae* (Yi Zhi Ren) are added. For frequent urination in the night, *Cortex Eucommiae* (Du Zhong) and *Radix Dipsaci* (Xu Duan) are added.

加减 泛恶欲吐者,加半夏、砂仁;食欲不振者,加山楂、谷芽;鸡鸣泄泻者,加肉豆蔻、益智仁;夜间尿频者,加杜仲、续断。

Shanghai doctor TANG Jifu's experience prescription: composed of 12 g of *Radix Codonopsis Pilosulae* (Dang Shen), 9 g of *Rhizoma Atractylodis Macrocephalae* (Bai Zhu), 12 g of *Poriae* (Fu Ling), 12 g of *polyporus* (Zhu

上海医家唐吉父经验方:党参 12 克,白术 9 克,猪茯苓各 12 克,白扁豆 12 克,泽泻 12 克,车前子 12 克,当归 9 克,川芎 9 克,夏

Ling), 12 g of *Semen Dolichoris Album* (Bai Bian Dou), 12 g of *Rhizoma Alismatis* (Ze Xie), 12 g of *Semen Plantaginis* (Che Qian Zi), 9 g of *Radix Angelicae Sinensis* (Dang Gui), 9 g of *Rhizoma Ligustici Chuanxiong* (Chuan Xiong), 12 g of *Spica Prunellae* (Xia Ku Cao) and 9 g of *Radix Bupleuri* (Chai Hu).

枯草 12 克,柴胡 9 克。

3 Other therapeutic methods

3.1 Chinese patent drugs

(1) *Stagnancy-Relieving Pills* (Yue Ju Wan): Take 10 g each time and three times a day, applicable to the treatment of liver qi stagnation syndrome.

(2) *Free Wanderer Pill* (Xiao Yao Wan): Take 10 g each time and three times a day, applicable to the treatment of blood asthenia and liver qi stagnation syndrome.

(3) *Ginseng, Poria and White Atractylodes Pill* (Shen Ling Bai Zhu Wan): Take 6 g each time and twice a day, applicable to the treatment of spleen asthenia syndrome.

2.2 Empirical and folk recipes

(1) 15 g of *Pericarpium Citri Tangerinae* (Chen Pi) and 15 g of *Cervi Cornu Degelatinatum* (Lu Jiao Shuang) are decocted with rice wine and water, in equal amount, for oral taking. This decoction is applicable to the treatment of distending pain in the breasts.

(2) 30 g of *Semen Coicis* (Yi Yi Ren), 15 g of *Poriae* (Fu Ling) and 10 pieces of Chinese dates are decocted for oral taking. This decoction is taken one dose a day in summer, applicable to the treatment of edema before menstruation.

(3) Shanghai doctor CAI Xiaosun's experience prescription: 12 g of *Radix Rehmanniae Cruda* (Sheng Di Huang), 9 g of *Fructus Corni* (Shan Zhu

3 其他疗法

3.1 中成药

(1) 越鞠丸:每次服 10 克,每日 3 次,适用于肝郁气滞证。

(2) 逍遥丸:每次服 10 克,每日 3 次,适用于血虚肝郁证。

(3) 参苓白术丸:每次服 6 克,每日 2 次,适用于脾虚证。

2.2 单验方

(1) 陈皮 15 克,鹿角霜 15 克,黄酒、水各半煎服,适用于经前乳房胀痛。

(2) 薏苡仁 30 克,茯苓 15 克,大枣 10 枚,水煎服,入夏后每日 1 剂,适用于经前浮肿。

(3) 上海医家蔡小荪经验方:生地黄 12 克,山茱萸 9 克,菊花 6 克,石决明 30 克,

Yu), 6 g of *Flos Chrysanthemi* (Ju Hua), 30 g of *Concha Haliotidis* (Shi Jue Ming), 9 g of *Bombyx Batryticatus* (Jiang Can), 9 g of *Fructus Tribuli* (Bai Ji Li), 9 g of *Radix Achyranthis Bidentatae* (Niu Xi) and 9 g of *Rhizoma Alismatis* (Ze Xie) are decocted with water for oral taking. This decoction is applicable to the treatment of headache during menstruation.

僵蚕9克,蒺藜9克,怀牛膝9克,泽泻9克,水煎服,适用于经行头痛。

(4) Shanghai doctor TANG Xiyuan's experience prescription : 12 g of *Astragali Complanati Semen* (Tong Ji Li), 12 g of *Fructus Tribuli* (Bai Ji Li), 12 g of *Semen Coat Glycine* (Hei Dou Yi), 12 g of *Fructus Lycii* (Gou Qi Zi), 12 g of *Radix Rehmanniae Cruda* (Sheng Di Huang), 12 g of *Chinese Angelica* (Chao Dang Gui), 6 g of *Stir-Fried Rhizoma Ligustici Chuanxiong* (Chao Chuan Xiong), 10 g of *Stir-Fried Radix Paeoniae Rubra* (Chao Chi Shao), 10 g of *Radix Paeoniae Alba* (Chao Bai Shao), 12 g of *Rhizoma Corydalis* (Yan Hu Suo), 12 g of *Curcumae Radix & Australis* (Guang Yu Jin), 18 g of *Ramulus Uncariae cum Uncis* (Gou Teng), 5 g of *Whellote Chrysanthemum* (Bai Ju Hua), 12 g of *Fructus Viticis* (Man Jing Zi) and 5 g of *Radix Glycyrrhizae Praeparata* (Zhi Gan Cao). This decoction is applicable to the treatment of headache during menstruation.

(4) 上海医家唐锡元经验方:潼蒺藜12克,白蒺藜12克,黑豆衣12克,枸杞子12克,生地黄12克,炒当归12克,炒川芎6克,炒赤芍10克,炒白芍10克,延胡索12克,广郁金12克,钩藤18克,白菊花5克,蔓荆子12克,炙甘草5克,适用于经行头痛。

Menopausal syndrome

绝经综合征

Menopausal syndrome refers mainly to a series of dysfunctions in autonomic nervous system due to ovarian failure before and after menopause, accompanied by neuropsychological symptoms, known as menopausal syndrome. In Chinese medicine, it is

绝经综合征是指妇女在绝经前后由于卵巢功能衰退引起的一系列以自主神经功能紊乱为主,伴有神经心理症状的一组症状。又称"绝

termed "various syndromes before and after menopause". It usually occurs in women aging from 45 to 55. The incidence rate is about 85%. About 25% cases are severe. The disease severity is greatly different in the individuals. In serious cases, treatment is necessary. This syndrome can also be induced by menopause after operation or actinotherapy or chemotherapy, in women of the non-menopausal phase.

The disease occurs mainly in women before and after menopause. It happens due to menopause induced by gradual decline of the kidney qi, gradual exhaustion of the reproductive substances, and deficiency in the Thoroughfare Vessel and Conception Vessel, and coming menstrual disorders, and it disappears with the decline of the reproductive ability. In this physiological transitional period, some women can not adapt themselves to this physiological changes, because of the reasons like constitution, delivery, disease, nutrition, work and rest, social environment, mental and spiritual factors, leading to this disease due to yin and yang imbalance. "The kidney is the pre-natal foundation." "In terms of migration among the five Zang organs, the kidney will surely be involved by disorders." Therefore, the dysfunction between the kidney yin and kidney yang will easily involve other Zangfu organs, and long-term disorders in the other Zangfu organs will certainly involve the kidney. The root cause of the syndrome lies in the kidney, and usually the heart, liver, spleen and other viscera, and meridians are affected, having the syndrome complicated. But because of frequent injury of blood from menstru-

经综合征”。中医称为“经断前后诸证”或“绝经前后诸证”。一般发生于45～55 岁之间，其发生率为 85%，较重者占 25%左右；发病程度个体差异较大，严重者需要治疗。非绝经期妇女因手术或放射、化疗等人工的方法致绝经后，也可引起本病。

本病的发生主要是妇女年届绝经前后，肾气渐衰，天癸将竭，冲任二脉虚衰，月经将失调而至绝经，生殖能力降低而至消失。在此生理转折时期，部分妇女由于体质、产育、疾病、营养、劳逸、社会环境、心理、精神因素等方面的原因，不能协调此生理变化，使得阴阳平衡失调而导致本病。“肾为先天之本”，又“五脏相移，穷必及肾”，故肾阴阳失调，每易波及其他脏腑，而其他脏腑病变，久则必然累及肾，故本病之本在肾，常累及心、肝、脾等多脏、多经，致使本病证候复杂。但因妇女一生经、孕、产、乳，数伤于血，往往是“有余于气，不足于血”，所以临床上以阴虚证居多。

ation, pregnancy, childbirth and lactation in the whole life of women, often "qi is surplus, and blood is insufficient". Therefore, yin deficiency syndrome is in majority clinically.

1 Key points for diagnosis

1.1 Medical history

It occurs in women aging from 45 to 55. If it occurs before 40 years old, premature ovarian failure should be considered. It is necessary to pay attention to special changes in work or life, history of psychological trauma, bilateral oophorectomy or radiation therapy.

1.2 Symptoms

The earliest symptoms include tidal feverish sensation, sweating and mood changes. Tidal feverish sensation occurs in the chest then flocks to the head, neck and face. Then sweating follows, feverish sensation is abated with sweating. The duration is uncertain, from a few seconds to a few minutes and the frequency of attack is indefinite too. Mood changes are manifested by irritability, sorrow, desiring to weep for no reason and losing self-control. In addition, there are dizziness, headache, palpitations, insomnia, lumbar and back pain, menstrual disorders. Late-stage symptoms are dry, burning hot, itching sensation in the vagina, urinary urgency and frequency or incontinence, and skin pruritus.

1.3 Examination

(1) Gynecological examinations: varying degrees of atrophy in vulva, vagina and uterus, decrease of vaginal secretion.

(2) Laboratory tests: Vaginal exfoliated cells

1 诊断要点

1.1 病史

发病年龄多在 45～55 岁，若在 40 岁以前发病者，应考虑为卵巢早衰。要注意发病前有无工作、生活的特殊改变；精神创伤史及双侧卵巢切除或放射治疗史。

1.2 症状

最早出现的症状常为潮热、汗出和情绪改变。潮热从胸前开始，涌向头部、颈部和面部，继而出汗，汗出热退，持续时间长短不定，短者数秒，长者数分钟，发作次数也多少不一；情绪改变表现为易激动，烦躁易怒，或无故悲伤欲哭，不能自我控制。此外，尚有头晕头痛，心悸失眠，腰酸背痛，月经紊乱等。晚期症状则有阴道干燥灼热，阴痒，尿频急或尿失禁，皮肤瘙痒等。

1.3 检查

（1）妇科检查：外阴、阴道、子宫不同程度的萎缩，阴道分泌物减少。

（2）实验室检查：阴道脱

smears examination shows decline of estrogen levels in varying degree, elevation of serum follicle stimulating hormone (FSH) and luteinizing hormone (LH), and decrease in estradiol (E_2), in significant reference for the diagnosis of this disease.

落细胞涂片检查显示雌激素水平不同程度的低落，血清卵泡刺激素(FSH)、黄体生成素(LH)水平增高，雌二醇(E_2)水平下降，对本病的诊断有参考意义。

2 Syndrome differentiation and treatment

2 辨证论治

Kidney asthenia is mostly the root cause of this syndrome, more asthenia and less sthenia. Even if the syndrome is of sthenia, it is often mingled with asthenia. The viscera involved are the heart, liver, spleen and kidney. Syndrome differentiation should be done in light of the clinical manifestations, menstruation and the conditions of the tongue and pulse, so as to make clear whether it is due to asthenia of kidney yin or kidney yang or disharmony between the heart and kidney or asthenia of both the heart and spleen or liver qi stagnation.

本病以肾虚为本，虚多实少，即便有实证，亦多为虚中夹实，纯实证不多见。累及的脏腑主要是心、肝、脾、肾。临证时应根据临床表现、月经情况、舌脉的变化，辨证其属肝肾阴虚、肾阳虚、心脾两虚，或是肝郁证等。

2.1 Yin asthenia syndrome of the liver and kidney

2.1 肝肾阴虚证

Main manifestations　Dizziness and tinnitus, flushed cheeks, occasional sweating, feverish sensation over the palms, soles and chest, insomnia and dreaminess, aching and weak sensation in the loins and knees, dryness and pruritus of skin, dry mouth and constipation, scanty yellowish urine, or scanty menstruation with red menses, or disturbance of menstrual cycle, sudden profuse uterine bleeding and dripping uterine bleeding in alternation, red tongue with scanty fur and thready and rapid pulse.

主要证候　绝经前后，眩晕耳鸣，潮红烘热，时有汗出，五心烦热，失眠多梦，腰膝酸软，皮肤干燥瘙痒，口干便结，尿少色黄，或月经先期量少，色红，或周期紊乱，崩漏交替，舌红苔少，脉细数。

Therapeutic methods　Nourishing the liver and kidney, fostering yin and suppressing yang.

治法　滋补肝肾，育阴潜阳。

Formulas and herbs　*Kidney Pills* (Zuo Gui Wan), composed of 10 g of *Radix Rehmanniae*

方药　代表方为左归丸；常用药如生地黄、熟地黄

Cruda (Sheng Di Huang), 10 g of *Radix Rehmanniae Praeparata* (Shu Di Huang), 10 g of *Fructus Lycii* (Gou Qi Zi), 10 g of *Fructus Corni* (Shan Zhu Yu), 20 g of *Rhizoma Dioscoreae* (Shan Yao), 10 g of *Poriae* (Fu Ling), 10 g of *Cortex Moutan Radicis* (Mu Dan Pi), 10 g of *Processed Plastrum Testudinis* (Zhi Gui Jia), 15 g of *Os Draconis* (Long Gu), 15 g of *Fructus Ligustri Lucidi* (Nü Zhen Zi) and 15 g of *Herba Ecliptae* (Mo Han Lian).

各10克，枸杞子10克，山茱萸10克，山药20克，茯苓10克，牡丹皮10克，炙龟甲10克，龙骨15克，女贞子15克，墨旱莲15克。

Modification For insomnia, *Caulis Polygoni Multiflori* (Ye Jiao Teng) and *Semen Zizyphi Spinosae* (Suan Zao Ren) are added. For dry mouth, *Radix Scrophulariae* (Xuan Shen) and *Ophiopogonis Radix* (Mai Dong) are added. For profuse sweating, *Fructus Schisandrae* (Wu Wei Zi) and *Tritici Fructus Levis* (Fu Xiao Mai) are added. For pruritus of skin, *Periostracum Cicadae* (Chan Tui) and *Cortex Dictamni Radicis* (Bai Xian Pi) are added. For constipation, *Semen Biotae* (Bai Zi Ren) and *Fructus Cannabis* (Huo Ma Ren) are added.

加减 若彻夜难眠者，加夜交藤、酸枣仁；口干者，加玄参、麦冬；多汗者，加五味子、浮小麦；皮肤瘙痒甚者，加蝉蜕、白鲜皮；便秘者，加柏子仁、火麻仁。

Shanghai doctor WANG Dazeng's experience prescription: 15 g of *Radix Rehmanniae Cruda* (Sheng Di Huang), 9 g of *Radix Scrophulariae* (Xuan Shen), 9 g of *Rhizoma Anemarrhenae* (Zhi Mu), 6 g of *Cortex Phellodendri* (Huang Bo), 15 g of *Radix Paeoniae Alba* (Bai Shao), 9 g of *Fructus Lycii* (Gou Qi Zi) and 9 g of *Chrysanthemi Flos* (Ju Hua).

上海医家王大增经验方：生地黄15克，玄参9克，知母9克，黄柏6克，白芍15克，枸杞子9克，菊花9克。

2.2 Kidney yang deficiency syndrome

Main manifestations Before and after menopause, dizziness, tinnitus, chilly body and cold limbs, aching and flaccid sensation in the loins and knees, cold abdomen, sagging sensation of vagina, frequent urination and profuse urine or urinary incontinence, profuse leukorrhea, menstrual disorder, light-colored and thin profuse or scanty men-

2.2 肾阳虚证

主要证候 经断前后，头晕耳鸣，形寒肢冷，腰酸膝软，腹冷阴坠，小便频数或失禁，带下量多，月经不调，量多或少，色淡质稀，精神萎靡，面色晦暗。舌淡，苔白滑，脉沉细而迟。

ses, dispiritedness, grayish complexion, pale tongue with whitish and slippery fur, deep, thready and slow pulse.

Therapeutic methods　Warming the kidney and invigorating yang, replenishing essence and nourishing blood.

治法　温肾壮阳，填精养血。

Formulas and herbs　*Vital Gate Pills* (You Gui Wan), composed of 10 g of *Colla Cornus Cervi* (Lu Jiao Jiao), 15 g of *Radix Codonopsis Pilosulae* (Dang Shen), 10 g of *Rhizoma Atractylodis Macrocephalae* (Bai Zhu), 10 g of *Fructus Psoraleae* (Bu Gu Zhi), 10 g of *Rhizoma Curculiginis* (Xian Mao), 10 g of *Epimedium davidii* (Yin yang Huo), 15 g of *Rhizoma Dioscoreae* (Shan Yao), 10 g of *Fructus Corni* (Shan Zhu Yu), 10 g of *Cortex Eucommiae* (Du Zhong) and 10 g of *Semen Cuscutae* (Tu Si Zi).

方药　代表方为右归丸；常用药如鹿角胶 10 克，党参 15 克，白术 10 克，补骨脂 10 克，仙茅 10 克，淫羊藿 10 克，山药 15 克，山茱萸 10 克，杜仲 10 克，菟丝子 10 克。

Modification　For morning diarrhea, *Roasting Radix Aucklandiae* (Wei Mu Xiang) and *Semen Myristicae* (Rou Dou Kou) are added. For frequent urination and incontinence of urine, *Fructus Alpiniae Oxyphyllae* (Yi Zhi Ren) and *Rosae Laevigatae Fructus* (Jin Ying Zi) are added. For distension in the epigastric and abdominal region, *Poriae* (Fu Ling) and *Fructus Amomi* (Sha Ren) are added. For swelling of limbs, *Radix Astragali* (Huang Qi), *Cortex Poria* (Fu Ling Pi) and *Radix Stephanie Tetrandrae* (Fang Ji) are added. For chest oppression, *Rhizoma Acori Graminei* (Shi Chang Pu) and *Radix Curcumae* (Yu Jin) are added.

加减　若晨起腹泻者，加煨木香、肉豆蔻；尿频失禁者，加益智仁、金樱子；脘腹作胀者，加茯苓、砂仁；四肢肿胀者，加黄芪、茯苓皮、防己；胸闷者，加石菖蒲、郁金。

2.3　Liver depression syndrome

2.3　肝郁证

Main manifestations　Before and after menopause, mental depression, anxiety, sentimentality, irritability, chest oppression, susceptibility to sig-

主要证候　绝经前后，精神抑郁，多愁善感，烦躁易怒，胸闷叹息，两胁胀痛，烘

hing, distending pain in hypochondria, feverish sweating, disturbance of menstruation, scanty menorrhea in the late stage of menstruation, in dark red color, red tongue with thin and white or thin and yellow fur as well as taut pulse.

热汗出，月经紊乱，后期量少，色暗红，舌红，苔薄白或薄黄，脉弦。

Therapeutic methods Soothing the liver to relieve stagnation, regulating qi to nourish yin.

治法 疏肝解郁，理气益阴。

Formulas and herbs *Free Wanderer Powder* (Xiao Yao San), composed of 10 g of *Radix Paeoniae Alba* (Bai Shao), 10 g of *Radix Angelicae Sinensis* (Dang Gui), 10 g of *Radix Bupleuri* (Chai Hu), 10 g of *Radix Rehmanniae Cruda* (Sheng Di Huang), 10 g of *Poriae* (Fu Ling), 10 g of *Radix Curcumae* (Yu Jin), 15 g of *Rhizoma Dioscoreae* (Shan Yao), 6 g of *Pericarpium Citri Tangerinae* (Chen Pi) and 5 g of *Radix Glycyrrhizae* (Gan Cao).

方药 代表方为逍遥散；常用药如白芍 10 克，当归 10 克，柴胡 10 克，生地黄 10 克，茯苓 10 克，郁金 10 克，山药 15 克，陈皮 6 克，甘草 5 克。

Modification For transformation of heat from liver stagnation, dysphoria, bitter taste in the mouth and dry throat, *Fructus Gardeniae* (Zhi Zi) and *Cortex Moutan Radicis* (Mu Dan Pi) are added. For anorexia and loose stool, *Rhizoma Atractylodis Macrocephalae* (Bai Zhu) and *Radix Pseudostellariae* (Tai Zi Shen) are added. For restless sleep in the night, *Dens Draconis* (Qing Long Chi) and *Semen Zizyphi Spinosae* (Suan Zao Ren) are added.

加减 若肝郁化热见烦热、口苦咽干者，加栀子、牡丹皮；纳少便溏者，加白术、太子参；夜寐欠宁者，加青龙齿、酸枣仁。

Shanghai doctor CAI Xiaosun's experience description, *Liver-Coursing and Depression-Resolving Prescription* (Shu Gan Kai Yu Fang): 10 g of *Chinese Angelica* (Chao Dang Gui), 10 g of *Rhizoma Atractylodis Macrocephalae* (Chao Bai Zhu), 12 g of *Poriae* (Fu Ling), 5 g of *Radix Bupleuri* (Chai Hu), 10 g of *Radix Paeoniae Alba* (Bai Shao), 10 g of *Radix Curcumae* (Yu Jin), 30 g of *Semen Tritici* (Huai Xiao Mai), 5 g of *Pericarpium Citri Reticulatae Viride* (Qing Pi), 5 g of

上海医家蔡小荪经验方（疏肝开郁方）：炒当归 10 克，炒白术 10 克，云茯苓 12 克，柴胡 5 克，白芍 10 克，广郁金 10 克，淮小麦 30 克，青皮、陈皮各 5 克，金铃子 10 克，生甘草 3 克。

Pericarpium Citri Tangerinae (Chen Pi), 10 g of *Toosendan Fructus* (Jin Ling Zi) and 3 g of *Glycyrrhizae Radix Cruda* (Sheng Gan Cao).

2.4 Syndrome of simultaneous asthenia of kidney yin and yang

Main manifestations Aversion to cold and wind or tidal feverish sensation and sweating, aching lumbs, lack of strength, dizziness, tinnitus, feverish sensation over the palms, soles and chest, disturbance of menstruation with profuse or scanty menses, red tongue with thin fur, deep and thready pulse.

Therapeutic methods Supplementing the kidney and supporting yang, enriching the kidney and nourishing the blood.

Formulas and herbs *Two Immortals Decoction* (Er Xian Tang) composed of 10 g of *Rhizoma Curculiginis* (Xian Mao), 10 g of *Epimedium davidii* (Yin Yang Huo), 12 g of *Radix Angelicae Sinensis* (Dang Gui), 10 g of *Radix Morindae Officinalis* (Ba Ji Tian), 10 g of *Cortex Phellodendri* (Huang Bo), 12 g of *Rhizoma Anemarrhenae* (Zhi Mu), 10 g of *Testudinis Carapax et Plastrum cum Liquido Fricti* (Zhi Gui Jia) and 12 g of *Fructus Ligustri Lucidi* (Nü Zhen Zi).

Modification For incessant vaginal bleeding, *Mastodi Ossis Fossilia Calcinata* (Duan Long Gu) and *Ostreae Concha Calcinata* (Duan Mu Li) are added. For aching in the loins, and lassitude as well as aversion to cold and cold limbs, *Fructus Psoraleae* (Bu Gu Zhi) and *Cortex Eucommiae* (Du Zhong) are added. For facial dropsy and foot edema, *Semen Coicis* (Yi Yi Ren) and *Maydis Stigma* (Yu Mi Xu) are added.

2.4 肾阴阳俱虚证

主要证候 经断前后，时而畏寒恶风，时而潮热汗出，腰酸乏力，头晕耳鸣，五心烦热，月经紊乱，量少或多。舌红，苔薄，脉沉细。

治法 补肾扶阳，滋肾养血。

方药 代表方为二仙汤；常用药如仙茅 10 克，淫羊藿 10 克，当归 12 克，巴戟天 10 克，黄柏 10 克，知母 12 克，炙龟甲 10 克，女贞子 12 克。

加减 若阴道流血不止者，加煅龙骨、煅牡蛎；腰酸乏力、畏寒肢冷者，加补骨脂、杜仲；面浮足肿者，加薏苡仁、玉米须。

3 Other therapeutic methods

3.1 Chinese patent drugs

(1) *Rehmannia Pills with Six Ingredients* (Liu Wei Di Huang Wan): Take 6 g each time and three times a day, applicable to the treatment of yin asthenia syndrome.

(2) *Lycium, Chrysanthemun and Rehmannia Pills* (Qi Ju Di Huang Wan): Take 1 pill each time and twice a day, applicable to the treatment of liver-kidney yin depletion syndrome.

(3) *Moutan and Gardenia Free Wanderer Pill* (Dan Zhi Xiao Yao Wan): Take 6-9 g each time and three times a day, applicable to the treatment of stagnant heat in the liver meridian.

(4) *Golden Chamber Kidney Qi Pills* (Jin Kui Shen Qi Wan): Take 4-5 g each time and twice a day, applicable to the treatment of kidney asthenia syndrome.

(5) *Kun Bao Pill* (Kun Bao Wan): Take 50 pills each time and twice a day, applicable to the treatment of liver-kidney yin asthenia syndrome.

(6) *Ginseng Spleen-Returning Pill* (Ren Shen Gui Pi Wan): Take 1 pill each time and twice a day, applicable to the treatment of syndrome of heart asthenia and insufficiency of qi and blood.

3.2 Empirical and folk recipes

(1) *Semen Zizyphi Spinosae and Bulbus Lilii Decoction* (Zao He Yin): 30 g of *Semen Zizyphi Spinosae* (Suan Zao Ren) is decocted in water. After removal of the residue, 50 g of fresh *Bulbus Lilii* (Bai He) is decocted in the decoction. The decoction is taken orally and the cooked *Bulbus Lilii* (Bai He) is eaten in the morning and evening respectively for restless sleep.

3 其他疗法

3.1 中成药

（1）六味地黄丸：每次 6 克，每日 3 次，适用于阴虚证。

（2）杞菊地黄丸：每次 1 丸，每日 2 次，适用于肝肾阴亏证。

（3）丹栀逍遥丸：每次 6～9 克，每日 3 次，适用于肝经郁热证。

（4）金匮肾气丸：每次 4～5 克，每日 2 次，适用于肾虚证。

（5）坤宝丸：每次 50 粒，每日 2 次，适用于肝肾阴虚证。

（6）人参归脾丸：每次 1 丸，每日 2 次，适用于心阴虚，气血不足证。

3.2 单验方

（1）枣合饮：酸枣仁 30 克，水煎后去渣，用药液煎煮鲜百合 50 克，熟后饮汤食百合，早晚分服，适用于夜寐不安者

(2) *Semen Tritici Decoction* (Huai Xiao Mai Yin): 30 g of *Semen Tritici* (Huai Xiao Mai) and 6 g of *Radix Glycyrrhizae* (Gan Cao) are decocted in water. After the removal of the residue, 5 Chinese dates and 5 dried longan pulps are decocted in the decoction with mild fire for oral taking for flushed cheeks.

(2) 淮小麦饮：淮小麦30克，甘草6克，加水煎汤，去渣留汁，加大枣5枚，桂圆5枚，文火煎煮饮用，适用于潮红烘热者。

(3) Shanghai doctor CAI Xiaosun's experience prescription, *Kan-Trigram and L-Trigram Instant Supplementation Prescription* (Kan Li Ji Ji Fang): 12 g of *Radix Rehmanniae Cruda* (Sheng Di Huang), 2 g of *Rhizoma Coptidis* (Chuan Lian), 9 g of *Semen Biotae* (Bai Zi Ren), 12 g of *Poriae* (Fu Ling), 3 g of *Radix Polygalae* (Yuan Zhi), 6 g of *Rhizoma Acori Tatarinowii* (Shi Chang Pu), 12 g of *Dens Draconis* (Long Chi), 9 g of *Asparagi Radix* (Tian Dong), 9 g of *Ophiopogon* (Mai Dong), 30 g of *Semen Tritici* (Huai Xiao Mai) and 3 g of *Fructus Schisandrae* (Wu Wei Zi).

(3) 上海医家蔡小荪经验方（坎离既济方）：生地黄12克，川连2克，柏子仁9克，朱茯苓12克，淡远志3克，九节菖蒲6克，龙齿12克，天冬9克，麦冬9克，淮小麦30克，五味子3克。

Chapter 2 Endometriosis and adenomyosis

第2章 子宫内膜异位症和子宫腺肌病

Endometriosis

Endometriosis means that the endometrium tissues with growing function appears on the other body parts outside the uterus. It is a common disease in women of childbearing age. The incidence rate is 10% to 15% and increases annually. As a hormone-dependent diseases, the morbidity in the women with late and less childbirth is significantly higher than women with more childbirth. After menopause, pregnancy, removal of both ovaries or in administration of hormones to inhibit ovarian function, endometrium will gradually shrink. The clinical manifestations are varied, and its lesions may involve any part of the body, in the pelvic cavity mostly. 65. 5% of the patients have obvious dysmenorrhea, and 30% to 40% patients are complicated with infertility too, in malignant transformation rate from 0.7% to 1%. It has a variety of clinical manifestations, in infiltration, metastasis, recurrence, and malignant biological behaviors. It is one of the most difficult and intractable gynecological diseases.

子宫内膜异位症

子宫内膜异位症是指具有生长功能的子宫内膜组织出现在子宫腔被覆内膜以外的身体其他部位。是育龄期女性常见病、多发病，发病率为 10%～15%，并且有逐年上升的趋势。作为一种激素依赖性疾病，生育晚、生育少的女性发病明显高于多生育者。绝经后、妊娠时、切除双侧卵巢后或使用激素抑制卵巢功能时，异位内膜会逐渐萎缩。临床表现多种多样，其病变部位可以累及全身任何部位，绝大多数位于盆腔内，其中 65.5%患者有明显的痛经，30%～40%合并不孕，恶变率为0.7%～1%。其临床表现形态多样性，且有浸润、转移和复发等恶性生物学行为，为妇科难治病之一。

According to the main clinical manifestations, such as abdominal pain during menstruation, non-menstrual pelvic pain, infertility, pelvic masses, it is attributed to the scope of "dysmenorrhea", "abdominal pain in women", "infertility", "abdominal mass" in Chinese Medicine. The main causes of the syndrome are attack of exogenous pathogens, emotion, and emotional upsets, which lead to obstruction of qi and blood in Thoroughfare and Conception Vessels, uterus, or malnutrition in the Thoroughfare and Conception Vessels, and uterus. The positions of the syndrome are in Thoroughfare and Conception Vessels and uterus, and the changes of the syndrome are in the blood, manifested by pain syndrome. Prolonged retention of blood stasis may transform into heat or lead to abdominal mass.

中医根据其主要的临床表现，如经行腹痛、非经期盆腔疼痛、不孕、盆腔肿块等，将之归属于"痛经""妇人腹痛""不孕""癥瘕"等门类。本病发生多因外邪入侵、情志、内伤等，导致冲任、胞宫气血阻滞，"不通则痛"；或冲任胞宫失于濡养，"不荣而痛"。其病位在冲任、胞宫，变化在气血，表现为痛证。瘀血留滞日久可以化热，亦可变生癥瘕等病。

1　Key points for diagnosis

1　诊断要点

1.1　Medical history

Secondary dysmenorrhea, sterility, uterine surgery, genital malformation, or cervical adhesions are often found in women of childbearing age.

1.1　病史

育龄期继发性痛经、不孕，或宫腔手术史，或有生殖器畸形、宫颈粘连等病史。

1.2　Symptoms

(1) Pelvic pain: Typical symptom is progressive secondary dysmenorrhea, which starts 1-2 days before menstruation, becomes most serious on the first day of menstruation. The pain mostly happens in the lower abdomen and lumbosacral region, radiating to vagina, perineum, anus or leg. It may be accompanied by prolapsing sensation in the anus and diarrhea. Some patients have chronic pelvic pain and coital pain, which are more obvious before menstruation and manifested by deep dyspareunia. If the chocolate cyst ruptures in endometriosis, it

1.2　症状

(1) 盆腔疼痛：典型症状为渐进性的继发性痛经，在经前 1～2 日开始，经期首日最剧烈，疼痛部位多为下腹部及腰骶部，放射至阴道、会阴、肛门或大腿。可伴有肛门下坠或腹泻。部分患者有慢性盆腔痛、性交痛等；性交痛在月经来潮前较明显，一般表现为深部性交痛；若卵巢巧克力囊肿破裂可引起突

may result in acute abdominal pain, accompanied by nausea, vomiting and distending and prolapsing sensation in anus, mostly before, after, or during menstrual period.

发性剧烈腹痛,伴恶心、呕吐和肛门坠胀,多发生在经期前后或经期。

(2) Menstrual disorder: 15% to 30% patients have increased menses amount, prolonged menstrual period, or premenstrual spotting bleeding.

(2) 月经失调:15%～30%患者有经量增多、经期延长或经前点滴出血。

(3) Sterility and miscarriage: 40% of patients are complicated with sterility, because the extensive adhesions around the ovaries and fallopian tubes influence the egg collection and transportation of the fallopian tubes, leading to the changes in the pelvic microenvironment and immune dysfunction. The ovulation disorders include luteinized unruptured follicle syndrome (LUFS) or inadequate luteal secretion. About 40% endometriosis patients have a spontaneous abortion.

(3) 不孕和流产:40%的患者合并不孕,主要由于卵巢、输卵管周围广泛粘连影响输卵管的拾卵与运输功能;盆腔内微环境改变和免疫功能异常;卵巢排卵障碍,包括未破裂卵泡黄素化综合征(LUFS)或黄体分泌不足等。内异症患者妊娠亦有约40%发生自然流产。

(4) Other symptoms: Intestinal endometriosis patients may suffer from abdominal pain, diarrhea or constipation, and even a cyclical small amount of hematochezia. Ectopic endometrium on bladder muscle wall can cause painful urination and frequent urination during menstruation. Cyclical pain or bleeding or enlarged lump may appear in the lesions of the patients with endometriosis outside of the pelvic cavity.

(4) 其他症状:肠道内异症患者可出现腹痛、腹泻或便秘,甚至有周期性少量便血;异位内膜侵犯膀胱肌壁可在经期引起尿痛和尿频;盆腔外内异症可在病变部位出现周期性疼痛或出血或块物增大。

1.3 Examination

1.3 检查

(1) Gynecological examination: Fixed and retroverted uterus, palpable painful nodules on the uterosacral ligament and lower portion of the posterior wall of the uterus, fixed and painful cystic mass linking with the uterus on the unilateral or bilateral uterine adnexa. If the lesion involving the rectovaginal septum, the bulged purple blue spots and small

(1) 妇科检查:子宫多后倾固定,直肠子宫陷凹、宫骶韧带或子宫后壁下段等部位扪及触痛性结节,一侧或双侧附件处扪到与子宫相连的囊性不活动包块,有轻压痛。若病变累及直肠阴道隔,可

nodules can be palpable and seen at the posterior vaginal fornix.

在阴道后穹隆部扪及甚至可看到隆起的紫蓝色斑点、小结节。

(2) Imageological examination: Vaginal or abdominal B ultrasound can determine the location and size of ovarian endometriosis cyst and its relationship with the uterus and surrounding organs.

（2）影像学检查：阴道或腹部B超可确定卵巢内异症囊肿的位置、大小以及与子宫和周围脏器的关系。

(3) Laparoscopy: It is currently the gold standard for the diagnosis of endometriosis, to detect the lesion and estimate the extent of disease.

（3）腹腔镜检查：是目前诊断内异症的金标准，可以发现病灶并且估计病变的范围。

(4) Laboratory tests: Serum CA125 may be increased. Serum anti-cardiolipin antibodies may be increased, but their specificity and sensitivity are low. Serum anti-endometrial antibodies are elevated, with high but not sensitive specificity.

（4）实验室检查：血清CA125可升高。血清抗心磷脂抗体可升高，但二者特异性和敏感性均不高。血清抗子宫内膜抗体升高，特异性高但不敏感。

2　Syndrome differentiation and treatment

2　辨证论治

The main syndrome of endometriosis is dysmenorrhea. "Seeking the causes principally and relieve pain assistantly" should be the basic method for diagnosis and treatment. For qi stagnation, rectify qi, remove stagnation and relieve pain. For yang asthenia, supplement the kidney and warm yang to relieve pain. For qi asthenia and blood asthenia, boost qi and nourish blood to relieve pain. For congealing cold, warm the meridians and disperse cold to relieve pain. For accumulated heat, clear away heat and dissolve stasis to relieve pain. For endometrial cysts or endometrial nodules, disperse accumulation, eliminate lump to relieve pain.

本病临床主证是痛经，应当以"求因为主，止痛为辅"的辨证论治为基本方法。气滞者理气行滞止痛；阳虚者补肾温阳止痛；气虚血虚者益气养血止痛；寒凝者温经散寒止痛；瘀热互结热者清热化瘀止痛；有内膜异位囊肿或内膜异位结节者可选用散结消癥止痛。

Pain caused by the disease is closely related to menstruation. The treatment should be stressed ac-

本病所致疼痛与月经关系密切，治疗中当注意月经

cording to the changes of qi and blood during different stages of menstrual cycle. For instance, in the early stage of menstruation, the treatment is mainly given to dissolve blood stasis, regulate menstruation and dredge the collaterals. During menstruation, the treatment is mainly given to activate blood, dissolve blood stasis and stop pain. In the later stage of menstruation, the treatment is mainly given to nourish and activate blood, and eliminate lumps. For prevention of post-operative recurrence, the treatment should be given to support the body constitution and dissolve blood stasis, and nourish the liver and kidney simultaneously for protecting the constitutional and gastric qi, properly by adding the herbs to benefit qi, nourish blood and protect the stomach. For the patients desiring for fertility, the treatment should be stressed to regulate menstruation, disperse blood stasis and dredge the collaterals.

周期的不同阶段气血运行变化，治有侧重。如经前期以化瘀、调经、通络为主；行经期以活血、化瘀、止痛为主；经后期以养血、活血、消癥为主。针对手术后预防复发的治疗，治以扶正化瘀，兼以滋养肝肾，顾护正气和胃气，酌加益气、养血和护胃之品。有生育要求的患者，着重调经、化瘀通络。

2.1 Syndrome of kidney asthenia and blood stasis

2.1 肾虚血瘀证

Main manifestations Abdominal pain during or after menstruation, scanty or profuse menorrhea, unsmooth menorrhea, blackish menses, or with blood clot, aching and weak sensation in the loins and knees, blackish complexion, or accompanied by sterility, grayish tongue or tongue with ecchymosis on the tongue edge, and thready and taut pulse.

主要证候 经行或经后腹痛，经量或多或少，经行不畅，经色紫暗，或有血块，腰酸腿软，面色黧黑，或伴不孕，舌质偏暗，或舌边有瘀点，脉细弦。

Therapeutic methods Replenishing the kidney and activating blood, resolving stasis and regulating menstruation.

治法 补肾活血，化瘀调经。

Formulas and herbs ① *Amber Powder* (Hu Po San), composed of 3 g of *Succini Pulvis* (Hu Po Fen) (to be taken separately), 12 g of *Radix*

方药 代表方：①琥珀散；常用药如琥珀粉（吞）3克，当归12克，赤芍12克，丹

Angelicae Sinensis (Dang Gui), 12 g of *Radix Paeoniae Rubra* (Chi Shao), 10 g of *Radix Salviae Miltiorrhizae* (Dan Shen), 6 g of *Rhizoma Ligustici Chuanxiong* (Chuan Xiong), 10 g of *Pollen Typhae* (Pu Huang) (to be wrapped for decocting), 10 g of *Trogopteri Faeces Frictum* (Chao Wu Ling Zhi), 10 g of *Semen Cuscutae* (Tu Si Zi), 10 g of *Epimedium davidii* (Xian Ling Pi, Yin Yang Huo), 6 g of *Cortex Cinnamomi* (Rou Gui), 10 g of *Rhizoma Zedoariae* (E Zhu) and 10 g of *Flos Carthami* (Hong Hua). ② *Fenugreek Pill* (Hu Lu Ba Wan), composed of 6 g of *Trigonellae Semen* (Hu Lu Ba), 12 g of *Radix Morindae Officinalis* (Ba Ji Tian), 12 g of *Herba Cistanchis* (Rou Cong Rong), 6 g of *Ramulus Cinnamomi* (Gui Zhi), 15 g of *Fructus Psoraleae* (Bu Gu Zhi), 10 g of *Fructus Cnidii* (She Chuang Zi), 6 g of *Fructus Aurantii Immaturus* (Zhi Shi), 12 g of *Radix Cyathulae* (Chuan Niu Xi), 9 g of *Rhizoma Zedoariae* (E Zhu), 9 g of *Aconiti Radix Lateralis Tosta* (Pao Fu Zi) and 9 g of *Fructus Foeniculi* (Xiao Hui Xiang).

参10克,川芎6克,蒲黄(包煎)10克,炒五灵脂10克,菟丝子10克,淫羊藿10克,肉桂6克,莪术10克,红花10克。②胡芦巴丸;常用药如胡芦巴6克,巴戟天12克,肉苁蓉12克,桂枝6克,补骨脂15克,蛇床子10克,枳实6克,川牛膝12克,莪术9克,炮附片9克,小茴香9克。

Modification for severe abdominal pain, *Olibanum Praeparatum* (Zhi Ru Xiang), *Myrrha Praeparata* (Zhi Mo Yao), *Toosendan Fructus Frictus* (Chao Chuan Lian Zi) and *Rhizoma Corydalis* (Yan Hu Suo) are added. For profuse menorrhea with blood clots, *Radix Notoginseng* (San Qi) is added. For scanty and unsmooth menstruation, *Radix Cyathulae* (Chuan Niu Xi) and *Lycopi Herba* (Ze Lan Ye) are added. For lumbago, *Cortex Eucommiae* (Du Zhong) and *Ramulus Loranthi* (Sang Ji Sheng) are added. For prolapsing and distending sensation in the anus, *Fructus Aurantii* (Zhi Qiao) and *Herba*

加减　若小腹痛甚者,加制乳香、制没药、炒川楝子、延胡索;经量多,挟有血块者,加三七;经行量少不畅者,加川牛膝、泽兰叶;腰痛者,加杜仲、桑寄生;肛门坠胀者,加枳壳、败酱草;卵巢有异位囊肿者,加败酱草、刘寄奴、石打穿、牡蛎、鳖甲等。

Patriniae (Bai Jiang Cao) are added. For ovarian endometrial cysts, *Herba Patriniae* (Bai Jiang Cao), *Herba Artemisiae Anomalae* (Liu Ji Nu), *Hedyotis Chrysotrichae Herba* (Shi Da Chuan), *Concha Ostreae* (Mu Li) and *Carapax Trionycis* (Bie Jia) are added.

2.2 Syndrome of cold coagulation and blood stagnation

Main manifestations Cold pain aggravated by pressure in lower abdomen, worse before or after menstruation, alleviated with warmth, even nausea, vomiting, scanty menorrhea, unsmooth menorrhea, difficulty in getting pregnancy, pale complexion, aversion to cold, cold limbs, pale or light-purplish tongue or tongue with ecchymosis on the tongue edge, deep and tense or deep, thready and unsmooth pulse.

Therapeutic methods Warming meridians to disperse cold, resolving stasis to dredge collaterals.

Formulas and herbs *Meridian-Warming Decoction* (Wen Jing Tang), composed of 10 g of *Radix Codonopsis Pilosulae* (Dang Shen), 10 g of *Radix Angelicae Sinensis* (Dang Gui), 5 g of *Rhizoma Ligustici Chuanxiong* (Chuan Xiong), 15 g of *Radix Salviae Miltiorrhizae* (Dan Shen), 10 g of *Radix Achyranthis Bidentatae* (Niu Xi), 6 g of *Cortex Cinnamomi* (Rou Gui), 6 g of *Fructus Foeniculi* (Xiao Hui Xiang), 6 g of *Rhizoma Zingiberis* (Gan Jiang), 10 g of *Rhizoma Zedoariae* (E Zhu), 12 g of *Radix Linderae* (Wu Yao), 6 g of *Folium Artemistae Argyi* (Ai Ye) and 10 g of *Amethyst* (Zi Shi Ying).

Modification For aversion to cold and cold limbs, *Radix Aconiti Praeparata* (Fu Zi) and *Cortex*

2.2 寒凝血滞证

主要证候 小腹冷痛拒按,经前或经行加剧,得热痛减,甚则恶心呕吐,经行量少,排出不畅,不易受孕,面色苍白,形寒怕冷,四肢不温,舌淡白或淡紫,或舌边有瘀点,脉沉紧或沉细涩。

治法 温经散寒,化瘀通络。

方药 代表方为温经汤;常用药如党参10克,当归10克,川芎5克,丹参15克,牛膝10克,肉桂6克,小茴香6克,干姜6克,莪术10克,乌药12克,艾叶6克,紫石英10克。

加减 若形寒怕冷、四肢不温者,加附子、肉桂;小

Cinnamomi (Rou Gui) are added. For lower abdominal distending pain, *Rhizoma Cyperi* (Xiang Fu) and *Fructus Aurantii* (Zhi Qiao) are added. For scanty and unsmooth menorrhea, *Herba Artemisiae Anomalae* (Liu Ji Nu) and *Semen Leonuri* (Chong Wei Zi) are added.

腹胀痛，加香附、枳壳；经行量少不畅者，加刘寄奴、茺蔚子。

2.3 Syndrome of qi stagnation and blood stasis

Main manifestations Lower abdominal distending pain, aggravated during or after menstruation, in profuse amount, and purplish red color, mingled with blood clots, abdominal pain alleviated after removal of blood clots, or in scanty amount, unsmooth menorrhea, distending pain in the breasts before menstruation, chest oppression and restlessness, or mental depression, prolapsing and distending sensation in the anus, purplish and blackish tongue or tongue with ecchymosis on the edge, taut or taut and thready pulse.

Therapeutic methods Regulating qi and activating the blood, resolving stasis and freeing the bowels.

Formulas and herbs *Free Wanderer Powder* (Xiao Yao San) *plus Sanguine Mansion Stasis-Expelling Decoction* (Xue Fu Zhu Yu Tang), composed of 10 g of *Radix Angelicae Sinensis* (Dang Gui), 6 g of *Rhizoma Ligustici Chuanxiong* (Chuan Xiong), 10 g of *Radix Paeoniae Rubra* (Chi Shao), 6 g of *Radix Bupleuri* (Chai Hu), 12 g of *Rhizoma Cyperi* (Xiang Fu), 10 g of *Toosendan Fructus Frictus* (Chao Chuan Lian Zi), 10 g of *Semen Persicae* (Tao Ren), 10 g of *Flos Carthami* (Hong Hua), 10 g of *Fructus Aurantii* (Zhi Qiao), 10 g of *Radix Achyranthis Bidentatae* (Niu Xi), 12 g of *Radix Salviae Miltiorrhizae* (Dan Shen) and 10 g of *Radix*

2.3 气滞血瘀证

主要证候 小腹胀痛拒按，经行或经后加剧，经量偏多，色紫红，挟有血块，血块排出后腹痛减轻，或经量偏少，排出不畅，经前乳房胀痛，胸闷烦燥，或精神抑郁不舒，肛门坠胀，舌紫暗，或边有瘀斑，脉弦或弦细。

治法 理气活血，化瘀通腑。

方药 代表方为逍遥散合血府逐瘀汤；常用药如当归10克，川芎6克，赤芍10克，柴胡6克，香附12克，炒川楝子10克，桃仁10克，红花10克，枳壳10克，牛膝10克，丹参12克，郁金10克。

Curcumae (Yu Jin).

Modification For severe lower abdominal pain, 3 g of *Olibanum Praeparatum* (Zhi Ru Xiang) and 3 g of *Myrrha Praeparata* (Zhi Mo Yao) are added. For prolapsing and distending sensation in the anus and tenesmus, *Radix Astragali* (Huang Qi), *Rhizoma Cimicifugae* (Sheng Ma) and *Radix Aucklandiae* (Mu Xiang) are added. For stagnant mass in the lower abdomen, *Rhizoma Sparganii Stoloniferi* (San Leng), *Rhizoma Zedoariae* (E Zhu), *Sargassum* (Hai Zao), *Ostreae Concha* (Mu Li) and *Spica Prunellae* (Xia Ku Cao) are added.

加减 若小腹痛甚者，加制乳香、制没药3克；肛门坠胀，里急后重者，加黄芪、升麻、木香；下腹有瘀块者，加三棱、莪术、海藻、牡蛎、夏枯草。

Shanghai doctor WANG Dazeng's experience prescription, *Compound Formula Rhubarb Decoction* (Fu Fang Da Huang Tang): 6 g of *Rhei Radix et Rhizoma Crudi* (Sheng Da Huang) (to be decocted later), 6 g of *Semen Persicae* (Tao Ren), 15 g of *Carapax Trionycis* (Bie Jia) and 1 g of *Succini Pulvis* (Hu Po Fen) (to be taken separately).

上海医家王大增经验方（复方大黄汤）：生大黄（后下）6克，桃仁6克，鳖甲15克，琥珀粉（分吞）1克。

2.4 Syndrome of heat stagnation and blood stasis

2.4 热郁血瘀证

Main manifestations Lower abdominal pain, aggravated during menstruation, fever or high fever during menstruation and gradual improvement after menstruation, profuse menorrhea at the beginning with red color and thick texture or with blood clots, bitter taste in the mouth and dry throat, retention of dry feces, yellowish urine and frequent urination, yellowish leukorrhea, coital pain, red tongue with thin and yellow fur, thready and rapid or thready and taut pulse.

主要证候 下腹疼痛，经行加剧，经期发热，甚或高热，经净后渐至正常，月经先期量多，色红，质稠，或有血块，口苦咽干，大便干结，小便色黄尿频，带下色黄，性交疼痛，舌质红，苔薄黄，脉细数或细弦数。

Therapeutic methods Activating blood and resolving blood stasis, clearing away heat and dissipating nodules.

治法 活血化瘀，清热散结。

Formulas and herbs *Heat-Clearing Four Agents*

方药 代表方为清经四

Decoction (Qing Jing Si Wu Tang), composed of 10 g of *Radix Angelicae Sinensis* (Dang Gui), 6 g of *Rhizoma Ligustici Chuanxiong* (Chuan Xiong), 10 g of *Radix Rehmanniae Cruda* (Sheng Di Huang), 10 g of *Radix Paeoniae Rubra* (Chi Shao), 10 g of *Cortex Moutan Radicis* (Mu Dan Pi), 12 g of *Caulis Sargentodoxae* (Da Xue Teng), 12 g of *Herba Patriniae* (Bai Jiang Cao), 10 g of *Toosendan Fructus Frictus* (Chao Chuan Lian Zi), 10 g of *Semen Persicae* (Tao Ren), 12 g of *Faeces Trogopterorum* (Wu Ling Zhi), 10 g of *Spica Prunellae* (Xia Ku Cao) and 10 g of *Fructus Crataegi* (Shan Zha).

物汤;常用药如当归10克,川芎6克,生地黄10克,赤芍10克,牡丹皮10克,红藤12克,败酱草12克,炒川楝子10克,桃仁10克,五灵脂12克,夏枯草10克,山楂10克。

Modification For dysphoria and susceptibility to rage, *Fructus Gardeniae* (Zhi Zi) and *Radix Scutellariae* (Huang Qin) are added. For low fever, *Cortex Lycii Radicis* (Di Gu Pi) and *Herba Artemisiae Chinghao* (Qing Hao) are added. For profuse menorrhea, *Radix Sanguisorbae*(Di Yu) and *Rhizome Dryopteris Gassirhizomae* (Guan Zhong Tan) are added. For constipation, *Radix et Rhizoma Rhei* (Da Huang) and *Fructus Aurantii Immaturus* (Zhi Shi) are added. For yellowish leukorrhagia, *Toonae Radicis Cortex* (Chun Gen Pi), *Rhizoma Smilacis Glabrae* (Tu Fu Ling) and *Cortex Phellodendri* (Huang Bo) are added.

加减 若心烦易怒者,加栀子、黄芩;伴有低热者,加地骨皮、青蒿;经量过多者,加地榆、贯众炭;大便秘结,加大黄、枳实;带多色黄者,加椿根皮、土茯苓、黄柏。

Shanghai doctor DAI Deying's experience prescription, *Sargentodoxa Prescription* (Hong Teng Fang): 30 g of *Caulis Sargentodoxae* (Da Xue Teng), 15 g of *Typhae Pollen* (Pu Huang), 30 g of *Concha Ostreae* (Mu Li), 20 g of *Rhizoma Corydalis* (Yan Hu Suo), 10 g of *Cortex Moutan Radicis* (Mu Dan Pi), 10 g of *Semen Persicae* (Tao Ren) and 15 g of *Rhizoma Cyperi* (Xiang Fu).

上海医家戴德英经验方(红藤方):红藤30克,蒲黄15克,牡蛎30克,延胡索20克,牡丹皮10克,桃仁10克,香附15克。

3 Other therapeutic methods:

3.1 Chinese patent drugs

(1) *Sevenfold Processed Cyperus Pill* (Qi Zhi Xiang Fu Wan): Take 6 g each time and twice a day, applicable to the treatment of qi stagnation and blood stasis syndrome.

(2) *Rhubarb and Ground Beetle Pills* (Da Huang Zhe Chong Wan): For water and honey pill, take 3 g each time, for small honey pill, 3-6 pills each time, for big honey pill, 1-2 pills each time, and twice a day, applicable to the treatment of blood stasis syndrome.

(3) *Binds-Dispersing and Pain-Stopping Capsule* (San Jie Zhen Tong Jiao Nang): Take 4 capsules each time and three times a day, applicable to the treatment of pattern of phlegm and static blood with qi stagnation.

3.2 Empirical and folk recipes

(1) *Lumbricus* (Di Long), *Scolopendra subspinipes* (Wu Gong), *Eupolyphaga seu Steleophaga* (Zhe Chong), *Cortex Cinnamomi* (Rou Gui) and *Lignum Aquilariae Resinatum* (Chen Xiang) in the equal amount are ground into powder. 3 g is taken each time and three times a day, applicable to the treatment of blood stasis syndrome.

(2) 3 g of *Radix Notoginseng* (San Qi), 20 g of *Radix Salviae Miltiorrhizae* (Dan Shen) and 2 eggs are decocted together in 300 ml water. When the eggs are well cooked, the shells are removed and the rest is put into the decoction to boil for some time. After the removal of the residue, the decoction and eggs are eaten. Take the decoction 2 days before menstruation, once a day for 5 days. This decoction

3 其他疗法

3.1 中成药

（1）七制香附丸：每次 6 克，每日 2 次，适用于气滞血瘀证。

（2）大黄䗪虫丸：水蜜丸每次 3 克，小蜜丸每次 3～6 丸，大蜜丸每次 1～2 丸，每日 2 次，适用于血瘀证。

（3）散结镇痛胶囊：每次 4 粒，每日 3 次，适用于痰瘀互结兼气滞证。

3.2 单验方

（1）地龙、蜈蚣、䗪虫、肉桂、沉香等分，研细末，每服 3 克，每日 3 次，适用于血瘀证。

（2）三七 3 克，丹参 20 克，加鸡蛋 2 枚，水 300 毫升同煮，蛋熟后去壳再煮片刻，去药渣，食蛋饮汤。月经前 2 日开始每天服 1 次，连服 5 日，适用于血瘀证。

is applicable to the treatment of blood stasis syndrome.

(3) Shanghai doctor CAI Xiaosun's experience prescription: 10 g of *Stir-Fried Chinese Angelica* (Chao Dang Gui), 12 g of *Radix Salviae Miltiorrhizae* (Dan Shen), 10 g of *Radix Cyathulae* (Chuan Niu Xi), 10 g of *Cyperi Rhizoma Praeparatum* (Zhi Xiang Fu), 6 g of *Rhizoma Ligustici Chuanxiong* (Chuan Xiong), 10 g of *Radix Paeoniae Rubra* (Chi Shao), 6 g of *Myrrha Praeparata* (Zhi Mo Yao), 12 g of *Rhizoma Corydalis* (Yan Hu Suo), 12 g of *Typhae Pollen* (Pu Huang), 10 g of *Faeces Trogopterorum* (Wu Ling Zhi) and 3 g of *Resina Draconis* (Xue Jie), applicable to the treatment of prolonged stasis.

（3）上海医家蔡小荪经验方：炒当归 10 克，丹参 12 克，川牛膝 10 克，制香附 10 克，川芎 6 克，赤芍 10 克，制没药 6 克，延胡索 12 克，蒲黄 12 克，五灵脂 10 克，血竭 3 克，适用于宿瘀内结。

(4) Shanghai doctor LUO Yijun's experience prescription: 10 g of *Radix Angelicae Sinensis Frictum* (Chao Dang Gui), 9 g of *Rhizoma Sparganii Stoloniferi* (San Leng), 9 g of *Rhizoma Zedoariae* (E Zhu), 12 g of *Radix Rehmanniae Cruda* (Sheng Di Huang), 12 g of *Radix Paeoniae Rubra* (Chi Shao), 9 g of *Trionycis Carapax cum Liquido Frictus* (Zhi Bie Jia), 30 g of *Spica Prunellae* (Xia Ku Cao), 12 g of *Fructus Lycii* (Gou Qi Zi) and 12 g of *Ramulus Loranthi* (Sang Ji Sheng), applicable to the treatment of accumulation of blood stasis and heat.

（4）上海医家骆益君经验方：炒当归 10 克，三棱 9 克，莪术 9 克，生地黄 12 克，赤芍 12 克，炙鳖甲 9 克，夏枯草 30 克，枸杞子 12 克，桑寄生 12 克，适用于瘀热壅积。

3.3 External therapy

Enema. Enema formulas for endometriosis composed of 30 g of *Rhizoma Zedoariae* (E Zhu), 30 g of *Spina Gleditsiae* (Zao Jiao Ci), 15 g of *Rhizoma Cimicifugae* (Sheng Ma) and 30 g of *Caulis Sargentodoxae* (Da Xue Teng). Apply enema, once a night and for 7 successive days after menstruation. Three months is a course of

3.3 外治法

灌肠法。内异灌肠方：莪术 30 克，皂角刺 30 克，升麻 15 克，红藤 30 克，保留灌肠，每晚 1 次，月经干净后连用 7 日。连用 3 个月为 1 个疗程。

treatment.

Adenomyosis

子宫腺肌病

Adenomyosis refers to invasion of endometrial glants and stroma into myometrium, accompanied by compensatory hypertrophy and hyperplasia of surrounding myometrium cells, previously called the intrinsic endometriosis. The disease mostly occurs in women after the age of 40, complicated with uterine fibroids at the same time in about half of the patients, complicated with endometriosis in about 15%-40% of patients. After postmenopause, the symptoms are relieved and the lesions shrink. According to clinical manifestations, adenomyosis pertains to the scope of "dysmenorrhea", "abdominal mass" and "irregular menstruation" in TCM.

子宫腺肌病是指具有子宫内膜腺体及间质侵入子宫肌层中，伴随周围肌层细胞的代偿性肥大和增生，以往曾称为内在性子宫内膜异位症。本病多发生于 40 岁以上的经产妇，约有半数患者同时合并子宫肌瘤，约 15%～40%合并子宫内膜异位症，绝经后症状缓解，病灶萎缩。子宫腺肌病根据临床表现，属中医学"痛经""癥瘕""月经不调"等范畴。

The disease is mainly caused by retention of blood stasis in the Thoroughfare and Conception Vessels as well as the uterus. Blood stasis is caused by qi stagnation due to emotional depression, inhibited flow of liver qi, obstructed activity of qi, unsmooth circulation of blood. Abdominal mass results from stagnation of qi and blood due to excessive intake of uncooked and cold foods before and during menstruation or attack by exogenous pathogenic cold, which coagulates blood. Constitutional asthenia of spleen qi and hypofunction in transporting blood will slow the flow of blood and gradually lead to blood stasis.

本病主要是瘀血内阻，结于胞宫所致。平素情志抑郁，肝气不舒，气机不利，血行不畅，气滞而血瘀；或经前、经期恣食生冷，或感受寒凉，血遇寒则凝，气血瘀滞，日久结块，形成癥瘕；或素体脾虚气弱，运血无力，血行迟滞，日久成瘀。

1 Key points for diagnosis

1 诊断要点

1.1 Medical history

1.1 病史

Most patients are more than 40 years old, with

多为 40 岁以上，经产或

multiparity or uterine surgery, orendometriosis.

有宫腔手术史，或有子宫内膜异位症病史。

1.2 Symptoms

Increased amount of menstruation and prolonged menstrual period (40% to 50%), progressive dysmenorrhea (35%). Pain occurs one week before the start of menstruation until the end of the menstruation, or bleeding and pain occur during menstruation. About 35% of patients are without any symptoms.

1.2 症状

经量增多、经期延长(40%～50%)，逐年加剧的进行性痛经(35%)，痛经常在经前一周开始持续到月经结束。或有月经中期出血、疼痛。约35%患者无任何症状。

1.3 Examinations

The uterus is present with even enlargement or localized nodulated apophysis, in hard texture and tenderness, without obvious in the two uterine adnexa. B ultrasonic examination indicates their regular enhanced echo in the myometrium, thickened muscle wall, no boundaries. Serum CA125 levels can be increased.

1.3 检查

子宫呈均匀性增大或有局限性结节隆起，质硬而有压痛，双附件无明显异常。B超检查可在子宫肌层见到不规则增强回声，肌壁增厚，无边界。血清CA125水平可升高。

2 Syndorme differentiation and treatment

The main clinical manifestation is blood stasis syndrome, sthenia syndrome at the beginning. But it may develop into a syndrome mingled with both asthenia and sthenia due to profuse menorrhea, prolonged period and long-term progressive loss of blood. Syndrome differentiation should be done based on the nature, location, degree and duration of pain, and the quantity, color and texture of menses, based on the conditions of the tongue and pulse as well as general manifestations, so as to decide whether the syndrome is of sthenia or a mixture of both sthenia and asthenia.

2 辨证论治

本病临床表现为血瘀证，初为实证，因月经量多，经期延长，日久失血较多，致虚实夹杂证。临床辨证时要根据疼痛的性质、部位、程度、持续时间及月经量、色、质的变化和舌脉及全身表现辨虚实孰多孰少，辨其为实证，还是虚实夹杂之证。

Dysmenorrhea usually occurs beforeor during menstruation. Lower abdominal cold pain or colic

痛经多发生于经前、经期。小腹冷痛或绞痛，得热

may be due to cold coagulation and blood stasis, if it gets improved with warmth. Lower abdominal distending pain accompanied by distending pain in the breasts, is due to cold coagulation and blood stasis. Prolapsing pain in the lower abdomen with scanty and light-colored menses as well as lassitude is due to qi asthenia and blood stasis.

稍减者,为寒凝血瘀;小腹胀痛并伴胸胁乳房胀痛者,属气滞血瘀;小腹疼痛下坠,月经量少色淡,倦怠乏力者,为气虚血瘀。

The treatment is mainly given to dissolve blood stasis and diminish abdominal masses. If the illness is due to cold coagulation and blood stasis, the treatment should be given to warm the meridians to disperse cold. If it is due to qi stagnation and blood stasis, the treatment should be given to promote qi flow and activate blood. If it is due to qi asthenia and blood stasis, the treatment should be given to nourish qi and activate blood.

治疗总以化瘀消癥为主,其中寒凝血瘀者,宜温经散寒;气滞血瘀者,又当行气活血;气虚血瘀者,则应以益气活血为法。

2.1 Syndrome of cold coagulation and blood stasis

2.1 寒凝血瘀证

Main manifestations Lower abdominal cold pain or colic worsened by pressure, or lower abdominal mass, profuse or scanty menses with purplish color and blood clot, abdominal pain alleviated after removal of blood clot, cold limbs, purplish and blackish tongue with ecchymosis and whitish and slippery fur, deep and taut or deep and tense pulse before menstruation.

主要症状 经期经前小腹冷痛或绞痛,按之痛甚,痛势剧烈,或下腹结块,月经量多或少,色紫暗,有血块,块下痛减,四肢厥冷,舌质紫暗,有瘀斑、瘀点,苔白滑,脉沉弦或沉紧。

Therapeutic methods Warming meridians and dispersing cold, resolving stasis and eliminating mass.

治法 温经散寒,化瘀消癥。

Formulas and herbs *Lesser Abdomen Stasis-Expelling Decoction* (Shao Fu Zhu Yu Tang), composed of 10 g of *Fructus Foeniculi* (Xiao Hui Xiang), 10 g of *Rhizoma Zingiberis* (Gan Jiang), 6 g of *Ramulus Cinnamomi* (Gui Zhi), 12 g of

方药 代表方为少腹逐瘀汤;常用药如小茴香 10 克,干姜 10 克,桂枝 6 克,赤芍 12 克,当归 10 克,川芎 6 克,三棱 10 克,莪术 10 克,乌

Radix Paeoniae Rubra (Chi Shao), 10 g of *Radix Angelicae Sinensis* (Dang Gui), 6 g of *Rhizoma Ligustici Chuanxiong* (Chuan Xiong), 10 g of *Rhizoma Sparganii Stoloniferi* (San Leng), 10 g of *Rhizoma Zedoariae* (E Zhu), 10 g of *Radix Linderae* (Wu Yao), 12 g of *Thallus Laminariae seu Eckloniae* (Kun Bu) and 5 g of *Glycyrrhizae Radix* (Gan Cao).

药 10 克，昆布 12 克，甘草 5 克。

Modification For nausea, vomiting, *Fructus Evodiae* (Wu Zhu Yu) and *Rhizoma Pinelliae* (Ban Xia) are added to warm the stomach and check vomiting. For diarrhea, *Semen Myristicae* (Rou Dou Kou), *Herba Agastachis* (Huo Xiang) and *Rhizoma Atractylodis Macrocephalae* (Bai Zhu) are added to fortify the spleen. For severe abdominal pain, cold limbs and sweating, *Capsicum Annuum* (Chuan Jiao) and *Radix Aconiti Preparata* (Zhi Chuan Wu) are added to relieve pain by the drugs of the warming and dredging action. For yang asthenia and internal cold, *Radix Ginseng* (Ren Shen), *Aconiti Radix Lateralis Tosta* (Pao Fu Zi) and *Epimedium davidii* (Xian Ling Pi) are added to warm and supplement the spleen and kidney.

加减　若恶心呕吐者，加吴茱萸、半夏温胃止呕；腹泻者，加肉豆蔻、藿香、白术健脾；腹痛甚，肢冷出汗者加川椒、制川乌温通止痛；阳虚内寒者，加人参、炮附片、仙灵脾温补脾肾。

2.2 Syndrome of qi stagnation and blood stasis

Main manifestations Unbearable lower abdominal pain before and during menstruation, aggravated by pressure, or lower abdominal mass, profuse menses with deep-red color and blood clot, slight alleviation of pain after removal of blood clot, premenstrual dysphoria and susceptibility to rage, distending pain in chest, hypochondria and breasts, blackish tongue or tongue with ecchymosis and taut pulse.

Therapeutic methods Activating the blood and dissolving blood stasis, rectifying qi and moving

2.2 气滞血瘀证

主要症状　经前经期小腹胀痛难忍，拒按，或下腹结块，月经量多，色暗红有血块，块下痛稍减，经前心烦易怒，胸胁乳房胀痛，舌质紫暗或有瘀斑瘀点，脉弦。

治法　活血化瘀，利气行滞。

stagnation.

Formulas and herbs *Sanguine Mansion Stasis-Expelling Decoction* (Xue Fu Zhu Yu Tang), composed of 8 g of *Radix Bupleuri* (Chai Hu), 10 g of *Cyperi Rhizoma Praeparatum* (Zhi Xiang Fu), 10 g of *Radix Cyathulae* (Chuan Niu Xi), 12 g of *Fructus Aurantii* (Zhi Qiao), 10 g of *Semen Persicae* (Tao Ren), 10 g of *Flos Carthami* (Hong Hua), 6 g of *Rhizoma Ligustici Chuanxiong* (Chuan Xiong), 10 g of *Rhizoma Corydalis* (Yan Hu Suo), 10 g of *Rhizoma Sparganii Stoloniferi* (San Leng), 10 g of *Rhizoma Zedoariae* (E Zhu), 12 g of *Faeces Trogopterorum* (Wu Ling Zhi) and 12 g of *Thallus Laminariae seu Eckloniae* (Kun Bu).

方药 代表方为血府逐瘀汤;常用药如柴胡 8 克,制香附 10 克,川牛膝 10 克,枳壳 12 克,桃仁 10 克,红花 10 克,川芎 6 克,延胡索 10 克,三棱 10 克,莪术 10 克,五灵脂 12 克,昆布 12 克。

Modification For abdominal pain before and during menstruation, *Myrrha Praeparata* (Zhi Mo Yao) and *Caulis Spatholobi* (Ji Xue Teng) are added to move qi, activate the blood and relieve pain. For profuse menorrhea, *Rhizoma Sparganii Stoloniferi* (San Leng) and *Rhizoma Zedoariae* (E Zhu) are deleted while *Herba Leonuri* (Yi Mu Cao), *Madder Carbonisatum* (Qian Cao Tan) and *Notoginseng Radix Pulverata* (San Qi Fen) are added to dissolve stasis and stanch blood.

加减 若经前经期腹痛已作,加制没药、鸡血藤以行气活血止痛;若经行量多,经期去三棱、莪术活血逐瘀之品,加益母草、茜草炭、三七粉以化瘀止血。

Shanghai doctor ZHU Nansun's experience prescription, *Membrane-Transforming Decoction* (Hua Me Tang): 20 g of *Typhae Pollen* (Pu Huang) (to be wrapped for decocting), 12 g of *Rhizoma Sparganii Stoloniferi* (San Leng), 12 g of *Rhizoma Zedoariae* (E Zhu), 3 g of *Resina Olibani* (Ru Xiang), 3 g of *Myrrha* (Mo Yao), 15 g of *Fructus Crataegi* (Shan Zha), 6 g of *Pericarpium Citri Reticulatae Viride* (Qing Pi) and 2 g of *Daemonoropis Resina Pulverata* (Xue Jie Fen) (to be swallowed).

上海医家朱南孙经验方(化膜汤):蒲黄(包煎)20 克,三棱 12 克,莪术 12 克,乳香 3 克,没药 3 克,山楂 15 克,青皮 6 克,血竭粉(吞服)2 克。

2.3 Syndrome of qi asthenia and blood stasis

Main manifestations Abdominal pain during or after menstruation, relieved by pressure and warmth, menses with light color and thin texture, prolapsing and distending sensation in the anus, lusterless facial complexion, fatigued spirit and lack of strength, loose stool, pale and enlarged tongue with tooth marks on the margins of the tongue, thready and taut or rough pulse.

Therapeutic methods Nourishing qi and activating blood, resolving stasis and relieving pain.

Formulas and herbs *Original-Lifting Brew* (Ju Yuan Jian) combined with *Great Guffaw Powder* (Shi Xiao San), composed of 15 g of *Radix Ginseng* (Ren Shen), 15 g of *Astragali Radix cum Liquido Fricta* (Zhi Huang Qi), 6 g of *Radix Glycyrrhizae Praeparata* (Zhi Gan Cao), 6 g of *Rhizoma Cimicifugae Frictum* (Chao Sheng Ma), 9 g of *Stir-Fried Rhizoma Atractylodis Macrocephalae* (Chao Bai Zhu), 15 g of *Pollen Typhae* (Pu Huang), 12 g of *Faeces Trogopterorum* (Wu Ling Zhi) and 2 g of *Notoginseng Radix Pulverata* (San Qi Fen).

Modification For severe abdominal pain, *Folium Artemistae Argyi* (Ai Ye), *Fructus Foeniculi* (Xiao Hui Xiang), *Aconiti Radix Lateralis Tosta* (Pao Fu Pian) and *Rhizoma Zingiberis* (Gan Jiang) are added to warm meridians and stop pain. For blood asthenia, *Caulis Spatholobi* (Ji Xue Teng) is added to nourish and activate blood. For kidney asthenia and aching lumbus and legs, *Radix Dipsaci* (Xu Duan) and *Ramulus Loranthi* (Sang Ji Sheng) are added to supplement the liver and kidney and strengthen sinew and bone.

2.3 气虚血瘀证

主要症状　经期或经后腹痛，喜按喜温，月经色淡质薄，肛门坠胀，面色少华，神疲乏力，大便不实。舌淡胖，边有齿痕，脉细弦或涩。

治法　益气活血，祛瘀止痛。

方药　代表方为举元煎合失笑散；常用药如人参15克，炙黄芪15克，炙甘草6克，炒升麻6克，炒白术9克，蒲黄15克，五灵脂12克，三七粉2克。

加减　若腹痛甚者，加艾叶、小茴香、炮附片、干姜以温经止痛；血虚者，加鸡血藤以养血活血；兼肾虚，症见腰腿酸软者，加续断、桑寄生以补肝肾强筋骨。

3 Other therapeutic methods

3.1 Chinese patent drugs

(1) *Corydalis Pain-Relieving Tablet* (Yan Hu Zhi Tong Pian): Take 4 tablets each time and three times a day, applicable to the treatment of qi stagnation and blood stasis syndrome.

(2) Mugwort and Cyperus Uterus-Warming Pill (Ai Fu Nuan Gong Wan): Take 10 g each time and three times a day, applicable to the treatment of cold coagulation and blood stasis syndrome.

3.2 Empirical and folk recipes

(1) 45 g of *Herba Leonuri* (Yi Mu Cao) and 15 g of *Rhizoma Corydalis* (Yan Hu Suo) are decocted together with 2 eggs in 600 ml of water. When the eggs are well cooked, the shells are removed and the rest is put into the decoction to boil for a while. After the removal of the residue, the decoction and eggs are taken, The decoction and eggs are taken 2 days before menstruation, once a day for 5 days, applicable to the treatment of qi stagnation and blood stasis syndrome.

(2) 30 g of *Semen Litchi* (Li Zhi He) and 30 g of *Fructus Anisi Stellati* (Hui Xiang) are baked black and ground into fine powder. 3 g is taken 3 days before menstruation with warm rice wine each time and twice a day, applicable to the treatment of cold coagulation and blood stasis syndrome.

(3) 30 g of *Radix Codonopsis Pilosulae* (Dang Shen), 10 g of *Radix Astragali* (Huang Qi) and 30 g of *Radix Salviae Miltiorrhizae* (Dan Shen) are decocted in 500 ml of water. After boiling, the herbs continue to be decocted with mild fire for 30 minutes. 30 g of brown sugar is added into the decoction. The decoction is

3 其他疗法

3.1 中成药

（1）延胡止痛片：每次服4片，每日3次，适用于气滞血瘀证。

（2）艾附暖宫丸：每次服10克，每日3次，适用于寒凝血瘀证。

3.2 单验方

（1）益母草45克，延胡索15克，鸡蛋2枚，上药加水600毫升同煮，蛋熟后去壳再煮片刻，去药渣，吃蛋饮汤。于月经前2日开始每天服1次，连服5日，适用于气滞血瘀证。

（2）荔枝核30克，茴香30克，将上2味炒黑，研极细末，每服3克，温酒送下，经前3天开始服，每天2次，服至经净，适用于寒凝血瘀证。

（3）党参30克，黄芪10克，丹参30克，将上药加水500毫升，煮沸后用微火煎30分钟取汁，加入红糖30克当茶饮，于经前3日开始，连服10日，适用于气虚血

taken as tea 3 days before menstruation, for 10 days, applicable to the treatment of qi asthenia and blood stasis syndrome.

瘀证。

3.3 External method of treatment

Enema with Chinese medicinal herbs: 15 g of *Radix Salviae Miltiorrhizae* (Dan Shen), 15 g of *Radix Paeoniae Rubra* (Chi Shao), 10 g of *Semen Persicae* (Tao Ren), 15 g of *Rhizoma Sparganii Stoloniferi* (San Leng), 15 g of *Rhizoma Zedoariae* (E Zhu), 15 g *Sargassum* (Hai Zao), 10 g *Eupolyphaga Steleophaga* (Tu bie chong), 10 g *Rhizoma corydalis* (Yan Hu Sao), 10 g *Fructus Toosendan* (Chuan Lian Zi), 15 g *Semen Litchi* (Li Zhi He), and 10 g of *Radix Aucklandiae* (Mu Xiang) are decocted into 100 ml liquid for edema, once a night. This therapy is effective for promoting qi flow to activate blood and expelling stasis to stop pain. For cold coagulation and blood stasis syndrome, 3 g of *Herba Asari* (Xi Xin) and 10 g of *Ramulus Cinnamomi* (Gui Zhi) are added for warming the meridians and dredging the collaterals.

3.3 外治法

中药保留灌肠:丹参15克,赤芍15克,桃仁10克,三棱15克,莪术15克,海藻15克,蛰虫10克,延胡索10克,川楝子10克,荔枝核15克,木香10克,浓煎100毫升,保留灌肠,每晚1次。行气活血,祛瘀止痛。若寒凝血瘀者,加细辛3克,桂枝10克,以温经通络。

Chapter 3 Sterility

第3章 不孕症

Sterility is a commonly encountered gynecological disease and takes place in 10% of the couples in the normal right age, in an annually increasing tendency. Its onset age is from 25 to 35. In the reproductive activities of the mankind, sterility can be caused, if any link of conception is influenced by the comprehensive and multiple factors.

不孕症是妇科临床常见疾病，在正常适龄夫妇中有10%左右发生不孕症，且有逐年上升趋势。其发病年龄多集中在25～35岁。在人类生殖活动过程中，由综合性的、多方面的因素影响了受孕的任何一环节，都可导致不孕症。

Primary sterility

原发性不孕症

No pregnancy in the couple living together for one year after marriage, in the normal sex and reproductive functions, without contraception is called primary sterility. In various causes of infertility, the factors from woman account for 40% to 55%. The ovulation disorder and tubal factor are most common, each of which accounts for about 30%.

The kidney governs reproduction, and stores essence. Only when kidney qi is superabundant, essence and blood are sufficient, sex hormones arrive, and menstruation comes on time, and two kinds of essence get integrated, can pregnancy be possible. Any factor that affects any link in this procedure

凡婚后夫妇同居，性生活正常，配偶生殖功能正常，未避孕未孕1年者，称为原发性不孕症。古称“全不产”。各种不孕的原因中，女方因素占40%～55%，其中以排卵障碍和输卵管因素最为常见，各占约30%。

肾主生殖而藏精气，当肾气盛，精血充沛，天癸至，月事以时下，两精相搏，则可受孕。反之，若由某些因素影响了上述任何一个环节，都会导致不孕。因此，不孕

may cause sterility. Therefore, sterility is closely related to the kidney. Asthenia of the kidney may lead to dysfunction of the liver, spleen and heart. The dysfunction of these viscera further leads to insufficiency of the liver and kidney, asthenia of both the spleen and kidney as well as disharmony between the heart and kidney, resulting in disturbance of qi and blood in the Thoroughfare and Conception Vessels and failure of the uterus in collecting essences for pregnancy.

与肾的关系最为密切。肾虚可导致肝、脾、心等脏腑功能失调,出现肝肾不足、脾肾两虚、心肾不交等证,并影响冲任气血失调,胞宫难以摄精成孕。

1 Key points for diagnosis

1 诊断要点

1.1 General condition

No pregnancy for over one year after marriage, while the couple is regular in sex life, without contraception. The physical examinations are stressed on the body shape, development of the second sexuality, and distribution of the public hair of the patients. Gynecological examination is done to see whether any abnormal development is in the sexual organs, etc.

1.1 一般情况

婚后 1 年以上,夫妇同居,性生活规律,未避孕而不受孕,体格检查着重于患者体型、第二性征发育、阴毛分布等;妇科检查判断有无性器发育异常等。

1.2 Laboratory and other tests

① Ovarian function test: BBT test can be used to check ovulation. For instance, uni-directional BBT indicates no ovulation, bidirectional BBT, temperature difference less than or equal to 0.3 ℃, or continuous high fever for less than 1-2 days, or gradual increase of body temperature indicate ovulation but hypofunction of yellow body. Smear examination of the exfoliated cells in the vagina: Simple action of or hypofunction of estrogen in the smear examination indicates no ovulation. Examination of cervical mucus: cervical scores are used for monitoring ovulation. ② Endocrinology examination: It is

1.2 实验室及其他检查

①卵巢功能测定:基础体温(BBT)可检测排卵情况,如 BBT 为单相型的则无排卵,如 BBT 为双相型,但温差小于或等于 0.3 ℃,或高温相持续时间小于 1～2 日,或体温上升缓慢,则提示为有排卵而黄体功能不足。阴道脱落细胞涂片检查:如表现单纯雌激素作用或雌激素功能低下则提示无排卵功能。宫颈黏液检查:以宫颈评分

performed to analyze whether the functions of ovary, pituitary gland and hypothalamus are abnormal, affecting ovulation. ③ B ultrasonic examination: It is used to understand whether there are any organic changes in the uterus and ovary and monitor the follicular development and ovulation. ④ Fallopian tube patency examination: Hystero salpingography is helpful for detecting the pathological changes of the uterus and the conditions of the oviduct. ⑤ Abdominoscopy and uterioscopy are helpful for direct observation of the pelvis and the uterus. ⑥ Immunoassay: It is used to detect sperm antibodies, the zona pellucida antibodies, endometrial antibodies, blocking antibodies and cytotoxic antibodies. ⑦ Karyotype analysis. ⑧ Some severe congenital defects and deformity in the sexual organs, and purely male's factor should be carefully differentiated. ⑨ CT or MRI examination: For suspected pituitary tumor, sella layered radiography and pelvic examination should be done. ⑩ Routine and quality analysis of male sperm.

监测排卵。②内分泌学检查:用以分析卵巢、垂体及下丘脑功能有无异常而影响排卵。③B超检查:可了解子宫、卵巢有无器质性病变及监测卵泡发育与排卵。④输卵管通畅检查:子宫输卵管造影术可了解宫腔病变及输卵管通畅程度。⑤腹腔镜、宫腔镜检查则可直观了解盆腔脏器及宫腔。⑥免疫试验:检测精子抗体、透明带抗体、子宫内膜抗体、封闭抗体和细胞毒抗体等。⑦染色体核型分析。⑧某些严重的先天性器官缺如及畸形或纯属男方原因者,应注意加以鉴别。⑨CT或MRI检查:对疑有垂体瘤时可做蝶鞍分层摄片,以及盆腔情况检查。⑩男方精液常规及质量分析。

2 Syndrome differentiation and treatment

For primary sterility, asthenia or sthenia should be differentiated according to the age of menarche, menstruation, the development of secondary sex characteristic and constitution. The late age of menarche, delayed menstruation, scanty amount, grayish color, and multiple blood clots, and distending pain in lower abdomen, aggravated by pressure belong to asthenia. The root cause lies in the kidney, but the influence from the liver, spleen, qi and blood is also very important. Clinically, they should

2 辨证论治

原发性不孕症应根据初潮年龄、月经带下的情况以及第二性征发育、体质状况等辨别虚实。初潮年龄较晚,行经落后,量少,色暗,多血块,小腹胀痛拒按,属实。其根本在于肾,但肝、脾、气血的影响也是非常重要的。临证应当注意辨别。

be carefully differentiated.

2.1 Syndrome of kidney qi asthenia

Main manifestations No pregnancy long after marriage, late age of menarche, delayed menstruation, scanty amount with light or grayish color, even amenorrhea, blackish complexion, aching in the loins and weakness of legs, sexual frigidity, leukorrhagia with thin texture, clear and profuse urine, loose stool, sparce public hair, small uterus, light-colored tongue with whitish fur, deep and thready pulse or deep and slow pulse.

Therapeutic methods Warming the kidney, replenishing essence, nourishing the Thoroughfare and Conception Vessels.

Formulas and herbs *Unicorn-Rearing Pill* (Yu Lin Zhu), composed of 15 g of *Radix Codonopsis Pilosulae* (Dang Shen), 10 g of *Poriae* (Fu Ling), 15 g of *Rhizoma Dioscoreae* (Shan Yao), 10 g of *Radix Rehmanniae Praeparata* (Shu Di Huang), 10 g of *Fructus Corni* (Shan Zhu Yu), 10 g of *Radix Angelicae Sinensis* (Dang Gui), 6 g of *Rhizoma Ligustici Chuanxiong* (Chuan Xiong), 10 g of *Radix Dipsaci* (Xu Duan), 10 g of *Semen Cuscutae* (Tu Si Zi), 10 g of *Cortex Eucommiae* (Du Zhong), 15 g of *Colla Cornus Cervi* (Lu Jiao Jiao) and 10 g of *Placenta Hominis* (Zi He Che).

Modification For severe lumbago and lower abdominal cold, *Fructus Foeniculi* (Xiao Hui Xiang), *Amethyst* (Zi Shi Ying) and *Epimedium davidii* (Xian Ling Pi) are added. For thin and profuse leukorrhea, *Semen Euryales* (Qian Shi) and *Rosae Laevigatae Fructus* (Jin Ying Zi) are added. For loose stool, *Semen Lablab Album* (Chao Bai Bian Dou), *Roasting Radix Aucklandiae* (Wei Mu

2.1 肾气亏损证

主要证候 婚后久不孕,月经初潮较晚,经期错后而至,量少色淡或暗,甚至经闭,面色晦暗黧黑,腰酸腿软,性欲淡漠,带下量多、清稀,小便清长,大便溏薄,妇科检查阴毛稀疏,子宫偏小,舌淡苔白,脉沉细或沉迟。

治法 温肾填精,补益冲任。

方药 代表方为毓麟珠;常用药如党参15克,茯苓10克,山药15克,熟地黄10克,山茱萸10克,当归10克,川芎6克,续断10克,菟丝子10克,杜仲10克,鹿角胶(霜)15克,紫河车10克。

加减 若腰酸如折,小腹清冷者,加小茴香、紫石英、淫羊藿;带下量多清稀者,加芡实、金樱子;大便溏薄者,加炒白扁豆、煨木香、炮姜;小便频数,加益智仁、桑螵蛸。

Xiang) and *Rhizoma Zingiberis Praeparata* (Pao Jiang) are added. For frequent urination, *Fructus Alpiniae Oxyphyllae* (Yi Zhi Ren) and *Ootheca Mantidis* (Sang Piao Xiao) are added.

Shanghai doctor CAI Xiaosun's experience prescription, *Kidney and Origin Fostering Prescription* (Yu Shen Pei Yuan Tang): 12 g of *Poriae* (Fu Ling), 10 g of *Radix Rehmanniae Cruda* (Sheng Di Huang), 10 g of *Radix Rehmanniae Praeparata* (Shu Di Huang), 10 g of *Rhizoma Curculiginis* (Xian Mao), 12 g of *Epimedium davidii* (Yin Yang Huo), 10 g of *Cervi Cornu Degelatinatum* (Lu Jiao Shuang), 10 g of *Fructus Ligustri Lucidi* (Nü Zhen Zi), 12 g of *Amethyst* (Zi Shi Ying), 10 g of *Radix Morindae Officinalis* (Ba Ji Tian), 12 g of *Ophiopogonis Radix* (Mai Dong) and 10 g of *Fructus Corni* (Shan Zhu Yu).

上海医家蔡小荪经验方(育肾培元方):茯苓12克,生地黄、熟地黄各10克,仙茅10克,仙灵脾12克,鹿角霜10克,女贞子10克,紫石英12克,巴戟天10克,麦冬12克,山茱萸10克。

2.2 Syndrome of liver and kidney insufficiency

2.2 肝肾不足证

Main manifestations No pregnancy long after marriage, delayed menstruation, scanty amount, light-colored or grayish menorrhea, even amenorrhea, emaciation, feverish sensation over palms, soles, and chest, dizziness, tinnitus, palpitation, insomnia, aching in the loins and weakness of legs, red tongue with scanty fur, taut pulse or thready and taut pulse.

主要证候 婚后久不怀孕,经期错后而至,量少色淡或暗,甚至经闭,形体消瘦,五心烦躁,头晕耳鸣,心悸失眠,腰酸腿软,舌质红,苔少,脉弦或细弦。

Therapeutic methods Boosting qi, nourishing blood, nourishing the liver and kidney.

治法 益气养血,滋补肝肾。

Formulas and herbs *Kidney Pills* (Zuo Gui Wan), composed of 12 g of *Radix Rehmanniae Praeparata* (Shu Di Huang), 12 g of *Rhizoma Dioscoreae* (Shan Yao), 9 g of *Fructus Corni* (Shan Zhu Yu), 10 g of *Semen Cuscutae* (Tu Si Zi), 12 g of *Fructus Lycii* (Gou Qi Zi), 9 g of *Radix Achyranthis Bidentatae* (Huai Niu Xi), 9 g of *Processed Plastrum Testudinis* (Zhi Gui Ban) and 10 g of

方药 代表方为左归丸;常用药如熟地黄12克,山药12克,山茱萸9克,菟丝子10克,枸杞子12克,怀牛膝9克,炙龟板9克,杜仲10克。

Cortex Eucommiae (Du Zhong).

Modification At the middle stage of menstruation, *Semen Leonuri* (Chong Wei Zi), *Herba Lycopi* (Ze Lan), *Radix Salviae Miltiorrhizae* (Dan Shen) and *Luffae Fructus Retinervus* (Si Gua Luo) are added to activate the blood, dredge the collaterals and boost ovulation. Before menstruation period, *Amethyst* (Zi Shi Ying), *Radix Morindae Officinalis* (Ba Ji Tian) and *Photiniae Folium* (Shi Nan Ye) are added to boost the kidney and warm the uterus, provide conditions for the implantation of the fertilized egg.

加减 经中期加用茺蔚子、泽兰、丹参、丝瓜络以活血通络，促排卵；经前期（黄体期）加用紫石英、巴戟天、石楠叶以益肾暖宫，为受精卵着床提供条件。

Shanghai doctor TANG Xiyuan's experience prescription: 12 g of *Stir-Fried Chinese Angelica* (Chao Dang Gui), 12 g of *Radix Rehmanniae Praeparata* (Shu Di Huang), 9 g of *Stir-Fried Rhizoma Ligustici Chuanxiong* (Chao Chuan Xiong), 9 g of *Stir-Fried Radix Paeoniae Alba* (Chao Bai Shao), 12 g of *Radix Dipsaci* (Xu Duan), 12 g of *Cortex Eucommiae* (Du Zhong), 12 g of *Ramulus Loranthi* (Sang Ji Sheng), 15 g of *Semen Cuscutae* (Tu Si Zi), 15 g of *Fructus Lycii* (Gou Qi Zi), 9 g of *Fructus Corni* (Shan Zhu Yu), 9 g of *Herba Cistanchis* (Rou Cong Rong), 6 g of *Pericarpium Citri Tangerinae* (Chen Pi) and 5 g of *Radix Glycyrrhizae* (Gan Cao).

上海医家唐锡元经验方：炒当归12克，熟地黄12克，炒川芎9克，炒白芍9克，续断12克，杜仲12克，桑寄生12克，菟丝子15克，枸杞子15克，山茱萸9克，肉苁蓉9克，陈皮6克，甘草5克。

2.3 Syndrome of qi and blood asthenia

Main manifestations No pregnancy long after marriage, scanty menorrhea with light color, or amenorrhea, sallow complexion, lusterless skin, physical weakness, low spirit, lassitude, dizziness, shortness of breath and palpitation, accompanied by maldevelopment of the uterus, light-colored tongue with white fur, thready and weak pulse.

Therapeutic methods Boosting and nourishing qi, activating blood and freeing menstruation.

Formulas and herbs *Eight Jewel Decoction* (Ba

2.3 气血虚弱证

主要证候 婚后多年不孕，月经量少色淡，或闭经，面色萎黄，肌肤不泽，形体虚弱，神疲乏力，头晕目眩，心悸气短，可伴子宫发育不良，舌淡苔白，脉细弱。

治法 益气养血，活血通经。

方药 代表方为八珍

Zhen Tang), composed of 15 g of *Radix Astragali* (Huang Qi), 12 g of *Radix Codonopsis Pilosulae* (Dang Shen), 10 g of *Rhizoma Atractylodis Macrocephalae* (Bai Zhu), 10 g of *Poriae* (Fu Ling), 20 g of *Rhizoma Dioscoreae* (Shan Yao), 10 g of *Radix Angelicae Sinensis* (Dang Gui), 6 g of *Rhizoma Ligustici Chuanxiong* (Chuan Xiong), 10 g of *Radix Paeoniae Alba* (Bai Shao), 10 g of *Radix Rehmanniae Praeparata* (Shu Di Huang), 12 g of *Fructus Ligustri Lucidi* (Nü Zhen Zi), 12 g of *Colla Corii Asini* (E Jiao) and 10 g of *Rhizoma Cyperi* (Xiang Fu).

汤;常用药如黄芪15克,党参12克,白术10克,茯苓10克,山药20克,当归10克,川芎6克,白芍10克,熟地黄10克,女贞子12克,阿胶12克,香附10克。

Modification For severe aching in the loins, *Dipsaci Radix* (Chuan Xu Duan), *Semen Cuscutae* (Tu Si Zi) and *Placenta Hominis* (Zi He Che) are added. For palpitation, *Semen Zizyphi Spinosae* (Suan Zao Ren) and *Radix Polygalae* (Yuan Zhi) are added. For restless sleep in the night, *Radix Polygoni Multiflori* (He Shou Wu) and *Caulis Polygoni Multiflori* (Ye Jiao Teng) are added. For aversion to cold and cold limbs, *Fructus Psoraleae* (Bu Gu Zhi) and *Aconiti Radix Lateralis Tosta* (Pao Fu Zi) are added.

加减 若腰酸甚者,加川续断、菟丝子、紫河车;心悸怔忡者,加酸枣仁、远志;夜寐欠安,加何首乌、夜交藤;畏寒肢冷,加补骨脂、炮附片。

Shanghai doctor LE Xiu zhen's experience prescription: 12 g of *Cervi Cornu Sectum* (Lu Jiao Pian), 12 g of *Dioscoreae Rhizoma* (Huai Shan Yao), 12 g of *Radix Dipsaci* (Xu Duan), 12 g of *Aconiti Radix Lateralis Tosta* (Pao Fu Zi), 12 g of *Epimedium davidii* (Xian Ling Pi), 6 g of *Rhizoma Acori Graminei* (Shi Chang Pu), 9 g of *Radix Codonopsis Pilosulae* (Dang Shen), 9 g of *Rhizoma Atractylodis Macrocephalae* (Bai Zhu), 9 g of *Radix Paeoniae Alba* (Bai Shao), 12 g *Radix Angelicae Sinensis* (Dang Gui), 12 g of *Radix Rehmanniae Praeparata* (Shu Di Huang), 6 g of *Rhizoma Ligustici Chuanxiong* (Chuan Xiong), 6 g of *Radix Glycyrrhizae Praeparata* (Zhi Gan Cao) and 6 g of *Placenta Hominis Pulverata* (Zi He Che Fen)(to be swallowed).

上海医家乐秀珍经验方:鹿角片12克(先),炒山药12克,续断12克,炮附片12克,仙灵脾12克,石菖蒲16克,党参9克,白术9克,白芍9克,当归12克,熟地黄12克,川芎6克,炙甘草6克,紫河车粉6克(后)。

2.4 Syndrome of liver and heart qi stagnation

Main manifestations No pregnancy long after marriage, mental upset, depression, irritability, irregular menstruation, scanty menorrhea with blackish color, or unsmooth menorrhea, or abdominal pain during menstruation, distending pain in the breasts before menstruation, discomfort in the chest and hypochondria, insomnia and dreaminess, deep-red tongue with thin and white fur, taut pulse or thready pulse.

Therapeutic methods Soothing the liver to relieve depression and regulating qi and blood.

Formulas and herbs *Depression-Opening Jade-Planting Decoction* (Kai Yu Zhong Yu Tang), composed of 12 g of *Radix Angelicae Sinensis* (Dang Gui), 12 g of *Radix Paeoniae Rubra* (Chi Shao), 12 g of *Radix Paeoniae Alba* (Bai Shao), 10 g of *Rhizoma Atractylodis Macrocephalae* (Bai Zhu), 10 g of *Poriae* (Fu Ling), 10 g of *Rhizoma Cyperi* (Xiang Fu), 6 g of *Pericarpium Citri Reticulatae Viride* (Qing Pi), 6 g of *Radix Bupleuri* (Chai Hu), 10 g of *Radix Curcumae* (Yu Jin), 6 g of *Fructus Meliae Toosendan* (Chuan Lian Zi), 10 g of *Rhizoma Corydalis* (Yan Hu Suo), 10 g of *Radix Salviae Miltiorrhizae* (Dan Shen) and 10 g of *Radix Achyranthis Bidentatae* (Niu Xi).

Modification For unsmooth menorrhea, *Flos Carthami* (Hong Hua), *Herba Leonuri* (Yi Mu Cao), *Fructus Crataegi* (Shan Zha) and *Herba Lycopi* (Ze Lan) are added. For distending pain and nodules in the breasts, *Folium Citri Reticulatae* (Ju Ye), *Semen Citri Reticulatae* (Ju He), *Fructus Trichosanthis* (Quan Gua Lou) and *Liquidambaris Fructus* (Lu Lu Tong) are added. For restlessness

2.4 心肝气郁证

主要证候 婚后多年不孕，精神不安，抑郁烦躁，月经先后不定期，量少色暗，或经行不畅，或经期腹痛，经前乳房胀痛，胸胁不舒，失眠多梦，舌质暗红，苔薄白，脉弦或细弦。

治法 疏肝解郁，调和气血。

方药 代表方为开郁种玉汤；常用药如当归 12 克，赤芍、白芍各 12 克，白术 10 克，茯苓 10 克，香附 10 克，青皮 6 克，柴胡 6 克，郁金 10 克，川楝子 6 克，延胡索 10 克，丹参 10 克，牛膝 10 克。

加减 若经行不畅者，加红花、益母草、山楂、泽兰；乳房胀痛结块者，加橘叶、橘核、全瓜蒌、路路通；烦躁易怒者，加栀子、丹皮、钩藤；头晕耳鸣，加女贞子、桑椹子。

and susceptibility to rage, *Fructus Gardeniae* (Zhi Zi), *Cortex Moutan Radicis* (Mu Dan Pi) and *Ramulus Uncariae cum Uncis* (Gou Teng) are added. For dizziness and tinnitus, *Fructus Ligustri Lucidi* (Nü Zhen Zi) and *Fructus Mori* (Sang Shen Zi) are added.

3 Other therapeutic methods:

3.1 Chinese patent drugs

(1) *An Kun Zan Yu Pill* (An Kun Zan Yu Wan): 1 pill each time and twice a day, applicable to the treatment of kidney qi asthenia syndrome.

(2) *Ding Kun Bolus* (Ding Kun Dan): 1 bolus each time after menstruation and twice a day, applicable to the treatment of kidney qi asthenia syndrome.

(3) *Mugwort and Cyperus Uterus-Warming Pill* (Ai Fu Nuan Gong Wan): 5 g each time and twice a day, applicable to the treatment of cold syndrome.

(4) *Menstruation-Regulating and Seed-Planting Pill* (Tiao Jing Zhong Zi Wan): 1 pill each time and twice a day, applicable to the treatment of kidney asthenia and blood stasis syndrome.

3.2 Empirical and folk recipes

(1) *Tremella Decoction* (Mu Er Tang), composed of 30 g of *Tremella* (Bai Mu Er), 8 g of *Colla Cornus Cervi* (Lu Jiao Jiao)and 15 g of *Rock Candy* (Bing Tang). *Tremella* (Bai Mu Er) is washed and cooked in proper amount of water. Then *Rock Candy* (Bing Tang) and *Colla Cornus Cervi* (Lu Jiao Jiao) are added into the decoction. This decoction is applicable to the treatment of kidney yin asthenia syndrome.

(2) 500 g of black-boned chicken, 60 g of

3 其他疗法

3.1 中成药

（1）安坤赞育丸：每次1丸，每日2次，适用于肾气亏损证。

（2）定坤丹：于经净后每次1丸，每日2次，适用于肾气亏损证。

（3）艾附暖宫丸：每次5克，每日2次，适用于寒证。

（4）调经种子丸：每次1丸，每日2次，适用于肾虚血瘀证。

3.2 单验方

（1）木耳汤：白木耳30克，鹿角胶8克，冰糖15克，将白木耳洗净，加水适量，煎熬后，加入鹿角胶和冰糖搅拌均匀，熬至烊化，适用于肾阴虚证。

（2）乌骨鸡500克，当归

Radix Angelicae Sinensis (Dang Gui) and 3 slices of ginger are decocted in water with proper amount of salt. The decoction is taken orally in seven days, applicable to the treatment of blood asthenia syndrome.

60克，生姜3片，盐适量，煎汤，分7日服，适用于血虚证。

(3) 100 g of *Placenta Hominis* (Zi He Che) is ground into powder and put into capsules for oral taking, applicable to the treatment of kidney asthenia syndrome.

(3) 紫河车100克打粉，装入胶囊，分次服，适用于肾虚证。

Secondary sterility

继发性不孕症

Failure to be pregnant without contraceptions in one year after last pregnancy is called secondary sterility. Secondary sterility is usually due to improper care during menstruation and after delivery, or intemperance in sexual life and invasion of pathogenic factors into the uterus to coagulate with blood leading to downward migration of blood stasis or damp-heat to block the uterine collaterals as well as the Thoroughfare and Conception Vessels, or due to emotional upsets, stagnation of liver qi, disharmony between qi and blood as well as obstruction of the Thoroughfare and Conception Vessels, leading to failure of two essences in mergence, or due to obesity, excessive intake of greasy and rich foods, leading to endogenous phlegm-dampness, and obstructing the Thoroughfare and Conception Vessels. It is similar to sterility caused by salpingitis, endometriosis and immune disorder in Western medicine.

曾孕育过，未避孕又1年以上未再受孕者，称为继发性不孕。继发性不孕的发生常因经期、产后摄生不慎，或房事不节，邪入胞宫，与血相搏结，以致瘀血或湿热下注，胞脉受阻，任脉不通，两精不能攒合而不孕。或因七情内伤，肝气郁结，疏泄失常，气血不和，冲任瘀滞而至不孕。或因素体肥胖，恣食膏粱厚味，以致痰湿内生，冲任胞脉闭塞，而致不能摄精成孕。相当于西医输卵管炎症造成的阻塞性不孕、子宫内膜异位症的不孕、免疫性不孕等。

1 Key points for diagnosis

1 诊断要点

1.1 General condition

1.1 一般情况

Failure to be pregnant without contraceptions

婚后曾有过妊娠，以后

in one year after last pregnancy, accompanied by irregular menstruation, premenstrual distention or distending pain in the breasts, dysmenorrhea, aching, prolapsing and distending pain in the loins and abdomen, abnormal changes of leukorrhea, mass in the abdomen, occasional low fever, sexual frigidity, dyspareunia, coital pain or anxiety, insomnia and depression.

未避孕连续 1 年未再受孕，常伴有月经失调及经前乳胀或胀痛，痛经，腰腹酸胀坠痛，带下异常，腹部有包块，时有低热，性欲淡漠，性交障碍，性交痛，或有焦虑、失眠、忧郁等精神异常表现。

1.2 Auxiliary examination

1.2 辅助检查

(1) Fallopian tube potency test: Hysterosalpingography is helpful for detecting morbid changes in the uterus and conditions of oviduct. Abdominoscopy and uteroscopy are helpful for direct observation of the pelvic organs, and inflammation and mass of the reproductive system inside the uterus.

(1) 输卵管通畅检查：子宫输卵管造影术可了解宫腔病变及输卵管通畅程度；腹腔镜、宫腔镜检查则可直观盆腔脏器及宫腔内有无生殖系统炎症、肿块等。

(2) B ultrasonic examination is helpful for understanding whether there are organic changes of the uterus and ovary, and detecting follicular development and ovulation.

(2) B 超检查：可了解子宫、卵巢有无器质性病变及监测卵泡发育与排卵。

(3) Hormone level test: To analyze whether there is any abnormality in the function of ovary, pituitary gland and hypothalamus, affecting ovulation.

(3) 内分泌水平测定：以分析卵巢、垂体及下丘脑功能有无异常而影响排卵。

(4) PCT tests the ability of semen in penetrating cervical mucus and its survival.

(4) 性交后试验(PCT)：以测试精子穿透宫颈黏液的能力与存活情况。

(5) Immunological examination of serum and cervical mucus is done to determine whether sterility is immune sterility or not.

(5) 血清及宫颈黏液免疫学检查：以确定是否为免疫性不孕。

2 Syndrome differentiation and treatment

2 辨证论治

The secondary sterility may be traced back to the history of pregnancy, abortion or other diseases that may cause sterility. It is usually marked by as-

继发性不孕症可追溯其妊娠或流产史，或有可致不孕的其他病史。常有本虚标

thenia in the constitution and sthenia in the symptoms or syndrome mixed with asthenia and sthenia. Clinically, by the four diagnostic methods of "Observation, Auscultation-Olfaction, Interrogation and Palpation" for diagnosing and inspecting diseases, the pathological situations are understood to make a careful differentiation and analysis. Based upon the principles of "checking the causative reason for deciding the therapy, treating the diseases for the original factors", the asthenia syndrome should be treated by the attacking method and the sthenia syndrome should be treated by the reinforcing method. For instance, if menstruation, leucorrhea and abdominal lump exist, it is appropriate to treat diseases first, before the attempt to regulate menstruation and promote fertilization. In combination of the therapy to benefit the kidney and regulate menstrual cycle, it is appropriate to benefit the kidney and nourish yin and blood, together with the herbal drugs to dredge the collaterals, in the later stage of menstruation. When yin and yang grow up in the early stage of menstruation, it is appropriate to seek from yin, and warm up the kidney and uterus.

实，或虚实夹杂之证，临证通过"望、闻、问、切"四种诊察疾病的手段，了解病情，作出仔细辨析，遵循"审因论治，治病求本"原则，实者攻之，虚者补之。如有经带癥瘕等症，宜先治疾病，再予调经种子。结合益肾调周疗法，经后期益肾滋阴养血，且配以通络之品；经前期阴生阳长，治宜阴中求阳，温肾暖宫。

2.1 Syndrome of qi stagnation and blood stasis

Main manifestations Having pregnant experience after marriage, sterility for years due to abortion, premature delivery and gynecological operation, delayed menstruation, scanty and unsmooth menorrhea with purplish and blackish color or with blood clot, often accompanied by dysmenorrhea, pain aggaravated by pressure in the lower abdomen, purplish and blackish tongue or with ecchymoses, taut and unsmooth pulse.

2.1 气滞血瘀证

主要证候 婚后曾受孕，因流产、早产及妇科手术后多年不孕，月经后期，量少不畅，经血紫黑，或有血块，常伴痛经，小腹胀痛拒按，舌紫暗，或有瘀点，脉弦涩。

Therapeutic methods Activating blood and resolving stasis, moving qi and freeing meridians.

Formulas and herbs Lesser Abdomen Stasis-Expelling Decoction (Shao Fu Zhu Yu Tang), composed of 12 g of *Radix Angelicae Sinensis* (Dang Gui), 10 g of *Radix Paeoniae Rubra* (Chi Shao), 6 g of *Rhizoma Ligustici Chuanxiong* (Chuan Xiong), 10 g of *Semen Persicae* (Tao Ren), 10 g of *Flos Carthami* (Hong Hua), 10 g of *Radix Cyathulae* (Chuan Niu Xi), 12 g of *Faeces Trogopterorum* (Wu Ling Zhi), 10 g of *Rhizoma Cyperi* (Xiang Fu), 10 g of *Radix Linderae* (Wu Yao), 10 g of *Fructus Aurantii* (Zhi Qiao), 15 g of *Radix Salviae Miltiorrhizae* (Dan Shen) and 12 g of *Rhizoma Corydalis* (Yan Hu Suo).

Modification For stabbing pain in lower abdomen, restlessness and susceptibility to rage before menstruation, *Radix Rehmanniae Praeparata* (Shu Di Huang) is deleted while *Radix Bupleuri* (Chai Hu) and *Radix Curcumae* (Yu Jin) are added. For aching lumbus and knees, insidious pain in abdomen, blood clot in menorrhea, *Caulis Sargentodoxae* (Da Xue Teng) is deleted while *Semen Cuscutae* (Tu Si Zi) and *Epimedium davidii* (Xian Ling Pi) are added. For thirst with dry throat and constipated stool, *Radix Rehmanniae Praeparata* (Shu Di Huang) is deleted while *Radix Rehmanniae Cruda* (Sheng Di Huang), *Cortex Moutan Radicis* (Mu Dan Pi) and *Radix Scutellariae* (Huang Qin) are added.

Shanghai doctor DAI Deying's experience prescription: composed of 9 g of *Semen Persicae* (Tao Ren), 6 g of *Flos Carthami* (Hong Hua), 10 g of *Radix Paeoniae Rubra* (Chi Shao), 12 g of *Typhae Pollen* (Pu Huang), 9 g of *Radix*

治法 活血化瘀，行气通络。

方药 代表方为少腹逐瘀汤；常用药如当归 12 克，赤芍 10 克，川芎 6 克，桃仁 10 克，红花 10 克，川牛膝 10 克，五灵脂 12 克，香附 10 克，乌药 10 克，枳壳 10 克，丹参 15 克，延胡索 12 克。

加减 若经前下腹刺痛，烦躁易怒者，去熟地黄，加柴胡、郁金；平素腰膝酸软，小腹隐痛，经行有块者，去红藤，加菟丝子、仙灵脾；口渴咽干，大便燥结者，去熟地黄，加生地黄、牡丹皮、黄芩。

上海医家戴德英经验方：桃仁 9 克，红花 6 克，赤芍 10 克，蒲黄 12 克，木香 9 克，地龙 9 克，黄芪 15 克，路路通 12 克，炙甘草 3

Aucklandiae (Mu Xiang), 9 g of *Lumbricus* (Di Long), 15 g of *Radix Astragali* (Huang Qi), 12 g of *Liquidambaris Fructus* (Lu Lu Tong), 3 g of *Radix Glycyrrhizae Praeparata* (Zhi Gan Cao), 12 g of *Rubiae Radix* (Qian Cao), 12 g of *Fructus Aurantii* (Zhi Qiao), 15 g of *Os Sepiellae seu Sepiae* (Hai Piao Xiao, Wu Zei Gu), 12 g of *Semen Coicis* (Yi Yi Ren), 30 g of *Caulis Sargentodoxae* (Hong Teng), 9 g of *Spina Gleditsiae* (Zao Jiao Ci) and 12 g of *Herba Salviae Chinensis* (Shi Jian Chuan).

克，茜草12克，枳壳12克，海螵蛸15克，薏苡仁12克，红藤30克，皂角刺9克，石见穿12克。

Shanghai doctor CHEN Danian's experience prescription: composed of 12 g of *Radix Angelicae Sinensis* (Dang Gui), 9 g of *Rhizoma Ligustici Chuanxiong* (Chuan Xiong), 9 g of *Rhizoma Cyperi* (Xiang Fu), 9 g of *Herba Lycopi* (Ze Lan), 9 g of *Flos Carthami* (Hong Hua), 12 g of *Radix Salviae Miltiorrhizae* (Dan Shen), 15 g of *Radix Achyranthis Bidentatae* (Niu Xi, Huai Niu Xi), 3 g of *Folium Artemistae Argyi* (Ai Ye), 12 g of *Radix Dipsaci* (Xu Duan), 15 g of *Herba Leonuri* (Yi Mu Cao) and 15 g of *Flos Rosae Chinensis* (Yue Ji Hua).

上海医家陈大年经验方：当归12克，川芎9克，香附9克，泽兰9克，红花9克，丹参12克，牛膝15克，艾叶3克，续断12克，益母草15克，月季花15克。

Shanghai doctor TANG Xiyuan's experience prescription: composed of 12 g of *Chinese Angelica* (Chao Dang Gui), 9 g of *Rhizoma Ligustici Chuanxiong* (Chao Chuan Xiong), 9 g of *Radix Paeoniae Rubra* (Chao Chi Shao), 9 g of *Herba Lycopi* (Ze Lan), 15 g of *Herba Leonuri* (Yi Mu Cao), 9 g of *Semen Persicae* (Tao Ren), 9 g of *Flos Carthami* (Hong Hua), 15 g of *Radix Cyathulae* (Chuan Niu Xi), 15 g of *Liquidambaris Fructus* (Lu Lu Tong), 6 g of *Pericarpium Citri Tangerinae* (Chen Pi) and 5 g of *Radix Glycyrrhizae* (Gan Cao).

上海医家唐锡元经验方：炒当归12克，炒川芎9克，炒赤芍9克，泽兰9克，益母草15克，桃仁9克，红花9克，川牛膝15克，路路通15克，陈皮6克，甘草5克。

2.2 Syndrome of interior retention of phlegm and dampness

2.2 痰湿内阻证

Main manifestations Sterility for years due to abortion after marriage, obesity, bright pale complexion, profuse and sticky leukorrhea, scanty and delayed menorrhea, or even amenorrhea, chest oppression and nausea, lassitude and fatigue, sexual

主要证候 婚后曾因流产而后多年不孕，形体肥胖，面色㿠白，头晕心悸，白带量多、质稠黏，月经后期量少，甚或闭经，胸闷泛恶，倦怠乏

frigidity, pale bulgy tongue with whitish greasy fur and slippery pulse.

力,性欲淡漠,舌淡胖,苔白腻,脉滑。

Therapeutic methods Drying up dampness and resolving phlegm, strengthening the spleen and regulating qi.

治法 燥湿化痰,健脾理气。

Formulas and herbs *Uterus-Activating Pill* (Qi Gong Wan), composed of 10 g of *Rhizoma Pinelliae* (Ban Xia), 10 g of *Rhizoma Atractylodis* (Cang Zhu), 10 g of *Rhizoma Atractylodis Macrocephalae* (Bai Zhu), 10 g of *Poriae* (Fu Ling), 10 g of *Pericarpium Citri Tangerinae* (Chen Pi), 10 g of *Massa Fermentata Medicinalis* (Shen Qu), 8 g of *Rhizoma Acori Graminei* (Shi Chang Pu), 6 g of *Cortex Magnoliae Officinalis* (Hou Pu), 10 g of *Rhizoma Cyperi* (Xiang Fu), 6 g of *Rhizoma Ligustici Chuanxiong* (Chuan Xiong), 10 g of *Radix Polygalae* (Yuan Zhi) and 15 g of *Sargassum* (Hai Zao).

方药 代表方为启宫丸;常用药如半夏 10 克,苍术 10 克,白术 10 克,茯苓 10 克,陈皮 10 克,神曲 10 克,石菖蒲 8 克,厚朴 6 克,香附 10 克,川芎 6 克,远志 10 克,海藻 15 克。

Modification For dizziness and headache, *Rhizoma seu Radix Notopterygii* (Qiang Huo) and *Fructus Tribuli* (Bai Ji Li) are added. For lumbago and tinnitus, *Cortex Eucommiae* (Du Zhong), *Fructus Psoraleae* (Bu Gu Zhi) and *Semen Cuscutae* (Tu Si Zi) are added. For chest oppression and anorexia, *Semen Coicis* (Yi Yi Ren) and *Herba Eupatorii* (Pei Lan) are added. For delayed menstruation with scanty menorrhea, *Semen Persicae* (Tao Ren) and *Flos Carthami* (Hong Hua) are added.

加减 若头晕头痛者,加羌活、白蒺藜;腰痛耳鸣者,加杜仲、补骨脂、菟丝子;胸闷、纳呆者,加薏苡仁、佩兰;月经错后量少者,加桃仁、红花。

2.3 Syndrome of downward migration of damp-heat

2.3 湿热下注证

Main manifestations Sterility for years, profuse and sticky leukorrhea with white or yellow color and foul smell, lowerabdominal pain, irregular menstruation, red tongue with yellow and greasy fur as well as taut and rapid pulse.

主要证候 多年不孕,带下量多,质地稠黏,色白或黄,时有臭味,少腹疼痛,月经失调,舌红,苔黄腻,脉弦数。

Therapeutic methods Clearing away heat and eliminating dampness, regulating the Thoroughfare and Conception Vessels.

Formulas and herbs *Mysterious Four Pill* (Si Miao Wan) combined with *Sargentodoxa and Patrinia Powder* (Hong Teng Bai Jiang San), composed of 10 g of *Cortex Phellodendri* (Huang Bo), 10 g of *Rhizoma Atractylodis* (Cang Zhu), 10 g of *Radix Achyranthis Bidentatae* (Niu Xi), 15 g of *Semen Coicis* (Yi Yi Ren), 15 g of *Caulis Sargentodoxae* (Hong Teng), 12 g of *Herba Patriniae* (Bai Jiang Cao), 10 g of *Poriae* (Fu Ling), 10 g of *Rhizoma Cyperi* (Xiang Fu), 10 g of *Rhizoma Corydalis* (Yan Hu Suo), 12 g of *Liquidambaris Fructus* (Lu Lu Tong), 15 g of *Herba Aristolochiae* (Tian Xian Teng) and 10 g of *Fructus Aurantii* (Zhi Qiao).

Modification For lower abdominal distending pain, *Olibanum Praeparatum* (Zhi Ru Xiang) and *Myrrha Praeparata* (Zhi Mo Yao) are added. For yellow and gray tongue fur and bitter taste in the mouth, *Rhizoma Arisaematis cum Bile* (Dan Nan Xing) and *Pericarpium Trichosanthis* (Gua Lou Pi) are added. For profuse leukorrhea, *Rhizoma Smilacis Glabrae* (Tu Fu Ling), *Rhizoma Alismatis* (Ze Xie) and *Toonae Radicis Cortex* (Chun Gen Pi) are added.

Shanghai doctor CAI Xiaosun's experience description: composed of 12 g of *Poriae* (Fu Ling), 2.5 g of *Ramulus Cinnamomi* (Gui Zhi), 4.5 g of *Radix Bupleuri Tip* (Chai Hu Qiao), 9 g of *Radix Paeoniae Rubra* (Chi Shao), 20 g of *Herba Patriniae* (Bai Jiang Cao), 9 g of *Cortex Moutan Radicis* (Mu Dan Pi), 20 g of *Commelinae Herba* (Ya Zhi Cao), 9 g of *Toosendan Fructus* (Jin Ling Zi), 15 g of *Caulis Sargentodoxae* (Da Xue Teng), 9 g of *Rhizoma Corydalis* (Yan Hu

治法　清化湿热，调理冲任。

方药　代表方为四妙丸合红藤败酱散；常用药如黄柏10克，苍术10克，牛膝10克，薏苡仁15克，红藤15克，败酱草12克，茯苓10克，香附10克，延胡索10克，路路通12克，天仙藤15克，枳壳10克。

加减　若小腹胀痛者，加制乳香、制没药；苔黄腻，口苦者，加胆南星、瓜蒌皮；带下过多者，加土茯苓、泽泻、椿根皮。

上海医家蔡小荪经验方：茯苓12克，桂枝2.5克，柴胡梢4.5克，赤芍9克，败酱草20克，牡丹皮9克，鸭跖草20克，金铃子9克，红藤15克，延胡索9克，怀牛膝9克。

Suo) and 9 g of *Radix Achyranthis Bidentatae* (Huai Niu Xi).

3 Other therapeutic methods

3.1 Chinese patent drugs

(1) *Tangkuei Pill* (Dang Gui Wan): Take 15 g each time and twice a day, applicable to the treatment of qi stagnation and blood stasis syndrome.

(2) *Eight-Gem Leonurus (Motherwort) Pill* (Yi Mu Ba Zhen Wan): Take 10 g each time and three times a day, applicable to the treatment of qi stagnation and blood stasis syndrome.

(3) *Gynecologic Qianjin Tablets* (Fu Ke Qian Jin Pian): Take 10 g each time and twice a day, applicable to the treatment of damp-heat syndrome.

3.2 Empirical and folk recipes

Shanghai doctor CAI Xiaosun's experience prescription: composed of 15 g of *Spina Gleditsiae* (Zao Jiao Ci), 9 g of *Semen Vaccariae* (Wang Bu Liu Xing Zi), 9 g of *Rosae Chinensis Flos* (Yue Ji Hua), 9 g of *Lumbricus* (Di Long) and 3 g of *Sliced Dalbergiae Lignum Pulveratum* (Jiang Xiang Pian), applicable to the treatment of obstruction, incomplete obstruction and hydrops of the fallopian tube. It should not be taken after mid-menstruation.

3.3 External therapy

(1) Enema: *Oviduct-Freeing Decoction* (Tong Guan Tang), composed of *Radix Angelicae Sinensis* (Dang Gui), *Radix Paeoniae Rubra* (Chi Shao), *Flos Carthami* (Hong Hua), *Herba Taraxaci* (Pu Gong Ying), *Spina Gleditsiae* (Zao Jiao Ci), *Herba Patriniae* (Bai Jiang Cao), *Caulis Sargentodoxae* (Da Xue Teng), *Semen Persicae* (Tao Ren), *Rhizoma Ligustici Chuanxiong* (Chuan Xiong), *Radix Bupleuri* (Chai Hu), *Rhizoma Cyperi* (Xiang

3 其他疗法

3.1 中成药

(1) 当归丸：每次服 15 克，每日 2 次，适用于气滞血瘀证。

(2) 益母八珍丸：每次服 10 克，每日 3 次，适用于气滞血瘀证。

(3) 妇科千金片：每次服 10 克，每日 2 次，适用于湿热证。

3.2 单验方

上海医家蔡小荪经验方：皂角刺 15 克，王不留行子 9 克，月季花 9 克，广地龙 9 克，降香片 3 克，适用于输卵管阻塞、不完全阻塞及积水者，月经中期以后不宜服用。

3.3 外治法

(1) 灌肠法：通管汤（当归、赤芍、红花、蒲公英、皂角刺、败酱草、红藤、桃仁、川芎、柴胡、香附、路路通各 15 克，加 300 毫升水，煎成 100 毫升），保留灌肠，每日 1 次，10 次为 1 个疗程，经期停用，可治疗因附件炎症、输卵管阻塞所致不孕症。

Fu) and *Liquidambaris Fructus* (Lu Lu Tong) (15 g for each). These herbs are decocted in 300 ml of water into 100 ml of decoction for enema. This treatment is given once a day and 10 times make up one course of treatment, applicable to the treatment of sterility due to inflammation of appendage and obstruction of oviduct. It should be suspended during menstruation.

(2) Hot compression: 20 g of *Radix Salviae Miltiorrhizae* (Dan Shen), 15 g of *Spina Gleditsiae* (Zao Jiao Ci), 30 g of *Herba Speranskia Tuberculata* (Tou Gu Cao), 20 g of *Cortex Cinnamomi* (Rou Gui), 20 g of *Flos Carthami* (Hong Hua), 10 g of *Radix Aconiti* (Chuan Wu), 10 g of *Radix Clematidis* (Wei Ling Xian), 6 g of *Myrrha* (Mo Yao), 6 g of *Resina Olibani* (Ru Xiang), 20 g of *Radix Paeoniae Rubra* (Chi Shao) and 20 g of *Radix Angelicae Sinensis* (Dang Gui) are ground into fine powder. The powder, after being steamed with a little alcohol, is applied to both sides of the abdomen. This compression is applied once a day and 40 minutes each time. 10 days make up one course of treatment.

(2) 热敷法:丹参 20 克,皂角刺 15 克,透骨草 30 克,肉桂 20 克,红花 20 克,川乌 10 克,威灵仙 10 克,没药 6 克,乳香 6 克,赤芍 20 克,当归 20 克,研成细末,滴少许白酒蒸后热敷于下腹两侧,每日 1 次,热敷约 40 分钟,10 日为 1 个疗程。

Chapter 4 Edeitis

第4章 生殖器官炎症

Pelvic inflammation

Pelvic inflammatory disease refers to the a group of infectious diseases of the genital tract in females, including endometritis, salpingitis, tuboovarian abscess, pelvic peritonitis, and salpingitis most commonly. Inflammation may be confined to one area, and can also involve several parts at the same time. Pelvic inflammatory disease occurs mostly in childbearing age. Before menarche, postmenopausal or unmarried persons rarely suffer form the disease. If it happens, it may be diffused inflammation from adjacent organs mostly. Acute pelvic inflammatory disease can cause diffuse peritonitis, sepsis, septic shock, can be life-threatening in severe cases. If acute pelvic inflammatory disease is not treated timely and correctly, it may be converted to sequelae of pelvic inflammatory disease, causing infertility, tubal pregnancy, chronic pelvic pain and rccurrcnt inflammation, etc.

The disease is usually caused by improper recuperation after delivery or abortion, improper sexual intercourse during menstruation or infection of pathogenic toxin and retention of damp-heat in the

盆腔炎性疾病

盆腔炎性疾病指女性上生殖道的一组感染性疾病，主要包括子宫内膜炎、输卵管炎、输卵管卵巢脓肿、盆腔腹膜炎，最常见的是输卵管炎。炎症可局限于一个部位，也可同时累及几个部位。盆腔炎性疾病大多发生在育龄期。初潮前、绝经后或未婚者很少发病，若发生也往往是邻近器官炎症的扩散。急性盆腔炎发展可引起弥漫性腹膜炎、败血症、感染性休克、严重者可危及生命；若急性盆腔炎未能得到及时正确的治疗，可转为盆腔炎性疾病后遗症，引起不孕、输卵管妊娠、慢性盆腔痛及炎症反复发作等。

本病多因产后或流产后摄生不慎，经期房事不节，感染邪毒，湿热邪毒瘀滞于子宫、胞脉、胞络所致。其主要

uterus and uterine collaterals. The main mechanism is the struggle between constitutional energy and evil, including dampness, heat, stasis and toxin in the uterus and uterine collaterals, resulting in inhibited movement of qi and blood, blood stasis, or retention of lumps in the uterus, extracellular medium, simmers into pus.

机理为湿、热、瘀、毒交结，邪正相争于胞宫、胞脉，邪与气血相搏结，致气血运行不畅，瘀血内阻，或在胞中结块，蕴积成脓。

1　Key points for diagnosis

1　诊断要点

1.1　Medical history

1.1　病史

The patients may have unclean sexual activity during menstruation and after childbirth, or gynecological surgery, or past genital tract inflammation.

可有经行、产后房室不洁，或妇科手术，或既往有生殖道炎症病史。

1.2　Symptoms

1.2　症状

There are lower abdominal pain, fever, increased vaginal discharge. Abdominal pain was persistent, aggravated after fatigue or sexual intercourse. The severe patients may have chills, high fever, headache. The onset of the disease during menstruation may causean increase in the amount and prolonged duration of menstruation. If peritonitis happens, there could be nausea, vomiting, abdominal distension, diarrhea. If absess is formed, there could be abdominal mass and local irritation symptoms, such as difficult urination, frequent urination, painful urination or bowel movement problems. If outside of peritoneum, there could be diarrhea, tenesmus.

主要有下腹痛，发热，带下增多。腹痛呈持续性，劳累或性交后加重；严重者有寒战、高热、头痛；月经期发病则引起经量增多、经期延长；若有腹膜炎，则可有恶心、呕吐、腹胀、腹泻；若有脓肿形成，可有下腹包块及局部刺激症状；如排尿困难、尿频、尿痛，或排便困难；若在腹膜外可致腹泻、里急后重。

1.3　Examinations

1.3　检查

(1) Gynecological examinations: Muscle tension in lower abdomen, tenderness, rebound tenderness; vaginal congestion, secretions in purulence, profuse amount and odor, cervical, lifting pain; u-

（1）妇科检查：下腹部肌紧张、压痛、反跳痛；阴道充血，分泌物呈脓血性，量多，有臭气；宫颈抬举痛；宫体稍

terus slightly-enlarged, tenderness, limitation of activity; tenderness on both sides of the uterus, or palpable mass, full posterior fornix with fluctuation in those with pelvic abscess in the lower position.

大,压痛,活动受限;子宫两侧压痛明显,或可触及包块;盆腔脓肿位置较低者,则后穹隆饱满,有波动感。

(2) Laboratory tests and other tests: ① blood routine tests: leukocytes and neutrophils increased; ② erythrocyte sedimentation rate > 20 mm/h; ③ cervical secretions: white blood cells are seen in smears, pathogens culture and drug sensitivity test; ④ B ultrasound: visible pelvic fluid or mass; ⑤ Culdocentesis: if ultrasound shows effusion in the womb rectum concave, pathogens may be detected through secretion culture of punctured pus. ⑥ laparoscopy: hyperemia of the tubal surface, edema in tubal wall, purulent exudate in fimbriated extremity and serosal surface of fallopian.

(2)实验室检查与其他检查:①血常规检查:白细胞总数及中性粒细胞增高;②血沉>20毫米/小时;③宫颈管分泌物:涂片检查见白细胞,病原体培养及药敏试验;④B超:可见盆腔积液或包块;⑤后穹窿穿刺:若B超显示子宫直肠陷凹积液,穿刺抽出脓液做分泌物培养可检测病原体。⑥腹腔镜:输卵管表面明显充血,输卵管管壁水肿,输卵管伞端或浆膜面有脓性渗出物。

2 Syndrome differentiation and treatment

The main symptom in pelvic inflammation is lower abdominal pain. Clinically syndrome differentiation should be done in light of the nature and degree of pain as well as the accompanying symptoms. Usually the syndrome with sudden onset and severe pain accompanied by chills and high fever pertains to heat and sthenia. While the syndrome with incomplete treatment, long duration or slow onset is marked by a mixture of cold and heat as well as asthenia and sthenia. Clinically, it is necessary to make a careful investigation.

2 辨证论治

本病的主症是下腹疼痛,临证应当根据疼痛的性质、程度及其伴有症状进行辨证论治。一般情况下,凡起病急,疼痛剧烈,伴寒战高热者,多属热属实;若未能彻底治疗,而病状缠绵不愈,或起病较缓者,往往寒热虚实混杂可见,临床当仔细审证。

Acute pelvic inflammation is characterized by acute onset, severe condition and fast transmission. The main causes are mainly toxic heat, plus damp-

急性盆腔炎发病急,病情重,传变快。病因以热毒为主,兼有湿、瘀。治法以清

ness and blood stasis. Therapeutic method is mainly clearing away heat and resolving toxin, assisted by dissipating dampness and dissolving blood stasis. The treatment must be prompt and complete, so as to avoid aggravating illness, threatening life, leaving sequelae or causing infertility, ectopic pregnancy, etc.

热解毒为主，祛湿化瘀为辅。治疗务求及时彻底，以免病势加重，危及生命；或遗留后遗症，反复发作，或导致不孕、异位妊娠等。

Sequelae of pelvic inflammatory disease is mainly residual toxin of evil heat in the Thoroughfare and Conception Vessels and uterus, struggling with qi and blood, and resulting in blood stasis. Therefore, blood stasis is the key, and the manifestations are mingled with deficiency and excess. By the major therapeutic methods to dispel blood stasis, it is appropriate to give the internal treatment and external treatment jointly, and take care of the constitution, by dispelling pathogens without injuring the constitution and by supporting the constitution without retaining pathogens. If the disease recurs and abscess or mass is formed, surgery may be considered, while the therapeutic effects are not satisfactory by drug treatment.

盆腔炎性疾病后遗症主要是邪热余毒残留于冲任、胞宫，与气血相搏结，聚结成瘀。故以血瘀为关键，证候虚实错杂。治疗则以祛瘀为大法，宜内外合治，并须顾及正气，注意祛邪而不伤正，扶正而不留邪。若反复发作，脓肿或包块形成，经药物治疗效果不佳者，可考虑手术治疗。

2.1 Syndrome of accumulation and exuberance of damp-heat

2.1 湿热壅盛证

Main manifestations Fever, aversion to cold, sweating, unpressable pain in the lower abdomen and sides of the lower abdomen, yellowish and pus-like leukorrhea, red tongue with yellow and greasy fur as well as slippery and rapid pulse.

主要证候 发热、畏寒、有汗，下腹部及少腹两侧疼痛、拒按，带下色黄如脓，苔黄腻质红，脉滑数。

Therapeutic methods Clearing away heat and draining dampness, resolving toxin and stasis.

治法 清利湿热，解毒化瘀。

Formulas and herbs *Rhubarb and Moutan Decoction* (Da Huang Mu Dan Tang), composed of 30 g of *Herba Patriniae* (Bai Jiang Cao), 30 g of

方药 代表方为大黄牡丹汤；常用药如败酱草 30 克，红藤 30 克，紫花地丁 30

Caulis Sargentodoxae (Hong Teng), 30 g of *Herba Violae* (Zi Hua Di Ding), 15 g of *Flos Lonicerae* (Jin Yin Hua), 15 g of *Fructus Forsythiae* (Lian Qiao), 10 g of *Radix et Rhizoma Rhei* (Da Huang), 15 g of *Semen Coicis* (Yi Yi Ren), 10 g of *Cortex Moutan Radicis* (Mu Dan Pi), 10 g of *Radix Paeoniae Rubra* (Chi Shao) and 10 g of *Semen Persicae* (Tao Ren).

克，金银花15克，连翘15克，大黄10克，薏苡仁15克，牡丹皮10克，赤芍10克，桃仁10克。

Modification For severe damp-heat marked by thirst without desire to drink water, chest oppression, nausea, yellow urine and yellow and greasy tongue fur, *Rhizoma Atractylodis* (Cang Zhu), *Cortex Phellodendri* (Huang Bo), *Semen Plantaginis* (Che Qian Zi), *Polyporus Umbellatus* (Zhu Ling) and *Rhizoma Alismatis* (Ze Xie) are added. For formation of mass, *Eupolyphaga seu Steleophaga* (Zhe Chong), *Resina Olibani* (Ru Xiang) and *Myrrha* (Mo Yao) are added.

加减 若湿热甚，见口渴不欲饮、胸闷、恶心、尿黄、苔黄腻等症状者，酌加苍术、黄柏、车前子、猪苓、泽泻；有包块者，加䗪虫、乳香、没药。

Shanghai doctor ZHU Nansun's experience prescription, *Dandelion, Violet, Sargentodoxa and Patrinia Anti-Inflammatory Decoction* (Pu Ding Teng Jiang Xiao Yan Tang): 20 g of *Herba Taraxaci* (Pu Gong Ying), 15 g of *Violae Herba cum Radice* (Di Ding), 20 g of *Caulis Sargentodoxae* (Da Xue Teng), 15 g of *Herba Patriniae* (Bai Jiang Cao), 15 g of *Typhae Pollen* (Pu Huang), 6 g of *Rhizoma Corydalis* (Yan Hu Suo), 12 g of *Fructus Meliae Toosendan* (Chuan Lian Zi), 15 g of *Herba Artemisiae Anomalae* (Liu Ji Nu), 12 g of *Rhizoma Sparganii Stoloniferi* (San Leng) and 12 g of *Rhizoma Zedoariae* (E Zhu).

上海医家朱南孙经验方（蒲丁藤酱消炎汤）加减：蒲公英20克，地丁草15克，红藤20克，败酱草15克，生蒲黄15克，延胡索6克，川楝子12克，刘寄奴15克，三棱12克，莪术12克。

2.2 Syndrome of qi stagnation and blood stasis

2.2 气滞血瘀证

Main manifestations Stabbing pain in the lower abdomen and sides of lower abdomen, even formation of mass, aching pain in the loins, irregular menstruation, profuse leukorrhea, lassitude, pur-

主要证候 下腹部及少腹两侧疼痛如针刺，甚至有包块，腰脊酸痛，月经失调，带下量多，精神疲惫，舌质紫

plish tongue or with ecchymoses, whitish thin tongue fur and taut and unsmooth pulse.

暗或瘀斑，苔薄白，脉弦涩。

Therapeutic methods Regulating qi and activating blood, dissolving stasis and relieving pain.

治法 理气活血，化瘀止痛。

Formulas and herbs *Tangerine Seed Pill* (Ju He Wan), composed of 10 g of *Semen Citri Reticulatae* (Ju He), 10 g of *Semen Litchi* (Li Zhi He), 10 g of *Radix Salviae Miltiorrhizae* (Dan Shen), 10 g of *Radix Paeoniae Rubra* (Chi Shao), 10 g of *Herba Aristolochiae* (Tian Xian Teng), 10 g of *Rhizoma Cyperi* (Xiang Fu), 10 g of *Fructus Meliae Toosendan* (Chuan Lian Zi) and 10 g of *Rhizoma Corydalis* (Chao Yan Hu Suo).

方药 代表方为橘核丸；常用药如橘核10克，荔枝核10克，丹参10克，赤芍10克，天仙藤10克，香附10克，川楝子10克，炒延胡索10克。

Modification For formation of mass, *Semen Persicae* (Tao Ren), *Flos Carthami* (Hong Hua), *Rhizoma Sparganii Stoloniferi* (San Leng), *Rhizoma Zedoariae* (E Zhu), *Poriae* (Fu Ling) and *Rhizoma Alismatis* (Ze Xie) are added accordingly.

加减 有包块者，酌加桃仁、红花、三棱、莪术、茯苓、泽泻。

2.3 Syndrome of asthenia of both spleen and kidney

2.3 脾肾两虚证

Main manifestations Insidious pain in the lower abdomen and both sides of lower abdomen, even aching pain in the lumbosacral region, profuse and thin leukorrhea, spiritual lassitude, cold limbs, loose stool, thin and greasy tongue fur as well as thready and deep pulse.

主要证候 下腹部及少腹两侧隐隐作痛，甚至牵及腰骶酸痛，带下量多清稀，精神疲倦，四肢不温，大便溏薄，舌苔薄腻，脉细沉。

Therapeutic methods Supporting right and dissolving dampness, freeing the meridians and relieving pain.

治法 扶正化湿，通络止痛。

Formulas and herbs *Vital Gate Pills* (You Gui Wan), composed of 20 g of *Rhizoma Dioscoreae* (Shan Yao), 15 g of *Cortex Eucommiae* (Du Zhong), 10 g of *Radix Morindae Officinalis* (Ba Ji Tian), 10 g of *Cortex Moutan* (Chao Mu Dan Pi),

方药 代表方为右归丸；常用药如山药20克，杜仲15克，巴戟天10克，炒丹皮10克，茯苓10克，鹿角片10克，香附10克，续断12

10 g of *Poriae* (Fu Ling), 10 g of *Cervi Cornu Sectum* (Lu Jiao Pian), 10 g of *Rhizoma Cyperi* (Xiang Fu), 12 g of *Radix Dipsaci* (Xu Duan) and 12 g of *Ramulus Loranthi* (Sang Ji Sheng).

克,桑寄生12克。

Modification For qi asthenia and collapsing distention, *Rhizoma Cimicifugae* (Sheng Ma) is added. For aching in the loins, *Ramulus Loranthi* (Sang Ji Sheng) and *Radix Clematidis* (Wei Ling Xian) are added; for forming mass, *Euonymi Ramulus* (Gui Jian Yu) and *Herba Lycopi* (Ze Lan) are added. For profuse leukorrhea, *Semen Euryales* (Qian Shi), *Rosae Laevigatae Fructus* (Jin Ying Zi) and *Os Sepiellae seu Sepiae* (Hai Piao Xiao) are added.

加减 若气虚坠胀者,加升麻;腰酸者,加桑寄生、威灵仙;有包块者,酌加鬼箭羽、泽兰;带下量多,加芡实、金樱子、海螵蛸。

Shanghai doctor CAO Lingxian's experience prescription: composed of 12 g of *Radix Bupleuri* (Chai Hu), 12 g of *Radix Angelicae Sinensis* (Dang Gui), 12 g of *Rhizoma Atractylodis Macrocephalae* (Bai Zhu), 12 g of *Semen Coicis* (Yi Yi Ren), 12 g of *Poriae* (Fu Ling), 12 g of *Fructus Meliae Toosendan* (Chuan Lian Zi), 12 g of *Flos Lonicerae* (Jin Yin Hua), 12 g of *Fructus Forsythiae* (Lian Qiao), 12 g of *Caulis Sargentodoxae* (Da Xue Teng), 12 g of *Herba Patriniae* (Bai Jiang Cao), 12 g of *Herba Taraxaci* (Pu Gong Ying), 12 g of *Eupolyphaga seu Steleophaga* (Zhe Chong), 6 g of *Scorpio* (Quan Xie), 12 g of *Radix Angelicae Pubescentis* (Du Huo), 12 g of *Radix Cynanchi Paniculati* (Xu Chang Qing) and 12 g of *Radix Astragali* (Huang Qi).

上海医家曹玲仙经验方加减:柴胡12克,当归12克,白术12克,薏苡仁12克,茯苓12克,川楝子12克,金银花12克,连翘12克,红藤12克,败酱草12克,蒲公英12克,蜃虫12克,全蝎6克,独活12克,徐长卿12克,黄芪12克。

3 Other therapeutic methods

3 其他疗法

3.1 Chinese patent drugs

3.1 中成药

(1) *Gynecologic Qianjin Tablets* (Fu Ke Qian Jin Pian): 6 tablets each time and three times a day, applicable to the treatment of accumulation and exuberance of dampheat.

(1) 妇科千金片:每次6片,每日3次,适用于湿热瘀阻证。

(2) *Gynecologic Inflammation-Fighting Capsule* (Kang Fu Yan Jiao Nang): 4 capsules each time and

(2) 抗妇炎胶囊:每次4粒,每日3次,适用于湿热下

three times a day, applicable to the treatment of pattern of transmission of downward.

(3) *Hua Hong Granules* (Hua Hong Ke Li): 10 g each time and three times a day, applicable to the treatment of transmission of downward.

(4) *Pelvic Inflammation Granules* (Pen Yan Jing Ke Li): 12 g each time and three times a day, applicable to the treatment of pattern of retention of dampheat, and blood stasis.

(5) *Sanguine Mansion Stasis-Expelling Oral Liquid* (Xue Fu Zhu Yu Kou Fu Ye): 10 ml each time and twice a day, applicable to the treatment of internal retention of static blood.

(6) *Cinnamon Twig and Poria Capsule* (Gui Zhi Fu Ling Ke Li): 3 capsules each time and three times a day, applicable to the treatment of syndrome of obstruction of static blood in the collaterals.

3.2 Empirical and folk recipes

(1) 30 g of fresh *Herba Taraxaci* (Pu Gong Ying) washed, cut into sections, is decocted in water. The decoction is taken orally as tea.

(2) Shanghai doctor CAI Xiaosun's experience description: composed of 12 g of *Radix Salviae Miltiorrhizae* (Dan Shen), 12 g of *Radix Stemonae* (Bai Bu), 9 g of *Semen Vaccariae* (Wang Bu Liu Xing Zi), 15 g of *Codonopsis Lanceolatae Radix* (Shan Hai Luo), 12 g of *Herba Houttuyniae* (Yu Xing Cao), 15 g of *Mahoniae Folium* (Gong Lao Ye), 12 g of *Spica Prunellae* (Xia Ku Cao), 12 g of *Spina Gleditsiae* (Zao Jiao Ci), 9 g of *Radix Achyranthis Bidentatae* (Huai Niu Xi), 9 g of *Radix Rehmanniae Cruda* (Sheng Di Huang) and 9 g of *Liquidambaris Fructus* (Lu Lu Tong), applicable to the

注证。

（3）花红颗粒：每次10克，每日3次，适用于湿热下注证。

（4）盆炎净颗粒：每次12克，每日3次，适用于湿热瘀阻证。

（5）血府逐瘀口服液：每次10毫升，每日2次，适用于瘀血内阻证。

（6）桂枝茯苓胶囊：每次3粒，每日3次，适用于瘀血阻络证。

3.2 单验方

（1）新鲜蒲公英30克洗净，切段，煎汤代茶。

（2）上海医家蔡小荪经验方：丹参12克，百部12克，王不留行9克，山海螺15克，鱼腥草12克，功劳叶15克，夏枯草12克，皂角刺12克，怀牛膝9克，生地黄9克，路路通9克，适用于结核性盆腔炎。

treatment of tuberculotic pelvic inflammation.

3.3 External therapy

(1) Enema: 30 g of *Flos Lonicerae* (Jin Yin Hua), 20 g of *Herba Taraxaci* (Pu Gong Ying), 20 g of *Herba Violae* (Zi Hua Di Ding), 30 g of *Caulis Sargentodoxae* (Hong Teng), 20 g of *Herba Patriniae* (Bai Jiang Cao), 20 g of *Fructus Forsythiae* (Lian Qiao), 15 g of *Rhizoma Sparganii Stoloniferi* (San Leng), 15 g of *Rhizoma Zedoariae* (E Zhu), 20 g of *Radix Salviae Miltiorrhizae* (Dan Shen) and 15 g of *Radix Paeoniae Rubra* (Chi Shao) are decocted in water into 100 ml of decoction. When cooled down to 30～50 ℃, it is used for enema. This treatment is given once a day and 10 times make up one course of treatment.

(2) External application: 20 g of *Resina Olibani* (Ru Xiang), 20 g of *Myrrha* (Mo Yao), 20 g of *Capsicum Annuum* (Chuan Jiao), 20 g of *Fructus Anisi Stellati* (Ba Jiao Hui Xiang) and 20 g of *Fructus Foeniculi* (Xiao Hui Xiang) are ground into fine powder and mixed up with flour. In application, the powder is mixed with a little sorghum wine, spread on a piece of gauze and fixed on the affected part of the abdomen. Then hot-water bag is compressed on it. This treatment is given twice a day and 10 days make up one course of treatment.

3.3 外治法

（1）灌肠疗法：金银花30克，蒲公英20克，紫花地丁20克，红藤30克，败酱草20克，连翘20克，三棱15克，莪术15克，丹参20克，赤芍15克，浓煎至100毫升，冷却至30℃～50℃，保留灌肠，每日1次，10日为1个疗程。

（2）外敷疗法：乳香20克，没药20克，降香末20克，川椒20克，大茴香20克，小茴香20克，上药研成细末，用面粉和匀，用时以高粱酒少许，调湿摊于沙布上，置于腹部痛处，其上用热水袋外敷，每日2次，10日为1个疗程。

Chapter 5 Leukorrhea diseases

第5章 带下病

Leukorrhea disease refers to significantly increased or decreased amount of vaginal discharge-with abnormal color, quality and odor, or accompanied by general or local symptoms. Leucorrhea of significantly increased amount is called leucorrhagia, leucorrhea of significantly decreased amount is increases during pregnancy, before and after menstruation, without abnormal color, quality and odor and discomfort, is a normal physiological phenomenon, not a disease.

Leudorrhea is mainly due to dampness. The main pathogenesis is related to the disorder of the Conception and Belt Vessels. Dampness is either exogenous or endogenous. Exogenous dampness refers to infection of external dampness, such as living in the wetlands, wading rain, ormenstrual or postpartum careless recuperation, resulting in the invasion of dampness. Endogenous dampness is mainly due to dysfunction in the spleen, kidney and liver, resulting in spleen vacuity with impaired transportation and transformation and internal water-dampness. Debilitation of kidney yang, abnormal qi transformation, and internal retention of water-dampness; liver qi stagnation rebelling spleen, down migration of liver fire with dampness of the spleen, can lead to leukorrhea diseases.

带下病是指带下量明显增多或减少，色、质、气味发生异常，或伴有全身或局部症状者。带下明显增多着称为带下过多，带下明显减少者，称为带下减少。妇女在经间期、经前期以及妊娠期带下稍增多，但无色、质、气味异常或不适，属正常生理现象，不作疾病而论。

本病的主要病因是湿。主要病机是任脉不固，带脉失约。湿邪有内外之别。外湿指外感之湿邪，如久居湿地，涉水淋雨，或经期产后摄生不慎，湿邪侵袭；内湿多由脾肾肝三脏功能失调，脾虚失运，水湿内生；肾阳虚衰，气化失常，水湿内停；肝郁侮脾，肝火挟脾湿下注，均可导致带下病。

1 Key points for diagnosis

1.1 Medical history

Residual blood during menstruation or after childbirth, improper recuperation or no inhibition in sex, or infection of evil toxin after gynecologic surgery.

1.2 Symptoms

Increased leukorrhea with abnormal color, quality and odor, accompanied by vulvar and vaginal itching, burning sensation and pain.

1.3 Examination

(1) Gynecological examination: vaginitis, pelvic inflammation and cervicitis may be found.

(2) Other tests: A large number of white blood cells, or trichomonas, candida and other pathogens may be seen in vaginal smear, cervical smear or culture. Cervical cytology can be given. Colposcopy or cervical biopsy may be performed if necessary to exclude malignancy.

2 Syndrome differentiation and treatment

Syndrome differentiation of leukorrhea concentrates on the analysis of the quantity, color, texture and odor of leukorrhea. Usually, dark (yellow, red or dark green) leukorrhea with thick and sticky texture and odor pertains to sthenia and heat. Light-colored (white, slight yellow) leukorrhea with thin texture and the smell of fish pertains to asthenia and cold. Leukorrhea is usually marked by mixture of asthenia and sthenia, and complete asthenia is seldom seen. The treatment focuses on elimination of dampness. Exogenous dampness is treated mainly by

1 诊断要点

1.1 病史

经期、产后余血未净，摄生不洁，或不禁房事，或妇产科手术后感染邪毒史。

1.2 症状

带下增多，色、质、气味异常，可伴有外阴、阴道瘙痒、灼热、疼痛等症。

1.3 检查

（1）妇科检查：可有阴道炎、宫颈炎或盆腔炎性疾病的体征。

（2）其他检查：阴道、宫颈分泌物涂片或培养可见大量白细胞，或滴虫、假丝酵母菌等病原体。可行宫颈细胞学检查，必要时阴道镜或宫颈活组织检查，以排除恶性病变。

2 辨证论治

带下辨证，首先在于辨别带下的量、色、质、气味异常。一般而言，带下色深（黄、赤、青绿），质黏稠，臭秽者，多属实、属热；带下色淡（白、淡黄），质稀，或有腥气者，多属虚、属寒。临床上往往是虚实夹杂多，全虚者少。治疗上着眼于“湿”，外湿者以清利为主，内湿者以调理肝脾肾为要，分别采用升阳、

the clearing and draining therapy, while endogenous dampness is dealt with mainly by regulating the liver, spleen and kidney by means of the yang-elevating, dampness-drying, and astringing therapy and clearing-draining method. If it is accompanied by genital pruritus, it can be treated with the combination of external therapy for clearing away heat, eliminating dampness and removing toxin, for enhancing the therapeutic effects. If middle-aged or old women with bloody leucorrhea, it is necessary to be alert to the possibility of cancer of the uterus or uterine cervix.

燥湿、固涩、清利诸法，伴有阴痒者可结合外治法，清热除湿解毒，才能提高疗效。若中老年女性出现血性白带，应警惕子宫或宫颈癌变的可能。

2.1 Syndrome of spleen asthenia

Main manifestations Profuse, whitish or light yellow, odorless and incessant leukorrhea with thick and sticky texture, pale white or withered yellow facial complexion, cold limbs, lassitude, anorexia and loose stool, swelling in feet, pale tongue with white and greasy fur as well as slow and weak pulse.

Therapeutic methods Strengthening the spleen and nourishing qi, elevating yang and eliminating dampness.

Formulas and herbs *Discharge-Ceasing Decoction* (Wan Dai Tang), composed of 10 g of *Stir-Fried Rhizoma Atractylodis Macrocephalae* (Chao Bai Zhu), 10 g of *Dioscoreae Rhizoma Frictum* (Chao Shan Yao), 10 g of *Radix Codonopsis Pilosulae* (Dang Shen), 10 g of *Radix Paeoniae Alba* (Bai Shao), 10 g of *Fried Rhizoma Atractylodis* (Chao Cang Zhu), 4 g of *Radix Glycyrrhizae Praeparata* (Zhi Gan Cao), 6 g of *Pericarpium Citri Tangerinae* (Chen Pi), 10 g of *Schizonepetae Flos Carbonisata* (Hei Jie Sui), 5 g of *Radix Bupleuri* (Chai Hu) and 10 g of *Semen Plantaginis* (Che Qian Zi) (to be

2.1 脾虚证

主要证候 带下量多，色白或淡黄，质黏稠，无臭气，绵绵不断，面色㿠白或萎黄，四肢不温，精神疲倦，纳少便溏，两足浮肿。舌淡苔白或腻，脉缓弱。

治法 健脾益气，升阳除湿。

方药 代表方为完带汤；常用药如炒白术 10 克，炒山药 10 克，党参 10 克，白芍 10 克，炒苍术 10 克，炙甘草 4 克，陈皮 6 克，黑芥穗 10 克，柴胡 5 克，车前子（包煎）10 克。

wrapped for decocting).

Modification For lumbago due to kidney asthenia, *Cortex Eucommiae* (Du Zhong) and *Semen Cuscutae* (Tu Si Zi) are added to secure the kidney qi. For abdominal pain due to congealing cold, *Rhizoma Cyperi* (Xiang Fu) and *Folium Artemistae Argyi* (Ai Ye) are added to warm the channels and relieve pain. For prolonged and incessant leukorrhea, *Rosae Laevigatae Fructus* (Jin Ying Zi), *Os Draconis* (Long Gu), *Semen Euryales* (Qian Shi) and *Os Sepiellae seu Sepiae* (Wu Zei Gu) are added to secure and astrinct leucorrhea. For several loose stools in a day, *Poriae* (Fu Ling), *Semen Dolichoris Album* (Bai Bian Dou) and *Nelumbinis Semen* (Lian Zi Rou) are added. For yellowish leukorrhea, *Dioscoreae Hypoglaucae seu Septemlobae Rhizoma* (Bi Xie), *Cortex Phellodendri* (Huang Bo) and *Semen Coicis* (Yi Yi Ren) are added. For abnormal smell, in combination of the formula for external treatment, by decoding *Fructus Cnidii* (She Chuang Zi), *Pericarpium Zanthoxyli* (Hua Jiao), *Cortex Phellodendri* (Huang Bo), *Rhizoma Coptidis* (Huang Lian) and *Radix Sophorae Flavescentis* (Ku Shen) to steam and wash the genital region.

加减 若肾虚腰痛者，加杜仲、菟丝子以固肾气；寒凝腹痛者，加香附、艾叶以温经止痛；若带下日久，滑脱不止者，加金樱子、龙骨、芡实、乌贼骨以固涩止带；若大便溏薄，日行数次者，加茯苓、白扁豆、莲子肉；带下色黄者，加萆薢、黄柏、薏苡仁；带下有异味者，配合外治方，用蛇床子、花椒、黄柏、黄连、苦参水煎熏洗阴部。

Shanghai doctro CHEN Pangen's experience prescription, *Discharge-Clearing Decoction* (Qing Dai Tang): 12 g of *Dioscoreae Rhizoma* (Huai Shan Yao), 12 g of *Os Draconis* (Long Gu), 12 g of *Concha Ostreae* (Mu Li), 10 g of *Os Sepiellae seu Sepiae* (Hai Piao Xiao), 12 g of *Rubiae Radix* (Qian Cao), 9 g of *Rhizoma Atractylodis Macrocephalae* (Bai Zhu), 15 g of *Rhizoma Smilacis Glabrae* (Tu Fu Ling) and 10 g of *Ginkgo Semen* (Bai Guo).

上海医家陈盘根经验方（清带汤）加减：怀山药12克，龙骨12克，牡蛎12克，海螵蛸10克，茜草12克，白术9克，土茯苓15克，白果10克。

Shanghai doctro CAI Xiaosun's experience prescription, *Spleen-Fortifying and Dampness-Dissolving Prescription* (Jian

上海医家蔡小荪经验方（健脾化湿方）：云茯苓12克，炒白术

Pi Hua Shi Fang): 12 g of *Poriae* (Fu Ling), 10 g of *Rhizoma Atractylodis Macrocephalae* (Chao Bai Zhu), 10 g of *Dioscoreae Rhizoma* (Huai Shan Yao), 12 g of *Coicis Semen Crudum* (Sheng Yi Yi Ren), 10 g of *Os Sepiellae seu Sepiae* (Hai Piao Xiao), 10 g of *Paeoniae Radix Alba & Hangzhouensis* (Hang Bai Shao) and 3 g of *Radix Angelicae Dahuricae* (Bai Zhi).

10克，怀山药10克，生薏苡仁12克，海螵蛸10克，杭白芍10克，白芷3克。

2.2 Syndrome of kidney yang asthenia

Main manifestations Profuse, transparent, cold, thin and incessant leukorrhea, severe aching sensation in the loins, cold sensation in the abdomen, clear and profuse urine, especially in the night, loose stool, pale tongue with thin and white fur, deep and slow pulse.

Therapeutic methods Warming the kidney, cultivating original qi and astringing and stopping leukorrhea.

Formulas and herbs *Internal Supplementation Pill* (Nei Bu Wan) composed of 10 g of *Cervi Cornu Pantotrichum* (Lu Rong), 10 g of *Semen Cuscutae* (Tu Si Zi), 10 g of *Astragali Complanati Semen* (Tong Ji Li), 10 g of *Radix Scutellariae* (Huang Qin), 10 g of *Fructus Tribuli* (Bai Ji Li), 5 g of *Cortex Cinnamomi* (Rou Gui) (to be decocted later), 10 g of *Ootheca Mantidis* (Sang Piao Xiao), 10 g of *Herba Cistanchis* (Rou Cong Rong) and 5 g of *Aconiti Radix Lateralis Tosta* (Pao Fu Zi).

Modification For diarrhea and loose stool, *Herba Cistanchis* (Rou Cong Rong) is deleted while *Fructus Psoraleae* (Bu Gu Zhi) and *Semen Myristicae* (Rou Dou Kou) are added to warm the spleen and kidney. For fulminant leukorrhea due to kidney deficiency, *Essence-Controlling Pills* (Gu Jin Wan) is used to nourish the spleen and kidney as well as to

2.2 肾阳虚证

主要证候 白带量多，清冷，质稀薄，终日淋漓不断，腰酸如折，小腹冷感，小便频数清长，夜间尤甚，大便溏薄。舌质淡，苔薄白，脉沉迟。

治法 温肾培元，固涩止带。

方药 代表方为内补丸；常用药如鹿茸10克，菟丝子10克，潼蒺藜10克，黄芪10克，白蒺藜10克，肉桂（后下）5克，桑螵蛸10克，肉苁蓉10克，炮附片5克。

加减 若腹泻便溏者，去肉苁蓉，酌加补骨脂、肉豆蔻以温脾肾；若肾虚不固，带下如崩者，可用固精丸以补脾肾、固奇经，药用牡蛎（先煎）10克，桑螵蛸10克，龙骨（先煎）10克，茯苓10克，五

consolidate the extraordinary meridians, composed of 10 g of *Concha Ostreae* (Mu Li) (to be decocted first), 10 g of *Ootheca Mantidis* (Sang Piao Xiao), 10 g of *Os Draconis* (Long Gu) (to be decocted first), 10 g of *Poriae* (Fu Ling), 10 g of *Fructus Schisandrae* (Wu Wei Zi), 10 g of *Semen Cuscutae* (Tu Si Zi) and 10 g of *Allii Tuberosi Semen* (Jiu Cai Zi).

味子10克，菟丝子10克，韭菜子10克。

2.3 Syndrome of kidney yin asthenia

Main manifestations Yellowish or yellowish and reddish leukorrhea with sticky texture and without odor, burning sensation in the vagina, feverish sensation over the palms, soles and chest, aching in the loins and tinnitus, dizziness and palpitation, red tongue with scanty fur, thready and rapid pulse.

Therapeutic methods Nourishing the kidney yin, clearing away heat and eliminating dampness.

Formulas and herbs *Modified Anemarrhena, Phellodendron, and Rehmannia Decoction* (Zhi Bo Di Huang Tang), composed of 10 g of *Radix Rehmanniae Praeparata* (Shu Di Huang), 10 g of *Fructus Corni* (Shan Zhu Yu), 10 g of *Rhizoma Dioscoreae* (Shan Yao), 10 g of *Rhizoma Alismatis* (Ze Xie), 10 g of *Poriae* (Fu Ling), 10 g of *Cortex Moutan Radicis* (Mu Dan Pi), 10 g of *Rhizoma Anemarrhenae* (Zhi Mu), 10 g of *Cortex Phellodendri* (Huang Bo), 10 g of *Semen Euryales* (Qian Shi) and 10 g of *Rosae Laevigatae Fructus* (Jin Ying Zi).

Modification For yin asthenia and fire exuberance, *Processed Plastrum Testudinis* (Zhi Gui Ban) and *Processed Cortex Lycii Radicis* (Zhi Di Gu Pi) are added to enrich yin and downbear fire. For accompanying damp-heat, *Herba Patriniae* (Bai Jiang Cao) and *Semen Coicis* (Yi Yi Ren) are added to

2.3 肾阴虚证

主要证候 带下色黄或兼赤，质黏无臭，阴户灼热，五心烦躁，腰酸耳鸣，头晕心悸，舌红苔少，脉细数。

治法 益肾滋阴，清热祛湿。

方药 代表方为知柏地黄汤；常用药如熟地黄10克，山茱萸10克，山药10克，泽泻10克，茯苓10克，牡丹皮10克，知母10克，黄柏10克，芡实10克，金樱子10克。

加减 若偏于阴虚火旺者，加炙龟版、炙地骨皮以滋阴降火；若挟湿热者，加败酱草、薏苡仁以清热利湿。

clear away heat and disinhibit dampness.

2.4 Syndrome of downward migration of damp-heat

Main manifestations Profuse, yellowish or purulent, sticky, thick, smelly leukorrhea, or white leukorrhea like bean dregs, pruritus in the vagina, chest oppression, poor appetite, bitterness and sliminess in the mouth, abdominal pain, scanty and brown urine, red tongue with yellow and greasy or thick fur, soft and rapid pulse.

Therapeutic methods Clearing away heat, draining dampness and stopping leukorrhea.

Formulas and herbs *Leukorrhea-Stopping Prescription* (Zhi Dai Fang), composed of 10 g of *Polyporus Umbellatus* (Zhu Ling), 10 g of *Poriae* (Fu Ling), 10 g of *Semen Plantaginis* (Che Qian Zi) (to be wrapped for decocting), 10 g of *Rhizoma Alismatis* (Ze Xie), 10 g of *Herba Artemisiae Scopariae* (Yin Chen), 10 g of *Radix Paeoniae Rubra* (Chi Shao), 10 g of *Cortex Moutan Radicis* (Mu Dan Pi), 10 g of *Fructus Gardeniae* (Zhi Zi), 10 g of *Cortex Phellodendri* (Huang Bo) and 10 g of *Radix Achyranthis Bidentatae* (Niu Xi).

Midification For downward migration of damp-heat from the liver meridian marked by profuse leukorrhea, yellow or yellow and green color like pus, sticky or frothy texture, foul odor, accompanied by pudendal pruritus and pain, dizziness, bitter taste in the mouth and dry throat, restlessness and susceptibility to rage, retention of dry feces, brown urine, red tongue with yellow and greasy fur, taut, slippery and rapid pulse, *Gentian Liver-Draining Decoction* (Long Dan Xie Gan Tang) can be used, composed of 3 g of *Gentianae Radix* (Long

2.4 湿热下注证

主要证候 带下量多，色黄或呈脓性，质黏稠，有臭气，或带下色白质黏如豆腐渣状，外阴瘙痒；胸闷纳呆，口苦而腻，或小腹作痛，小便短赤。舌红，苔黄腻或厚，脉濡略数。

治法 清热利湿止带。

方药 代表方为止带方；常用药如猪苓10克，茯苓10克，车前子（包煎）10克，泽泻10克，茵陈10克，赤芍10克，牡丹皮10克，栀子10克，黄柏10克，牛膝10克。

加减 若肝经湿热下注者，症见带下量多，色黄或黄绿如脓，质黏稠或呈泡沫状，有臭气，伴阴部痒痛，头晕目眩，口苦咽干，烦躁易怒，便结尿赤，舌红苔黄腻，脉弦滑而数，宜用龙胆泻肝汤清热除湿，药用龙胆草3克，柴胡5克，栀子10克，黄芩10克，车前子（包煎）10克，木通6克，泽泻10克，生地黄10克，

Dan Cao), 5 g of *Radix Bupleuri* (Chai Hu), 10 g of *Fructus Gardeniae* (Zhi Zi), 10 g of *Radix Scutellariae* (Huang Qin), 10 g of *Semen Plantaginis* (Che Qian Zi) (to be wrapped for decocting), 6 g of *Caulis Akebiae* (Mu Tong), 10 g of *Rhizoma Alismatis* (Ze Xie), 10 g of *Radix Rehmanniae Cruda* (Sheng Di Huang), 10 g of *Radix Angelicae Sinensis* (Dang Gui), 4 g of *Radix Glycyrrhizae* (Gan Cao), 10 g of *Radix Sophorae Flavescentis* (Ku Shen) and 3 g of *Rhizoma Coptidis* (Huang Lian). For relative predomination of dampness marked by profuse leukorrhea with white color like bean dregs or coagulated milk, pudendal pruritus, chest oppression and anorexia, red tongue with yellow and greasy fur, slippery and rapid pulse, *Fish Poison Yam Dampness-Percolating Decoction* (Bi Xie Shen Shi Tang) can be used to clear away heat and drain dampness as well as to expel wind and resolve turbid substance. This prescription is composed of 10 g of *Dioscoreae Hypoglaucae seu Septemlobae Rhizoma* (Bi Xie), 10 g of *Semen Coicis* (Yi Yi Ren), 10 g of *Cortex Phellodendri* (Huang Bo), 10 g of *Poria* (Fu Ling), 10 g of *Cortex Moutan Radicis* (Mu Dan Pi), 10 g of *Rhizoma Alismatis* (Ze Xie), 10 g of *Talcum* (Hua Shi), 10 g of *Rhizoma Atractylodis* (Cang Zhu) and 10 g of *Herba Agastachis* (Huo Xiang).

当归 10 克，甘草 4 克，苦参 10 克，黄连 3 克。若湿浊偏重者，症见带下量多，色白，如豆渣状或乳凝状，阴部瘙痒，胸闷纳差，舌红苔黄腻，脉滑数，宜用萆薢渗湿汤以清热利湿，疏风化浊，药用萆薢 10 克，薏苡仁 10 克，黄柏 10 克，茯苓 10 克，牡丹皮 10 克，泽泻 10 克，滑石 10 克，苍术 10 克，藿香 10 克。

2.5 Syndrome of accumulation of heat toxin

Main manifestations Profuse leukorrhea, yellow and green color like pus, or red and white color, or multicolors, sticky and greasy texture or like pus, smelly odor, or putrid smelling, abdominal pain, aching pain in the lumbosacral region, bitter taste in the mouth, dry throat, dysphoria, dizzi-

2.5 热毒蕴结证

主要证候 带下量多，黄绿如脓，或赤白相兼，或五色杂下，质黏腻，或如脓样，有臭气，或腐臭难闻，小腹作痛，腰骶酸痛，口苦咽干，烦热头晕，大便干结或臭秽，小

ness, retention of dry feces or with smelly odor, scanty and brown urine, red tongue with yellow or yellow and greasy fur, slippery and rapid pulse.

便短赤。舌红，苔黄或黄腻，脉滑数。

Therapeutic methods Clearing away heat and resolving toxin.

治法 清热解毒。

Formulas and herbs *Five Ingredients Detoxifying Drink* (Wu Wei Xiao Du Yin), composed of 15 g of *Herba Taraxaci* (Pu Gong Ying), 10 g of *Flos Lonicerae* (Jin Yin Hua), 15 g of *Flos Chrysanthemi Indici* (Ye Ju Hua), 10 g of *Violae Herba* (Zi Hua Di Ding), 10 g of *Semiaquilegiae Radix* (Tian Kui Zi), 15 g of *Herba Hedyotis Diffusae* (Bai Hua She She Cao) and 6 g of *Rhizoma Atractylodis Macrocephalae* (Bai Zhu).

方药 代表方为五味消毒饮；常用药如蒲公英 15 克，金银花 10 克，野菊花 15 克，紫花地丁 10 克，天葵子 10 克，白花蛇舌草 15 克，白术 6 克。

3 Other therapeutic methods

3 其他疗法

3.1 Chinese patent drugs

3.1 中成药

(1) *Gynecologic Inflammation-Fighting Capsule* (Kang Fu Yan Jiao Nang): 4 capsules each time and three times a day, applicable to the treatment of syndrome of downward migration of damp-heat.

（1）抗妇炎胶囊：每次 4 粒，每日 3 次，适用于湿热下注证。

(2) *Thousand Gold Leukorrhea-Stopping Pills* (Qian Jin Zhi Dai Wan): 6-9 g each time and twice or three times a day, applicable to the treatment of syndrome of spleen and kidney asthenia accompanied by dampness.

（2）千金止带丸：每次 6～9 克，每日 2～3 次，适用于脾肾虚挟湿证。

(3) *Gynecologic Inflammation-Calming Capsule* (Fu Yan Ping Jiao Nang): Slip into vagina, 2 capsules each time and once a day, applicable to the treatment of downward migration of damp-heat.

（3）妇炎平胶囊：每次 2 粒，阴塞，每日 1 次，适用于湿热下注证。

(4) *Vagina-Clearing and Washing Liquor* (Jie Er Yin Xi Ye): Mix with warm water, clean and wash the vulva, 10 ml each time and once a day, 7 days for a course of treatment, applicable to the

（4）洁尔阴洗液：每次 10 毫升，温开水混匀，擦洗外阴，每日 1 次，7 日为 1 个疗程，适用于湿热下注证。

treatment of syndrome of downward migration of damp-heat.

3.2 Empirical and folk recipes

(1) 15 g of *Celosiae Cristatae Flos Albus* (Bai Ji Guan Hua) is decocted for oral taking, applicable to the treatment of leukorrhagia due to spleen asthenia complicated by dampness.

(2) 60 g of *Semen Coicis* (Yi Yi Ren) and 60 g of *Semen Euryales* (Qian Shi) are decocted in water with proper amount of rice, sesame oil and salt, applicable to the treatment of spleen asthenia syndrome with cold and dampness.

(3) *Aspidii Rhizoma* (Guan Zhong) and *Os Sepiellae seu Sepiae* (Hai Piao Xiao) in equal portion are ground into powder for oral taking with rice wine, 10 g each time and twice a day. This treatment is applicable to damp-heat and spleen asthenia syndrome.

(4) 30 g of *Herba Leonuri* (Yi Mu Cao) and 30 g of *Fructus Ziziphi Jujubae* (Hong Zao) are decocted for oral taking, applicable to the treatment of spleen asthenia syndrome.

(5) 50 g of *Dioscoreae Rhizoma* (Huai Shan Yao) and 30 g of *Rosae Laevigatae Fructus* (Jin Ying Zi) are decocted for oral taking, applicable to the treatment of spleen asthenia and retention of dampness.

(6) Shanghai doctor HU Qinkui's experience description: Spleen-Fortifying, Dampness-Eliminating and Leukorrhea-Stopping Prescription (Jian Pi Chu Shi Zhi Dai Fang): 12 g of *Radix Astragali* (Huang Qi), 12 g of *Radix Codonopsis Pilosulae* (Dang Shen), 12 g of *Rhizoma Atractylodis Macrocephalae* (Bai Zhu), 12 g of *Rhizoma Dioscoreae*

3.2 单验方

（1）白鸡冠花15克，水煎服，适用于脾虚挟湿带下证。

（2）薏苡仁60克，芡实60克，米适量共煮，加麻油、食盐调味，适用于脾虚寒湿证。

（3）贯众、海螵蛸各等分，研细末，每次10克，黄酒送服，每日2次，适用于湿热脾虚证。

（4）益母草30克，大红枣30克，水煎服，适用于脾虚证。

（5）怀山药50克，金樱子30克，水煎服，适用于脾虚湿滞证。

（6）上海医家胡溱魁经验方（健脾除湿止带方）：黄芪12克，党参12克，白术12克，山药12克，茯苓12克，生、熟薏苡仁各15克，山药12克，车前子12克，牡蛎30克，乌贼骨15克，芡实12克，

(Shan Yao), 12 g of *Poriae* (Fu Ling), 15 g of *Coicis Semen Crudum* (Sheng Yi Yi Ren), 15 g of *Cooked Semen Coicis* (Shu Yi Yi Ren), 12 g of *Semen Plantaginis* (Che Qian Zi), 30 g of *Concha Ostreae* (Mu Li), 15 g of *Os Sepiellae seu Sepiae* (Hai Piao Xiao, Wu Zei Gu), 12 g of *Semen Euryales* (Qian Shi) and 9 g of *Celosiae Cristatae Flos Albus* (Bai Ji Guan Hua), applicable to the treatment of leukorrhagia due to spleen vacuity with impaired transportation and transformation, downward migrantion of water and dampness fall and insecurity of Belt Vessel.

鸡冠花 9 克，适用于脾虚失运，水湿下陷，带脉不固之带下病。

3.3 External therapy

(1) Fumigation and washing lotion: 15 g of *Carpesii Fructus* (He Shi), 15 g of *Radix Sophorae Flavescentis* (Ku Shen), 15 g of *Radix Clematidis* (Wei Ling Xian), 12 g of *Angelicae Sinensis Radicis Extremitas* (Dang Gui Wei), 15 g of *Fructus Cnidii* (She Chuang Zi) and 10 g of *Radix Euphorbiae Ebracteolatae* (Lang Du) are decocted in 3,000 ml of water. After boiling, the residue is removed. The decoction is used to fumigate and wash the pudendum. To improve the effect, the bile of 1-2 pig gallbladder can be put into the decoction before washing. This decoction is applicable to the treatment of attack by exogenous dampness and insects. This treatment should not be used if there is pudendal ulceration.

(2) Sitting bathing: 15 g of *Fructus Cnidii* (She Chuang Zi), 10 g of *Pericarpium Zanthoxyli* (Hua Jiao), 10 g of *Alumen* (Ming Fan), 15 g of *Radix Sophorae Flavescentis* (Ku Shen) and 15 g of *Radix Stemonae* (Bai Bu) are decocted into decoction for fumigation and then bathing in it. This treatment is

3.3 外治法

（1）熏洗法：鹤虱 15 克，苦参 15 克，威灵仙 15 克，归尾 12 克，蛇床子 15 克，狼毒 10 克，加水 3 000 毫升，煮沸去渣，趁热熏洗阴部，临洗时加 1～2 枚猪胆汁更佳，适用于外感湿虫者，外阴溃疡者勿用。

（2）坐浴法：蛇床子 15 克，花椒 10 克，明矾 10 克，苦参 15 克，百部 15 克，煎汤趁热先熏后坐浴，适用于滴虫性阴道炎，若阴痒破溃者，则去花椒。

applicable to trichomonal vaginitis. If pudendal pruritus is ulcerated, *Pericarpium Zanthoxyli* (Hua Jiao) in the prescription should be deleted.

(3) HU Qinkui's experience prescription (washing prescription for genital itch): 30 g of *Cortex Phellodendri* (Huang Bo), 30 g of *Kochiae Fructus* (Di Fu Zi), 30 g of *Radix Stemonae* (Bai Bu), 30 g of *Fructus Cnidii* (She Chuang Zi), 10 g of *Alumen Dehydratum* (Ku Fan) and 30 g of *Radix Sophorae Flavescentis* (Ku Shen) are wrapped and decocted in water, for fumigation, washing and sitting bathing, 1 dose a day, applicable to the treatment of leukorrhagia due to damp-heat or genital itch syndrome.

(3) 胡溱魁经验方(阴痒外洗方):黄柏 30 克,地肤子 30 克,百部 30 克,蛇床子 30 克,枯矾 10 克,苦参 30 克,用上药布包水煎,熏洗坐浴,每日 1 剂,适用于湿热带下或阴痒症。

Chapter 6 Pregnancy diseases

第6章 妊娠病

Abortion

Abortion refers to stoppage of pregnancy within 28 weeks and with the weight of the fetus less than 1,000 g. Abortion occurring within 12 weeks after pregnancy is called early abortion, while abortion occurring from 12 weeks to less than 28 weeks is known as late abortion. Abortion may be either natural or artificial. Only natural abortion is discussed in this section. The incidence of abortion accounts for 10%-15% of total pregnancy, 80% of which is early abortion.

During pregnancy, if fetal qi is damaged, presenting vaginal bleeding, lower abdominal pain, aching lumbus, or even disappearance of the fetal origin, repeated pregnancy and abortion during menstruation, they are called insecurity of the fetal origin, including threatened abortion, restless fetus, abortion, miscarriage, retention of dead fetus, habitual abortion and other diseases. Slight and occasional bleeding from vagina after pregnancy, or dripping vaginal bleeding without aching lumbus and lower abdominal pain is called threatened abortion. Aching lumbus and lower abdominal pain or prolapsing sensation in the lower abdomen with slight

流　产

流产是指妊娠不足28周、胎儿体重不足1 000克而终止者。流产发生在妊娠12周前称为早期流产，发生在妊娠12～28周者称晚期流产；流产又可分自然流产和人工流产。本章节仅阐述自然流产，其发病率约占全部妊娠的10%～15%，其中80%以上为早期流产。

妊娠期间，胎气受损，出现阴道流血，下腹痛，腰酸，甚或胎元自殒，屡孕屡堕等的一类疾病，统称胎元不固，包括胎漏、胎动不安、堕胎、小产、胎死不下、滑胎等病。妊娠期，阴道少量流血，时下时止，或淋漓不断，而无腰酸腹痛者，称为“胎漏”，亦称“胞漏”或“漏胎”等。若妊娠期间出现腰酸腹痛或小腹下坠，或伴有少量阴道出血者，为胎动不安。凡妊娠12周

bleeding from vagina is restless fetus. Abortion occurring within 12 weeks after pregnancy is called miscarriage, while abortion occurring from 12 weeks to less than 28 weeks, with formed fetus and natural death, is called late miscarriage. Death in uterus, failing to deliver is called retention of dead fetus. Repeated abortion or miscarriage more than three times is called habitual abortion.

内，胚胎自然殒堕者，称为"堕胎"；妊娠12～28周内，胎儿已成形而自然殒堕者，称为"小产"。胎死胞中，不能自行产出者，称为"胎死不下"，亦称"胎死不能出"。凡堕胎、小产连续发生3次或以上者，称为"滑胎"，亦称"数堕胎"。

Threatened abortion and restless fetus is the harbinger of abortion and miscarriage. It is called threatened abortion in western medicine. If miscarriage is prevented, the pregnancy may continue. If the disease develops, abortion is inevitable. It is called inevitable abortion in western medicine. Retention of dead fetus is called missed abortion in western medicine. Miscarriage is called habitual abortion in western medicine.

胎漏、胎动不安是堕胎、小产的先兆，西医学称之为"先兆流产"；若安胎成功则可继续正常妊娠，若病情发展，胎堕难留，西医称之为"难免流产"；胎死胞中而不下，西医学称之为"过期流产""稽留流产"；滑胎，西医学称之为"习惯性流产"。

This problem happens due to two reasons of the parent body and fetus. Fetus origin: Because of insufficiency of essence in the couple, two kinds of essences could unite, but the fetal origin is insecure, leading to abortion. If due to defect in the fetus origin, the fetus is unable to be firm and easy to cause abortion. Parent body: because of constitutional weakness, insufficiency of the kidney qi, or consumption of the kidney essence due to intemperance in sexual life, or because of deficiency in qi and blood, impact of fetus by pathogenic heat, or complication with other diseases after pregnancy, the fetus is disturbed, leading to abortion. Besides, falling, sprain, contusion, operation and certain drugs may also lead to abortion.

本病的发生有母体与胎儿两方面原因。胎元方面：夫妇之精气不足，两精虽能结合，但胎元不固，以致流产。若因胎元有缺陷，胎多不能成实而易陨堕。母体方面：因素体虚弱，肾气不足，或因房事不节，耗损肾精，或由气血虚弱，或因邪热动胎，或受孕之后兼或其他疾病，干扰胎气，以致流产。此外，跌仆闪挫、手术和药物的影响也可引起流产。

1 Key points for diagnosis

1.1 Basic conception

During pregnancy, slight occasional vaginal bleeding and restless movement of the fetus are described "threatened abortion". Aching sensation in the loins, distenting and prolapsing sensation and pain in the abdomen, or accompanied by slight vaginal bleeding, is termed "restless fetus". If abortion occurs frequently and the examination of the husband is normal, it is known as habitual abortion.

1.2 Examination

(1) Pregnancy test is positive. B ultrasonic examination indicates normal fetal movement and fetal heart beat, and in match with menopause but vaginal bleeding is helpful for diagnosis.

(2) Chromosome examination excludes hereditary factors.

2 Syndrome differentiation and treatment

Clinically, abortion is classified into four types: insufficiency of kidney qi, asthenia of qi and blood, interior disturbance of blood heat and external injury of the collaterals. Based upon the major method to tonify the kidney, secure the Thoroughfare and Conception Vessels this problem is treated according to different situation by the methods to reinforce qi, nourish blood, tranquilize the heart and calm the mind, strengthen the spleen and harmonize the stomach, clear away heat and prevent miscarriage respectively. After proper treatment with Chinese herbs, if vaginal bleeding is controlled and abdominal pain disappears, pregnancy can continue mostly. If vaginal bleeding continues in large

1 诊断要点

1.1 基本概念

妊娠期间，阴道少量下血，时下时止为“胎漏”；腰酸腹部胀坠作痛，或伴有少量出血称为“胎动不安”。屡孕屡堕，男方检查正常者为“滑胎”。

1.2 检查

(1) 妊娠试验呈阳性反应，B 超检查胎动、胎心搏动正常，并与停经月份相符而见阴道出血者，有助于确立诊断。

(2) 染色体检查排除遗传因素所致。

2 辨证论治

流产临床上主要分为肾气不足证、气血亏虚证、血热内扰证及外伤损络证。本病的治疗，以补肾固冲任安胎为大法，并根据不同情况分别采用补气养血、宁心安神、健脾和胃、清热安胎等法。经过中医药治疗，阴道出血迅速控制，腹痛消失，多能继续妊娠。若继续出血量多、腰酸、腹痛加剧则胎元难安，又当急以去胎益母。

volume, with worsened aching in the loins and abdomen, the measures should be taken to remove the fetus to protect the mother.

2.1 Syndrome of insufficiency of kidney qi

Main manifestations Aching sensation in the loins and abdominal pain during pregnancy, stirring fetus and prolapsing sensation, or slight vaginal bleeding with light color, dizziness and tinnitus, aching knees, frequent urination, or several experiences of abortion, pale tongue with white fur, deep, thready and slippery pulse.

Therapeutic methods Supplementing kidney and qi, securing the Thoroughfare Vessel and calming the fetus.

Formulas and herbs *Fetal Longevity Pill* (Shou Tai Wan), composed of 10 g of *Semen Cuscutae* (Tu Si Zi), 15 g of *Ramulus Loranthi* (Sang Ji Sheng), 10 g of *Dipsaci Radix Fricta* (Chao Xu Duan), 10 g of *Cortex Eucommiae* (Du Zhong), 9 g of *Rhizoma Dioscoreae* (Shan Yao), 9 g of *Rhizoma Atractylodis Macrocephalae* (Bai Zhu), 15 g of *Radix et Rhizoma Boehmeriae* (Zhu Ma Gen), 10 g of *Colla Corii Asini* (E Jiao)(to be melted) and 5 g of *Fructus Amomi* (Sha Ren) (to be decocted later).

Modification For kidney yin deficiency, accompanied by feverish sensation in the chest palms and soles, red face and lips, dry mouth and throat, red tongue with little fur, thready, slippery and rapid pulse, *Radix Rehmanniae Praeparata* (Shu Di Huang), *Fructus Corni* (Shan Zhu Yu), *Cortex Lycii Radicis* (Di Gu Pi), *Polygonati Odorati Rhizoma* (Chao Yu Zhu) and *Herba Ecliptae* (Han Lian Cao) are added to nourish yin and clear away heat, secure the Thoroughfare Vessel and quiet the fetus. For

2.1 肾气不足证

主要证候 妊娠期间腰酸腹痛,胎动下坠,或伴阴道少量流血,色暗淡,头晕耳鸣,两膝酸软,小便频数,或曾屡有堕胎,舌淡,苔白,脉沉细而滑。

治法 补肾益气,固冲安胎。

方药 代表方为寿胎丸;常用药如菟丝子10克,桑寄生15克,炒续断10克,杜仲10克,山药9克,白术9克,苎麻根15克,阿胶(烊冲)10克,砂仁(后下)5克。

加减 若肾阴虚者,兼有手足心热,面赤唇红,口燥咽干,舌红少苔,脉细滑而数,加熟地黄、山茱萸、地骨皮、炒玉竹、旱莲草以滋阴清热,固冲安胎;若肾阳虚者,兼腰痛如折,畏寒肢冷,小便清长,面色晦暗,舌淡苔白滑,脉沉细而迟,治宜补肾助阳,固冲安胎,方用补肾安胎

kidney yang asthenia, severe low back pain, aversion to cold and cold limbs, profuse clear urine, somber facial complexion, pale tongue with white and slippery fur, deep, thready and slow pulse, *Kidney-Supplementing and Fetus-Quieting Decoction* (Bu Shen An Tai Yin) is used to supplement the kidney and assist yang, secure the Thoroughfare Vessels and quiet the fetus, composed of 12 g of *Radix Ginseng* (Ren Shen), 6 g of *Rhizoma Atractylodis Macrocephalae* (Bai Zhu), 12 g of *Cortex Eucommiae* (Du Zhong), 12 g of *Radix Dipsaci* (Xu Duan), 9 g of *Fructus Alpiniae Oxyphyllae* (Yi Zhi Ren), 3 g of *Colla Corii Asini* (E Jiao), 6 g of *Folium Artemistae Argyi* (Ai Ye), 12 g of *Semen Cuscutae* (Tu Si Zi), 12 g of *Fructus Psoraleae* (Bu Gu Zhi) and 12 g of *Rhizoma Cibotii* (Gou Ji). For accompanying serious qi asthenia with prolapsing sensation, *Radix Codonopsis Pilosulae* (Dang Shen) and *Radix Astragali* (Huang Qi) are added. For insufficiency of the spleen and stomach accompanied by abdominal distension, flatus and loose stool, *Radix Codonopsis Pilosulae* (Dang Shen), *Caulis Perillae* (Zi Su Geng) and *Roasting Radix Aucklandiae* (Wei Mu Xiang) are added. For dysphoria and insomnia, *Ramulus Uncariae cum Uncis* (Gou Teng), *Ziziphi Spinosi Semen Frictum* (Chao Zao Ren) and *Poria cum Ligno Hospite* (Fu Shen) are added.

饮,人参 12 克,白术 6 克,杜仲 12 克,续断 12 克,益智仁 9 克,阿胶 3 克,艾叶 6 克,菟丝子 12 克,补骨脂 12 克,狗脊 12 克;兼气虚下坠甚者,酌加党参、黄芪;脾胃不足者,兼见腹胀矢气,大便溏,加党参、紫苏梗、煨木香;心烦不得眠者,加钩藤、炒枣仁、茯神。

2.2 Syndrome of qi and blood asthenia

Main manifestations Aching sensation in the loins and abdominal pain, prolapsing sensation in the abdomen, slight vaginal bleeding with light color and thin texture, dizziness, fatigue, shortness of breath, laziness to speak, palpitation, insomnia, pale facial complexion, pale tongue with thin fur,

2.2 气血虚弱证

主要证候 妊娠期间腰酸腹痛,小腹空坠,阴道少量流血,色淡质稀,头晕眼花,精神倦怠,气短懒言,心悸失眠,面色晄白,舌淡,苔薄,脉缓滑。

slow and slippery pulse.

Therapeutic methods Supplementing qi and nourishing blood, strengthening the kidney and calming the fetus.

治法 补气养血,固肾安胎。

Formulas and herbs ① *Fetus Origin Decoction* (Tai Yuan Yin), composed of 10 g of *Radix Codonopsis Pilosulae* (Dang Shen), 10 g of *Rhizoma Atractylodis Macrocephalae* (Bai Zhu), 10 g of *Radix Paeoniae Alba* (Bai Shao), 10 g of *Radix Rehmanniae Praeparata* (Shu Di Huang), 10 g of *Colla Corii Asini* (E Jiao), 10 g of *Cortex Eucommiae* (Du Zhong), 15 g of *Radix Astragali* (Huang Qi), 6 g of *Pericarpium Citri Tangerinae* (Chen Pi) and 5 g of *Radix Glycyrrhizae Praeparata* (Zhi Gan Cao). ② *Rock of Taishan Fetus-Quieting Powder* (Tai Shan Pan Shi San), composed of 3 g of *Radix Ginseng* (Ren Shen), 6 g of *Radix Astragali* (Huang Qi), 6 g of *Rhizoma Atractylodis Macrocephalae* (Bai Zhu), 2 g of *Radix Glycyrrhizae Praeparata* (Zhi Gan Cao), 3 g of *Radix Angelicae Sinensis* (Dang Gui), 2 g of *Rhizoma Ligustici Chuanxiong* (Chuan Xiong), 3 g of *Radix Paeoniae Alba* (Bai Shao), 3 g of *Radix Rehmanniae Praeparata* (Shu Di Huang), 3 g of *Radix Dipsaci* (Xu Duan), 6 g of *Oryzae Glutinosae Semen* (Nuo Mi), 3 g of *Radix Scutellariae* (Huang Qin) and 1.5 g of *Fructus Amomi* (Sha Ren).

方药 代表方:①胎元饮;常用药如党参 10 克,白术 10 克,白芍 10 克,熟地黄 10 克,阿胶 10 克,杜仲 10 克,黄芪 15 克,陈皮 6 克,炙甘草 5 克。②泰山磐石散;常用药如人参 3 克,黄芪 6 克,白术 6 克,炙甘草 2 克,当归 3 克,川芎 2 克,白芍 3 克,熟地黄 3 克,续断 3 克,糯米 6 克,黄芩 3 克,砂仁 1.5 克。

Modification For profuse vaginal bleeding, *Os Sepiellae seu Sepiae* (Wu Zei Gu) and *Artemisiae Argyi Folium Carbonisatum* (Ai Ye Tan) are added. For loose stool, *Fructus Amomi* (Sha Ren), *Roasted Radix Aucklandiae* (Wei Mu Xiang) and *Fructus Oryzae Germinatus* (Chao Gu Ya) are added. For palpitation and insomnia, *Radix Polygalae* (Zhi

加减 若阴道下血量多者,酌加乌贼骨、艾叶炭;大便溏泄者,加砂仁、煨木香、炒谷芽;心悸失眠者,加炙远志、炒枣仁、合欢皮。

Yuan Zhi), *Semen Ziziphi Spinosae* (Chao Zao Ren) and *Cortex Alibiziae* (He Huan Pi) are added.

Shanghai doctor CHEN Danian's experience prescription, composed of 10 g of *Radix Codonopsis Pilosulae* (Dang Shen), 10 g of *Rhizoma Atractylodis Macrocephalae* (Bai Zhu), 9 g of *Poriae* (Fu Ling), 10 g of *Cortex Eucommiae* (Du Zhong), 15 g of *Ramulus Loranthi* (Sang Ji Sheng), 12 g of *Oryzae Glutinosae Semen* (Nuo Mi) and 7 *Fructus Ziziphi Jujubae* (Hong Zao).

上海医家陈大年经验方加减:党参10克,白术10克,茯苓9克,杜仲10克,桑寄生15克,糯米12克,红枣7枚。

2.3 Syndrome of blood heat

Main manifestations Dark red or bright red-vaginal bleeding during pregnancy, aching lumbus and lower abdominal pain, restless fetus and prolapsing sensation, dysphoria and insomnia, thirst with preference of cold drinking, constipation, brown urine, red tongue with yellow fur, slippery and rapid pulse.

Therapeutic methods Nourishing yin and clearing away heat, cooling blood and calming fetus.

Formulas and herbs ① *Yin-Protecting Decoction* (Bao Yin Jian), composed of 10 g of *Radix Rehmanniae Cruda* (Sheng Di Huang), 10 g of *Radix Rehmanniae Praeparata* (Shu Di Huang), 10 g of *Rhizoma Dioscoreae* (Shan Yao), 10 g of *Radix Paeoniae Alba* (Bai Shao), 10 g of *Radix Astragali* (Huang Qi), 10 g of *Radix Dipsaci* (Xu Duan), 6 g of *Phellodendri Cortex Frictus* (Chao Huang Bo), 9 g of *Sanguisorbae Radix Carbonisata* (Di Yu Tan) and 15 g of *Radix et Rhizoma Boehmeriae* (Zhu Ma Gen). ② *Chinese Angelica Powder* (Dang Gui San), composed of 9 g of *Radix Angelicae Sinensis* (Dang Gui), 9 g of *Radix Scutellariae* (Huang Qin), 9 g of *Radix Paeoniae Alba* (Bai Shao), 9 g of *Rhizoma Ligustici Chuanxiong* (Chuan Xiong) and 15 g of

2.3 血热证

主要证候　妊娠期阴道下血,血色深红或鲜红,腰酸腹痛,胎动下坠,心烦少寐,渴喜冷饮,便秘溲赤,舌红苔黄,脉滑数。

治法　滋阴清热,凉血安胎。

方药　代表方:①保阴煎;常用药如生地黄10克,熟地黄10克,山药10克,白芍10克,黄芪10克,续断10克,炒黄柏6克,地榆炭9克,苎麻根15克。②当归散;常用药如当归9克,黄芩9克,白芍9克,川芎9克,白术15克。

Rhizoma Atractylodis Macrocephalae (Bai Zhu).

Modification For profuse vaginal bleeding, *Colla Corii Asini* (E Jiao), 10 g of *Ecliptae Herba* (Han Lian Cao), *Sanguisorbae Radix Carbonisata* (Di Yu Tan) and *Processed Plastrum Testudinis* (Zhi Gui Ban) are added. For dysphoria and insomnia, *Burnt Fructus Gardeniae* (Jiao Zhi Zi), *Ramulus Uncariae cum Uncis* (Gou Teng), *Rhizoma Coptidis* (Huang Lian), *Plumula Nelumbinis* (Lian Zi Xin) and *Fructus Schisandrae* (Wu Wei Zi) are added.

加减 若下血较多者，酌加阿胶、旱莲草 10 克，地榆炭、炙龟版；心烦、失眠多梦者，可选择加焦栀子、钩藤、黄连、莲子心、五味子等。

2.4 Syndrome of fall and traumatic injury

Main manifestations During pregnancy, falls, sudden sprain, pain in the loins and abdomen, restless fetus and prolapsing sensation, vaginal bleeding, lassitude, slippery and weak pulse.

Therapeutic methods Nourishing qi and blood, Strengthening the kidney and calming the fetus.

Formulas and herbs *Modified Holy Cure Decoction Addictive* (Jia Wei Sheng Yu Tang), composed of 10 g of *Chinese Angelica* (Chao Dang Gui), 10 g of *Radix Paeoniae Alba* (Bai Shao), 10 g of *Radix Rehmanniae Praeparata* (Shu Di Huang), 15 g of *Radix Codonopsis Pilosulae* (Dang Shen), 15 g of *Radix Astragali* (Huang Qi), 10 g of *Cortex Eucommiae* (Du Zhong), 10 g of *Radix Dipsaci* (Xu Duan), 5 g of *Fructus Amomi* (Sha Ren) (to be decocted later), 10 g of *Colla Corii Asini* (E Jiao) and 10 g of *Artemisiae Argyi Folium Carbonisatum* (Ai Ye Tan).

Modification For profuse vaginal bleeding, *Radix Angelicae Sinensis* (Dang Gui) is deleted while *Colla Corii Asini* (E Jiao) and *Artemisiae Argyi Folium Carbonisatum* (Ai Ye Tan) are added to stop bleeding and calm fetus. For dysphoria and

2.4 跌仆外伤证

主要证候 妊娠期间跌仆闪挫，继而腰腹疼痛，胎动下坠，或伴阴道流血，精神倦怠，脉滑无力。

治法 益气养血，固肾安胎。

方药 代表方为加味圣愈汤；常用药如炒当归 10 克，白芍 10 克，熟地黄 10 克，党参 15 克，黄芪 15 克，杜仲 10 克，续断 10 克，砂仁（后下）5 克，阿胶 10 克，艾叶炭 10 克。

加减 若阴道流血量多者，去当归，酌加阿胶、艾叶炭以止血安胎；烦热口渴，苔黄燥者，加黄连、钩藤；腰酸神疲乏力者，加桑寄生。

thirst as well as yellow and dry tongue fur, *Rhizoma Coptidis* (Huang Lian) and *Ramulus Uncariae cum Uncis* (Gou Teng) are added. For aching sensation in the loins and spiritual lassitude, *Ramulus Loranthi* (Sang Ji Sheng) is added.

3 Other therapeutic methods

3.1 Chinese patent drugs

(1) *Kidney-Enriching and Fetus-Fostering Pill* (Zi Shen Yu Tai Wan): Take with salt water or honey water, 5 g each time and three times a day, applicable to the treatment of spleen and kidney asthenia syndrome.

(2) *Fetus-Safeguarding Pill* (Bao Tai Wan): 1 pill each time and twice a day, applicable to the treatment of insufficiency of qi and blood, insecurity of kidney qi.

(3) *Fetus-Quieting Leonurus Pill* (An Tai Yi Mu Wan): 9 g each time and twice a day, applicable to the treatment of spleen and kidney asthenia, insufficiency of qi and blood.

(4) *Fetal Longevity Pill* (Shou Tai Wan): 20 pills each time and twice a day, applicable to the treatment of kidney asthenia syndrome.

3.2 Empirical and folk recipes

(1) *Fetus Heat Decoction* (Tai Re Tang): 30 g of *Radix et Rhizoma Boehmeriae* (Zhu Ma Gen), 12 g of *Basis Folii Nelumbinis* (He Ye Di) and 9 g of *Caumen Biotae* (Ce Bai Ye) are decocted for oral taking, applicable to the treatment of blood heat syndrome.

(2) *Fetus-Safeguarding Powder* (Bao Tai San): 6 g of *Cortex Eucommiae* (Du Zhong), 6 g of *Radix Dipsaci* (Xu Duan), 6 g of *Semen Cuscutae* (Tu Si

3 其他疗法

3.1 中成药

（1）滋肾育胎丸：每次5克，每日3次，淡盐水或蜂蜜水送服，适用于脾肾两虚证。

（2）保胎丸：每次1丸，每日2次，适用于气血不足、肾气不固证。

（3）安胎益母丸：每次9克，每日2次，适用于脾肾两虚、气血不足证。

（4）寿胎丸：每次20丸，每日2次，适用于肾虚证。

3.2 单验方

（1）胎热汤：苎麻根30克，荷叶蒂12克，侧柏叶9克，水煎服，适用于血热证。

（2）保胎散：杜仲6克，续断6克，菟丝子6克，桑寄生6克，艾叶6克，共为细末，

Zi), 6 g of *Ramulus Loranthi* (Sang Ji Sheng) and 6 g of *Folium Artemistae Argyi* (Ai Ye) are ground into fine powder for oral taking, 3 g each time and twice a day in the morning and evening, applicable to the treatment of liver and kidney asthenia syndrome.

每次3克,每日早、晚各1次,适用于肝肾亏损证。

(3) *Fetus-Safeguarding Priscription* (Bao Tai Fang): 15 g of *Radix Codonopsis Pilosulae* (Dang Shen), 15 g of *Radix Astragali* (Huang Qi), 15 g of *Rhizoma Atractylodis Macrocephalae* (Bai Zhu), 15 g of *Radix Dipsaci* (Xu Duan), 15 g of *Fructus Rubi* (Fu Pen Zi), 15 g of *Semen Cuscutae* (Tu Si Zi), 15 g of *Cortex Eucommiae* (Du Zhong), 10 g of *Rhizoma Cimicifugae* (Sheng Ma) and 10 g of *Colla Cornus Cervi* (Lu Jiao Jiao) are decocted for oral taking, applicable to the treatment of spleen and kidney asthenia syndrome.

(3) 保胎方:党参15克,黄芪15克,白术15克,续断15克,覆盆子15克,菟丝子15克,杜仲15克,升麻10克,鹿角胶10克,水煎服,适用于脾肾亏虚证。

(4) 15 g of *Folium Nelumbinis* (He Ye) and 6 g of *Alumen* (Bai Fan) are decocted with 3 eggs of red shell for oral taking, applicable to the treatment of fetal heat syndrome.

(4) 荷叶15克,白矾6克,红皮鸡蛋3个,水煎煮,去药渣分服,适用于胎热证。

(5) Shanghai doctor CAI Xiaosun's experience prescription, *Kidney-Fostering, Spleen-Fortifying and Fetus-Quieting Prescription* (Yu Shen Jian Pi An Tai Fang): 10 g of *Semen Cuscutae* (Tu Si Zi), 12 g of *Eucommiae Cortex Frictus* (Chao Du Zhong), 10 g of *Ramulus Loranthi* (Sang Ji Sheng), 12 g of *Radix Dipsaci* (Xu Duan), 12 g of *Rhizoma Boehmeriae* (Zhu Ma Gen), 12 g of *Radix Codonopsis Pilosulae* (Dang Shen), 12 g of *Poriae* (Fu Ling), 10 g of *Radix Rehmanniae Cruda* (Sheng Di Huang), 10 g of *Atractylodis Macrocephalae Rhizoma Frictum* (Chao Bai Zhu) and 10 g of *Caulis Perillae* (Zi Su Geng).

(5) 上海医家蔡小荪经验方(育肾健脾安胎方):菟丝子10克,炒杜仲12克,桑寄生10克,续断12克,苎麻根12克,党参12克,茯苓12克,生地黄10克,炒白术10克,紫苏梗10克。

(6) Shanghai doctor HU Qinkui's experience prescription, *Fetus-Safeguarding Priscription* (Bao Tai Fang): 12 g of *Cortex Eucommiae* (Du Zhong), 12 g of *Radix Dipsaci* (Xu Duan), 12 g of *Ramulus Loranthi* (Sang Ji Sheng), 15 g of *Semen Cuscutae* (Tu Si Zi), 12 g of *Radix Codonopsis Pilosulae* (Dang Shen), 12 g of *Rhizoma Atractylodis Macrocephalae* (Chao Bai Zhu), 6 g of *Rhizoma Cimicifugae* (Sheng Ma), 10 g of *Pollen Typhae* (Pu Huang) and *Colla Corii Asini* (E Jiao), 10 g of *Radix Scutellariae* (Chao Huang Qin), 10 g of *Crinis Carbonisatus* (Xue Yu Tan) and 12 g of *Radix Sanguisorbae Carbonisata* (Di Yu Tan), applicable to the treatment of habitual abortion.

(6) 上海医家胡溱魁经验方(保胎方):杜仲12克,续断12克,桑寄生12克,菟丝子15克,党参12克,炒白术12克,升麻6克,蒲黄炒阿胶10克,炒黄芩10克,血余碳10克,地榆炭12克,主治漏胎或习惯性流产。

Heterotopic pregnancy

异位妊娠

Heterotopic pregnancy refers to nidation of the fertilized ovum outside the uterus, one of the common gynecological acute abdominal condition. Clinically, heterotopic pregnancy is classified into oviducal pregnancy, ovary pregnancy, abdominal pregnancy and cervical pregnancy, among which oviducal pregnancy is most commonly encountered and accounts for about 95% of heterotopic pregnancy and about 75% of it happens in the ampullar region.

异位妊娠是指受精卵在子宫体腔以外着床发育,是妇科常见的急腹症之一。临床上分为输卵管妊娠、卵巢妊娠、腹腔妊娠、宫颈妊娠等,以输卵管妊娠为最常见,占异位妊娠发生率的95%左右,发生部位以壶腹部多见,约占75%。

According to acute sharp abdominal pain and massive hemorrhage in the abdominal cavity, heterotopic pregnancy is similar to "abdominal pain during pregnancy", "blood stasis in the lower abdomen" and "abdominal mass" in TCM. Heterotypic pregnancy is usually caused by retention of stasis in the lower abdomen, unsmooth circulation of qi and

根据本病急性剧烈腹痛及腹腔内大量出血的特点,与中医学"妊娠腹痛""少腹瘀血""癥瘕"等病证相似。其发病多因少腹宿有瘀滞,冲任不畅,孕卵未能移行子宫;或先天肾气不足或气虚

blood in the Thoroughfare and Conception Vessels, failure of the fertilized ovum to migrate to the uterus, or by insufficiency of prenatal kidney qi or forceless transportation failing to transport the fertilized ovum to the uterus. Before the unbroken stage of the tubal pregnancy, the pathogenesis is mainly the blockage of fetus origin in the collateral in the bifurcations of uterus. As the disease progresses, when the obstructed collateral break, resulting in hemorrhage in the lower abdomen and blockage of the blood. If blood stasis is obstructed in the lower abdomen for long tiem, it can be accumulated to lump.

运送无力，孕卵不能及时运达子宫等因素有关。在输卵管妊娠未破损期，病机以胎元阻滞胞宫两歧之脉络为主。当病情进展，瘀滞之脉络破损时，则阴血内溢于少腹，阻滞血脉，不通则痛。若瘀阻少腹日久，亦可结而成癥。

1　Key points for diagnosis

1.1　Medical history

Most patients have a history of amenorrhea, a small number of patients with no obvious history of amenorrhea. Patients may have pelvic inflammatory disease, infertility and so on, or a history of pelvic, uterine surgery.

1.2　Symptoms

amenorrhea, abdominal pain, irregular vaginal bleeding, syncope and coma due to acute abdominal hemorrhage and sharp abdominal pain in some patient, tenderness and obvious rebound pain in the lower abdomen as well as bile shifting dullness by percussion.

1.3　Gynecological examination

Fullness and tenderness in the posterior fornix, evident raising and shaking pain in the neck of uterus, slight enlargement and softness of the uterus, floating sensation in the uterus, tumescent mass palpable in one side or in the posterior side of the ute-

1　诊断要点

1.1　病史

多有停经史，也有少数患者无明显停经史。可有盆腔炎、不孕症等病史，或盆腔、宫腔手术史。

1.2　症状

停经、腹痛、阴道不规则出血，部分患者由于腹腔内急性出血和剧烈腹痛引起昏厥与休克。出血量多时下腹部压痛及反跳痛明显，叩诊有移动性浊音。

1.3　妇科检查

阴道后穹窿饱满，触痛；宫颈有明显举痛和摇摆痛；子宫稍大而软，有漂浮感；子宫一侧或后方可触及肿块；后穹窿穿刺可抽出不凝血。

Xiang) and 6 g of *Myrrha Praeparata* (Zhi Mo Yao).

Modification For constipation and abdominal distention as well as yellow and greasy tongue fur, *Radix et Rhizoma Rhei* (Da Huang) and *Fructus Aurantii Immaturus* (Zhi Shi) are added. For complication with cold and heat, yellow, white greasy and thick tongue fur, *Radix et Rhizoma Rhei* (Da Huang) and *Cortex Cinnamomi* (Rou Gui) are added.

加减　大便秘结，腹胀，苔黄腻者，加生大黄、枳实；寒热夹杂，苔黄白腻厚者，加生大黄、肉桂。

2.2 Syndrome of blood stasis

Mian manifestations: Abortion or rupture of oviducal pregnancy, mild interior hemorrhage, stable blood pressure, distending pain aggravated by pressure in the lower abdomen, tenderness and rebound pain, slight vaginal bleeding and thready and slow pulse.

Therapeutic methods Activating blood and resolving stasis, regulating qi and stopping pain.

Formulas and herbs *No. 1 Prescription for Heterotypic Pregnancy* (Gong Wai Yun Yi Hao Fang), composed of 15 g of *Radix Salviae Miltiorrhizae* (Dan Shen), 10 g of *Radix Paeoniae Rubra* (Chi Shao), 9 g of *Semen Persicae* (Tao Ren), 10 g of *Radix Cyathulae* (Chuan Niu Xi), 3 *Scolopendra subspinipes* (Wu Gong), 10 g of *Faeces Trogopterorum* (Wu Ling Zhi) and 9 g of *Rhizoma Cyperi Praeparata* (Zhi Xiang Fu).

Modification For profuse bleeding, *Yunnan White Powder* (Yun Nan Bai Yao) and *Notoginseng Radix Pulverata* (Shen San Qi Fen) (to be swallowed) are added, twice or three times a day.

2.2 血瘀证

主要证候　输卵管妊娠流产或破裂，内出血量不多，血压平稳，腹痛腹胀拒按，有压痛及反跳痛，有少量阴道流血，脉细缓。

治法　活血化瘀，理气止痛。

方药　代表方为宫外孕Ⅰ号方；常用药如丹参15克，赤芍10克，桃仁9克，川牛膝10克，蜈蚣3条，五灵脂10克，制香附9克。

加减　出血多者，加云南白药或参三七粉吞服，每日2～3次。

2.3 Syndrome of blood stasis

Main manifestations Hematoma and mass in

2.3 血瘀证

主要证候　腹腔血肿包

the abdomen, gradual alleviation of abdominal pain, prolapsing sensation and distention in the lower abdomen or desire for defection, stoppage of vaginal bleeding and thready and unsmooth pulse.

块形成，腹痛逐渐减轻，有下腹坠胀或便意感，阴道出血停止，脉细涩。

Therapeutic methods Breaking stasis and eliminating abdominal mass.

治法 破瘀消癥。

Formulas and herbs *No. 2 Prescription for Heterotypic Pregnancy* (Gong Wai Yun Er Hao Fang), composed of 12 g of *Radix Salviae Miltiorrhizae* (Dan Shen), 10 g of *Radix Paeoniae Rubra* (Chi Shao), 6 g of *Resina Olibani* (Ru Xiang), 6 g of *Myrrha* (Mo Yao), 9 g of *Semen Persicae* (Tao Ren), 10 g of *Rhizoma Sparganii Stoloniferi* (San Leng), 10 g of *Rhizoma Zedoariae* (E Zhu) and 6 g of *Eupolyphaga seu Steleophaga* (Zhe Chong).

方药 宫外孕Ⅱ号方：常用药如丹参12克，赤芍10克，乳香6克，没药6克，桃仁9克，三棱10克，莪术10克，䗪虫6克。

Modification For infection, *Flos Lonicerae* (Jin Yin Hua), *Fructus Forsythiae* (Lian Qiao), *Caulis Sargentodoxae* (Da Xue Teng) and *Herba Patriniae* (Bai Jiang Cao) are added. For constipation, *Radix et Rhizoma Rhei* (Da Huang) and *Folium Cassiae* (Fan Xie Ye) are added.

加减 有感染者，加金银花、连翘、红藤、败酱草；便秘，加生大黄、番泻叶。

3 Other therapeutic methods

3 其他疗法

3.1 Chinese patent drugs

3.1 中成药

(1) *Rhubarb and Ground Beetle Pills* (Da Huang Zhe Chong Wan): 1 pill each time and twice a day, applicable to the treatment of heterotopic pregnancy due to blood stasis.

(1) 大黄䗪虫丸：每次1丸，每日2次，适用于血瘀证之异位妊娠。

(2) *Great Guffaw Powder* (Shi Xiao San): Taken orally 6-9 g each time and once or twice a day with vinegar or rice wine, applicable to the treatment of heterotopic pregnancy without rupture or old heterotopic pregnancy.

(2) 失笑散：每次6～9克，每日1～2次，醋或黄酒冲服，适用于未破损期或陈旧性异位妊娠。

3.2 Empirical and folk recipes

(1) *Collateral-Activating Miraculous Effect Elixir* (Huo Luo Xiao Ling Dan) composed of 9-15 g of *Radix Salviae Miltiorrhizae* (Dan Shen), 6-9 g of *Radix Paeoniae Rubra* (Chi Shao), 3-6 g of *Resina Olibani* (Ru Xiang), 3-6 g of *Myrrha* (Mo Yao) and 6-9 g of *Semen Persicae* (Tao Ren). These herbs are decocted with water, applicable to the treatment of unruptured heterotopic pregnancy due to blood stasis.

(2) *Collateral-Activating Miraculous Effect Elixir in Addition* (Jia Wei Huo Luo Xiao Ling Dan), composed of 15 g of *Radix Salviae Miltiorrhizae* (Dan Shen), 12 g of *Radix Paeoniae Rubra* (Chi Shao), 6 g of *Resina Olibani* (Ru Xiang), 6 g of *Myrrha* (Mo Yao), 6 g of *Rhizoma Sparganii Stoloniferi* (San Leng), 6 g of *Rhizoma Zedoariae* (E Zhu), 30 g of *Radix Achyranthis Bidentatae* (Niu Xi), 9 g of *Semen Persicae* (Tao Ren), 18 g of *Semen Malvae* (Dong Kui Zi), 2 *Scolopendra subspinipes* (Wu Gong) and 10 g of *Eupolyphaga seu Steleophaga* (Zhe Chong), decocted with water, applicable to the treatment of unruptured heterotopic pregnancy due to blood stasis.

(3) 3-6 g of Radix Ginseng Rubra (Hong Shen) slices or powder for oral taking, applicable to the treatment of ruptured heterotopic pregnancy due to qi asthenia and blood loss.

(4) 3 g of powder of *Radix Notoginseng Pulverata* (San Qi Fen) for oral taking, applicable to the treatment of ruptured heterotopic pregnancy with massive bleeding.

3.2 单验方

(1) 活络效灵丹：丹参9～15克，赤芍6～9克，乳香3～6克，没药3～6克，桃仁6～9克，水煎服，适用于未破损期血瘀证异位妊娠。

(2) 加味活络效灵丹：丹参15克，赤芍12克，乳香6克，没药6克，三棱6克，莪术6克，牛膝30克，桃仁9克，冬葵子18克，蜈蚣2条，䗪虫10克，水煎服，适用于未破损期血瘀证异位妊娠。

(3) 红参片或红参粉3～6克，吞服，适用于已破损期气虚血脱证异位妊娠。

(4) 三七粉3克，吞服，适用于已破损期出血多之异位妊娠。

Morning sickness

Morning sickness refers to nausea, vomiting, anorexia or even postcibal vomiting during pregnancy.

Morning sickness in usually caused by upward adverse flow of qi from the Thoroughfare Vessel and failure of gastric qi to descend in the early period of pregnancy, or by original asthenia of gastric qi, or frequent restlessness and susceptibility to rage and heat transformed from liver qi stagnation, or by asthenia of spleen yang leading to interior retention of phlegm and fluid as well as upward attack of qi from the Thoroughfare Vessel with liver fire into the stomach; or by upward adverse flow of qi from the Thoroughfare Vessel with phlegm and fluid.

1 Key points for diagnosis

1.1 Clinical manifestation

(1) With a history of absence of menstruation, vomiting, anorexia or postcibal vomiting, usually occurring in the first three months of pregnancy.

(2) Frequent vomiting, anorexia, even leading to malaise, listlessness, obvious emaciation, dry skin and mucous membranes, sunken eyes, weight loss, and decreased blood pressure, fever, jaundice, lethargy and coma in severe cases.

1.2 Laboratory tests

① pregnancy testis positive. ② ketone bodies is an important indicator of diagnosis of metabolic aci-

妊娠恶阻

妊娠恶阻是指妊娠期间，反复出现恶心呕吐，进食受阻，甚则食入即吐。该病又称为“妊娠呕吐”“阻病”“子病”等。

本病多因妊娠早期冲脉之气上逆，胃失和降所致。若胃气素虚，或平素性燥多怒，肝郁化热，或脾阳素虚，痰饮内停，冲气挟肝火上逆犯胃，或冲气挟痰饮上逆所致。

1 诊断要点

1.1 临床表现

（1）有停经史，呕吐厌食或食入即吐，多发生在3个月内。

（2）呕吐发作频繁，厌食，甚则可导致全身乏力，精神萎靡，明显消瘦，全身皮肤和黏膜干燥，眼球凹陷，体重下降，严重者可出现血压降低，体温升高，黄疸，嗜睡和昏迷。

1.2 实验室检查

①妊娠试验阳性。②尿酮体是诊断妊娠呕吐引起代

dosis caused by pregnant vomiting. ③ Determination of peripheral red blood cell count, hematocrit, hemoglobin, carbon dioxide combining with power CO_2CP, potassium, sodium, chlorine, etc., as well as liver and kidney function, electrocardiogram.

谢性酸中毒的重要指标。③测定外周血红细胞计数、血细胞压积、血红蛋白、二氧化碳结合力，钾、钠、氯等，以及肝肾功能、心电图等。

2 Syndrome differentiation and treatment

2 辨证论治

Based upon the character, color, texture and smell of vomitus, in combination of general symptoms, tongue and pulse diagnosis, syndrome differentiation is processed for comprehensive analysis, in order to identify cold, heat, deficiency and excess. The major therapeutic method is fundamentally decided to regulate qi, harmonize the middle energizer, bring down counterflow, and stop vomiting. It is necessary to pay attention to diet and emotional regulation, and appropriate to use the drugs in moderate property, instead of the drugs in acid, dry, ascending and dispersing property.

辨证主要根据呕吐物的性状、色、质、气味，结合全身证候、舌脉进行综合分析，以辨其寒、热、虚、实。治疗大法以调气和中，降逆止呕为主。并应注意饮食和情志的调节，用药宜平和，忌辛燥、升散之品。

2.1 Syndrome of stomach asthenia

2.1 胃虚证

Main manifestations In early pregnancy, nausea, vomiting, postcibal vomiting, bland taste in the mouth, vomiting of clear saliva, poor appetite, abdominal distention, dizziness, lassitude, pale tongue with white fur, slow, slippery and weak pulse.

主要证候 妊娠早期，恶心呕吐，甚则食入即吐，口淡，呕吐清涎，纳呆腹胀，头晕体倦，舌淡，苔白，脉缓滑无力。

Therapeutic methods Strenghthening the spleen and harmonizing the stomach, descending adverse flow of qi to stop vomiting.

治法 健脾和胃，降逆止呕。

Formulas and herbs *Costus Root and Amomum with Six Nobles Decoction* (Xiang Sha Liu Jun Zi Tang), composed of 10 g of *Radix Codonopsis Pilosulae* (Dang Shen), 10 g of *Rhizoma Atractylodis Macrocephalae* (Bai Zhu), 3 g of *Radix Glycyrrhizae* (Gan Cao), 6 g of *Rhizoma Pinelliae*

方药 代表方为香砂六君子汤；常用药如党参 10 克，白术 10 克，甘草 3 克，制半夏 6 克，陈皮 6 克，茯苓 10 克，广藿香 5 克，砂仁 5 克，紫苏叶 5 克，炒竹茹 9 克，生姜

Praeparata (Zhi Ban Xia), 6 g of *Pericarpium Citri Tangerinae* (Chen Pi), 10 g of *Poriae* (Fu Ling), 5 g of *Herba Pogostemonis* (Guang Huo Xiang), 5 g of *Fructus Amomi* (Sha Ren), 5 g of *Folium Perillae* (Zi Su Ye), 9 g of *Caulis Bambusae in Taeniam* (Chao Zhu Ru), 3 slices of *Rhizoma Zingiberis Recens* (Sheng Jiang) and 3 *Fructus Ziziphi Jujubae* (Hong Zao).

3片,大枣3枚。

Modification For asthenia-cold of the spleen and stomach, *Flos Caryophylli* (Ding Xiang) and *Semen Amomi Cardamomi* (Bai Dou Kou) are added. For yin injury by severe vomiting, with the symptoms of dry mouth and constipation, *Radix Aucklandiae* (Mu Xiang), *Fructus Amomi* (Sha Ren) and *Poriae* (Fu Ling) are deleted while *Rhizoma Polygonati Odorati* (Yu Zhu), *Ophiopogonis Radix* (Mai Dong), *Herba Dendrobii* (Shi Hu) and *Sesami Semen Nigrum* (Hu Ma Ren) are added.

加减 若脾胃虚寒者,酌加丁香、白豆蔻;若吐甚伤阴,症见口干便秘,去木香、砂仁、茯苓,加玉竹、麦冬、石斛、胡麻仁。

2.2 Syndrome of liver-stomach disharmony

2.2 肝胃不和证

Main manifestations In early pregnancy, vomiting of acid fluid or bitter fluid, fullness and oppression in the chest and hypochondrium, belching and sighing, dizziness, blurred vision, bitter taste in the mouth and dry throat, thirst with preference for cold drinks, reddish tongue with yellow fur, slippery and taut pulse.

主要证候 妊娠早期,呕吐酸水或苦水,胸胁满闷,嗳气叹息,头晕目眩,口苦咽干,渴喜冷饮,舌红,苔黄,脉弦滑。

Therapeutic methods Clearing the liver and harmonizing the stomach, descending adverse flow of qi and stopping vomiting.

治法 清肝和胃,降逆止呕。

Formulas and herbs ① *Gallbladder-Warming Decoction in Addition* (Jia Wei Wen Dan Tang), composed of 6 g of *Pericarpium Citri Tangerinae* (Chen Pi), 6 g of *Rhizoma Pinelliae Praeparata* (Zhi Ban Xia), 6 g of *Caulis Bambusae in Taeniam*

方药 代表方:①加味温胆汤;常用药如陈皮6克,制半夏6克,炒竹茹6克,茯苓10克,甘草3克,炒枳实9克,黄芩9克,黄连5克,麦冬

(Chao Zhu Ru), 10 g of *Poriae* (Fu Ling), 3 g of *Radix Glycyrrhizae* (Gan Cao), 9 g of *Fructus Aurantii Immaturus* (Chao Zhi Shi), 9 g of *Radix Scutellariae* (Huang Qin), 5 g of *Rhizoma Coptidis* (Huang Lian), 10 g of *Ophiopogonis Radix* (Mai Dong), 15 g of *Rhizoma Phragmitis* (Lu Gen) and 3 slices of *Rhizoma Zingiberis Recens* (Sheng Jiang). ②*Perilla Leaf and Coptis Decoction* (Su Ye Huang Lian Tang) composed of 9 g of *Folium Perillae* (Zi Su Ye), 6 g of *Rhizoma Coptidis* (Huang Lian), 9 g of *Rhizoma Pinelliae* (Ban Xia), 9 g of *Caulis Bambusae in Taeniam* (Zhu Ru) and 6 g of *Pericarpium Citri Tangerinae* (Chen Pi).

10克，芦根15克，生姜3片。②苏叶黄连汤；常用药如紫苏叶9克，黄连6克，半夏9克，竹茹9克，陈皮6克。

Modification　For injury of body fluid due to excessive vomiting, feverish sensation over the palms, soles and chest, red tongue and dry mouth, *Herba Dendrobii* (Shi Hu) and *Rhizoma Polygonati Odorati* (Yu Zhu) are added to nourish yin and clear away heat. For constipation, *Sesami Semen Nigrum* (Hu Ma Ren) is added to lubricate intestines to promote defection.

加减　若呕吐甚伤津，五心烦热，舌红口干者，酌加石斛、玉竹以养阴清热；便秘者，酌加胡麻仁以润肠通便。

2.3　Syndrome of phlegm retention

2.3　痰滞证

Main manifestations　In early pregnancy, vomiting of sputum and saliva, fullness and oppression in the chest and diaphragm, anorexia, bland and greasy taste in the mouth, dizziness, blurred vision, palpitation and shortness of breath, pale and bulgy tongue, white and greasy tongue fur, and slippery pulse.

主要证候　妊娠早期，呕吐痰涎，胸膈满闷，不思饮食，口中淡腻，头晕目眩，心悸气短，舌淡胖，苔白腻，脉滑。

Therapeutic methods　Resolving phlegm and eliminating dampness, descending adverse flow of qi and stopping vomiting.

治法　化痰除湿，降逆止呕。

Formulas and herbs　*Minor Pinellia Decoction Plus Poria Decocotion* (Xiao Ban Xia Jia Fu Ling Tang), composed of 6 g of *Rhizoma Pinelliae*

方药　代表方为小半夏加茯苓汤；常用药如制半夏6克，陈皮6克，茯苓10克，生

Praeparata (Zhi Ban Xia), 6 g of *Pericarpium Citri Tangerinae* (Chen Pi), 10 g of *Poriae* (Fu Ling), 3 slices of *Rhizoma Zingiberis Recens* (Sheng Jiang), 6 g of *Herba Pogostemonis* (Guang Huo Xiang), 9 g of *Caulis Bambusae in Taeniam* (Chao Zhu Ru), 6 g of *Flos Magnoliae Officinalis* (Hou Po Hua), 10 g of *Fructus Oryzae Germinatus* (Chao Gu Ya) and 10 g of *Fructus Hordei Germinatus* (Chao Mai Ya).

姜3片,广藿香6克,炒竹茹9克,川朴花6克,炒谷芽10克,炒麦芽10克。

Modification For hypofunction of the spleen and stomach and interior exuberance of phlegm and dampness, *Rhizoma Atractylodis* (Cang Zhu) and *Rhizoma Atractylodis Macrocephalae* (Bai Zhu) are added. For vomiting of clear fluid, cold sensation in the body and limbs as well as pale complexion, *Flos Caryophylli* (Ding Xiang) and *Semen Amomi Cardamomi* (Bai Dou Kou) are added. For vomiting of yellowish fluid, dizziness, dysphoria and preference for sour and cold foods due to heat, *Radix Scutellariae* (Huang Qin), *Rhizoma Anemarrhenae* (Zhi Mu) and *Radix Peucedani* (Qian Hu) are added.

加减 若脾胃虚弱痰湿内盛者,酌加苍术、白术;兼寒者,症见呕吐清水,形寒肢冷,面色苍白,加丁香、白豆蔻;若挟热者,症见呕吐黄水,头晕心烦,喜食酸冷,酌加黄芩、知母、前胡。

3 Other therapeutic methods

3 其他疗法

3.1 Chinese patent drugs

3.1 中成药

(1) *Coptis and Evodia Pills* (Zuo Jin Wan): 3-6 g each time and twice a day, applicable to the treatment of syndrome of liver-stomach disharmony.

(1) 左金丸:每次3～6克,每日2次,适用于肝胃不和证。

(2) *Costus Root and Amomum with Six Nobles Pill* (Xiang Sha Liu Jun Wan): 6-9 g each time and twice or three times a day, applicable to the treatment of syndrome of hypofunction of the spleen and stomach.

(2) 香砂六君丸:每次6～9克,每日2～3次,适用于脾胃虚弱证。

(3) *Pulse-Engendering Capsule* (Sheng Mai Yin Jiao Nang): 3 capsules each time and three times a day, applicable to the treatment of syndrome of as-

(3) 生脉饮胶囊:每次3粒,每日3次,适用于气阴两亏证。

thenia of qi and yin.

(4) *Two Matured Ingredients Pill* (Er Chen Wan): 9-15 g each time and twice a day, applicable to the treatment of syndrome of phlegm retention.

(4) 二陈丸：每次 9～15 克，每日 2 次，适用于痰湿阻滞证。

3.2 Empirical and folk recipes

3.2 单验方

(1) *Loquat Leaf Tea* (Pi Pa Ye Cha): 15 g of *Folium Eriobotryae* (Pi Pa Ye) (removal of the hair) and 30 g of *Terra Flava Usta* (Fu Long Gan) (to be wrapped) are decocted in water. The decoction is taken orally as tea, applicable to the treatment of stomach asthenia syndrome.

(1) 枇杷叶茶：生枇杷叶(去毛)15 克，伏龙肝(布包) 30 克，水煎后代茶频呷，适用于胃虚证。

(2) 9 g of *Caulis Bambusae in Taeniam* (Zhu Ru) and 3 g of *Pericarpium Citri Tangerinae* (Chen Pi) are decocted in water for oral taking, applicable to the treatment of phlegm-dampness syndrome.

(2) 竹茹 9 克，陈皮 3 克，水煎服，适用于痰湿证。

(3) 30-90 g of *Terra Flava Usta* (Fu Long Gan) (to be wrapped) is decocted in water. The clear decoction is for oral taking in 3-5 times, applicable to the treatment of syndrome of asthenia-cold in the spleen and stomach.

(3) 伏龙肝 30～90 克，布包水煎，澄清液分 3～5 次服，适用于脾胃虚寒证。

(4) 1 cup of *Truncus Sacchari* (Gan Zhe) juice and 4-5 drops of *Rhizoma Zingiberis Recens* (Sheng Jiang) juice are mixed together and taken a little each hour, applicable to the treatment of syndrome of hypofunction of the spleen and stomach.

(4) 甘蔗汁 1 杯，生姜汁 4～5 滴，每隔 1 小时服少许，适用于脾胃虚弱证。

(5) 10 g of *Radix Scutellariae* (Huang Qin) and 50 g of *Fructus Lycii* (Gou Qi Zi) are soaked in boiling water for oral taking, applicable to the treatment of morning sickness due to various factors.

(5) 黄芩 10 克，枸杞子 50 克，沸水泡后频饮，适用于各证恶阻。

(6) Shanghai doctor CAI Xiaosun's experience prescription, *Center-Harmonizing and Pregnancy-Protecting Prescription* (He Zhong Bao Yun Fang): 12 g of *Poriae* (Yun Ling), 5 g of *Rhizoma Pinelliae Preparata* (Jiang Ban Xia), 6 g of *Caulis*

(6) 上海医家蔡小荪经验方(和中保孕方)：云茯苓 12 克，姜半夏 5 克，姜竹茹 6 克，桑寄生 10 克，炒白术 10 克，淡子芩 10 克，苏梗 10 克，

Bambusae in TaeniamPreparata (Jiang Zhu Ru), 10 g of *Ramulus Loranthi* (Sang Ji Sheng), 10 g of *Rhizoma Atractylodis Macrocephalae* (Chao Bai Zhu), 10 g of *Radix Scutellariae* (Zi Qin), 10 g of *Caulis Perillae* (Su Geng), 5 g of *Pericarpium Citri Tangerinae* (Chen Pi) and 10 g of *Rhizoma Boehmeriae* (Zhu Ma Gen).

陈皮5克,苎麻根10克。

(7) Shanghai doctor HU Qinkui's experience prescription, *Spleen-Fortifying, Liver-Coursing and Vomiting-Stopping Prescription* (Jian Pi Shu Gan Zhi Tu Fang): 12 g of *Rhizoma Atractylodis Macrocephalae cum Terra Frictum* (Tu Chao Bai Zhu), 12 g of *Rhizoma Dioscoreaecum Terra Frictum* (Tu Chao Shan Yao), 10 g of *Caulis Bambusae in TaeniamPreparata* (Jiang Zhu Ru), 10 g of *Herba Agastachis* (Huo Xiang), 10 g of *Caulis Perillae* (Zi Su Geng), 6 g of *Pericarpium Citri Tangerinae* (Chen Pi), 6 g of *Fructus Citri* (Xiang Yuan), 5 g of *Flos Mume* (Lu Mei Hua), 5 g of *Flos Citri Sarcodactyli* (Fo Shou Hua), 3 g of *Fructus Amomi* (Sha Ren) and 2 slices of *Rhizoma Zingiberis Recens* (Sheng Jiang), applicable to the treatment of morning sickness during pregnancy.

(7)上海医家胡溱魁经验方(健脾疏肝止吐方):土炒白术12克,土炒山药12克,姜竹茹10克,藿香10克,紫苏梗10克,陈皮6克,香橼皮6克,绿梅花5克,佛手花5克,砂仁3克,生姜2片,主治妊娠恶阻。

Pregnancy-induced hypertension syndrome

妊娠高血压综合征

Pregnancy-induced hypertension syndromeis characterized by hypertension, edema and proteinuria occurring 20 weeks after pregnancy. It severely affects maternal and fetus health, and is one of the major reasons to induce maternal and perinatal infant's mortality. According to their clinical fea-

妊娠高血压疾病以妊娠20周以后高血压、蛋白尿、水肿为特征,严重影响母婴健康,是引起孕产妇和围产儿死亡的重要原因之一。可根据其不同阶段的临床特征,

tures during different stages, it may be treated based on edema in pregnancy, dizziness in pregnancy and eclampsia gravidarum in TCM.

参照子肿、子晕和子痫论治。

This syndrome is usually caused by worsened weakness of the body after pregnancy, or by constitutional asthenia of the spleen and kidney yang, dysfunction of the spleen and liver, in the warming ability and in transforming and transporting dampness, leading to retention of fluid and dampness and edema in the skin and the four limbs, described as the spleen deficiency and liver hyperactivity. The gradual growth of the fetus can hinder the ascending and descending ability in qi activity. If the water passage is dysfunctional, water and dampness would overflow in the muscles and skin, leading to “edema during pregnancy”. If yin is deficient in the liver and kidney originally, and essence and blood are insufficient, when blood is accumulated after pregnancy to nourish the fetus, essence and blood would be more deficient, leading to “nausea in pregnancy”, while yin blood fails to preserve yin and the liver yang is hyperactive. In severe condition, if the liver fails to be nourished, the liver wind stirs internally, or disturbs upward with phlegm and fire, or attacks the clear orifice with deficient wind, resulting in “eclampsia gravidarum”.

本病多因脏气本虚，受孕后愈虚；或因素体脾肾阳虚，肝脾失调，不能温煦、运化水湿，以致水湿停滞，泛于肌肤、四肢，脾虚肝旺；胎体渐长，则可阻碍气机升降，水道不利，水湿泛于肌肤，发为“子肿”。如若素体肝肾阴虚，精血不足，妊娠后血聚以养胎，精血愈虚，阴血不敛阳，肝阳上亢谓之“子晕”；甚则肝失所养，肝风内动，或挟痰火上扰，或虚风上犯清窍而成“子痫”。

1 Key points for diagnosis

1 诊断要点

1.1 Clinical manifestation

1.1 临床表现

(1) The symptoms gradually occur after 20 weeks of pregnancy, such as dizziness, distention of head and headache, blurred vision, edema above the ankle and scanty urine. Sudden vertigo and fall, loss of consciousness, staring eyes, lockjaw, spasm

（1）妊娠20周后逐渐出现头晕目眩，头胀而痛，视物昏花，踝部以上水肿，小便短少；妊娠晚期及新产后，可突然眩晕仆倒，昏不知人，两目

of limbs, opisthotonos or even coma in the late stage of pregnancy and just after labor.

(2) Accompanied by hypertension in different degree, edema or proteinuria of mild, medium and severe degrees after 20 weeks of pregnancy.

1.2 Examination

Blood and urine tests, test of liver functions, fundus examination, electrocardiography and examination of placenta functions and fetal maturity are helpful for diagnosis.

1.3 Differentiation

This syndrome should be differentiated from pregnancy complicated with primary hypertension, chronic nephritis and pheochromocytoma. Eclampsia gravidarum should be differentiated from epilepsy, cerebral hemorrhage, hysteria and convulsion of hands and feet.

2 Syndrome differentiation and treatment

Clinically, this syndrome is classified into pattern of yin asthenia and liver hyperactivity, pattern of spleen asthenia and liver hyperactivity, pattern of wind-fire and phlegm-fire. The therapeutic principle is soothing the liver and suppressing yang. The therapeutic methods are used based upon the pathological situation respectively to nourish yin and descend adverse flow of qi, regulate qi and resolve phlegm, and nourish qi and invigorate blood.

2.1 Syndrome of yin asthenia and liver hyperactivity

Main manifestations Dizziness, poor sleep, aching sensation in the loins, palpitation, shortness of breath, flushed complexion, accompanied by hypertension, proteinuria, edema of lower limbs, red

上视，牙关紧闭，四肢抽搐，角弓反张，甚至昏迷不醒等。

(2) 妊娠20周后伴不同程度的高血压、水肿或蛋白尿，分为轻、中、重三度。

1.2 检查

如血液、尿液检查，肝肾功能测定，眼底检查，心电图，胎盘功能，胎儿成熟度检查等有助于诊断。

1.3 鉴别

本病须与妊娠合并原发性高血压、慢性肾炎、嗜铬细胞瘤等相鉴别；子痫还应与癫痫、脑溢血、癔病、手足搐搦症相鉴别。

2 辨证论治

本病临床主要分为阴虚肝旺证、脾虚肝旺证、风火证及痰火证。治疗以平肝潜阳为基本原则，根据病情分别采用滋阴潜降、理气化痰、益气养血法等。

2.1 阴虚肝旺证

主要证候 妊娠晚期头晕目眩，寐差，腰酸，心悸气短，面色潮红，伴见高血压，蛋白尿，下肢浮肿，舌红或

sion of limbs, lockjaw, staring eyes, opisthotonos, feverish palms and soles, flushed cheeks and coarce breathing, red or deep-red tongue with thin yellow fur, taut, thready and rapid or taut and powerful pulse.

临产及新产后,突然眩晕,四肢抽搐,牙关紧闭,目睛直视,腰背反张,手足心热,颧赤息粗,舌红或绛,苔薄黄,脉弦细而数或弦劲有力。

Therapeutic methods Stopping wind and suppressing yang, soothing the liver and clearing away heat from the heart.

治法 熄风潜阳,平肝清心。

Formulas and herbs *Antelope's Horn and Cat's Claw Decoction* (Ling Jiao Gou Teng Tang), composed of 0.6 g of *Cornu Saigae Tataricae Pulveratum* (Ling Yang Jiao Fen) (to be swallowed), 20 g of *Ramulus Uncariae cum Uncis* (Gou Teng) (to be decocted later), 12 g of *Folium Mori* (Sang Ye), 9 g of *Flos Chrysanthemi* (Ju Hua), 9 g of *Bulbus Fritillariae Cirrhosae* (Chuan Bei Mu), 30 g of *Radix Rehmanniae Recens* (Xian Sheng Di), 9 g of *Rhizoma Acori Graminei* (Shi Chang Pu), 9 g of *Concretio Siliceae Bambusae* (Tian Zhu Huang) and 30 g of *Concha Haliotidis* (Shi Jue Ming) (to be decocted early).

方药 代表方为羚角钩藤汤;常用药如羚羊角粉(吞服)0.6克,钩藤(后下)20克,桑叶12克,菊花9克,川贝母9克,鲜生地30克,石菖蒲9克,天竺黄9克,石决明(先煎)30克。

Modification For exuberant fire in the liver and heart, *Gentianae Radix* (Long Dan Cao), *Rhizoma Coptidis* (Huang Lian), *Folium Ilicis* (Ku Ding Cha) and *Spica Prunellae* (Xia Ku Cao) are added. For syncope and profuse phlegm, *Concretio Siliceae Bambusae* (Tian Zhu Huang), *Rhizoma Arisaematis cum Bile* (Dan Nan Xing) and *Radix Polygalae* (Zhi Yuan Zhi) are added.

加减 如心肝火旺盛者,加龙胆草、黄连、苦丁茶、夏枯草;挟有昏迷痰多者,加天竺黄、胆南星、炙远志。

2.4 Phlegm-fire syndrome

2.4 痰火证

Main manifestations In the late stage of pregnancy, about to give birth and postpartum, headache, chest oppression, sudden syncope, lockjaw, frothy drooling, rough breathing, sputum rale,

主要证候 妊娠晚期,或临产及新产后,头痛胸闷,突然昏仆不知人,牙关紧闭,口流痰涎,息粗痰鸣,烦躁不

restlessness, palpitation, nervousness, poor sleep at night, red tongue with yellow, greasy and thick fur, slippery and rapid pulse.

已，惊悸不安，入夜寐差，舌偏红，舌苔黄腻而厚，脉滑数。

Therapeutic methods Clearing away heat and expelling phlegm, resuscitating brain and tranquilizing spirit.

治法 清热豁痰，开窍安神。

Formulas and herbs *Peaceful Palace Bovine Bezoar Pills* (An Gong Niu Huang Wan), composed of 0.3 g of *Calculus Bovis Pulverata* (Niu Huang Fen) (to be swallowed), 9 g of *Radix Scutellariae* (Huang Qin), 9 g of *Rhizoma Coptidis* (Huang Lian), 9 g of *Fructus Gardeniae* (Zhi Zi), 9 g of *Rhizoma Acori Graminei* (Shi Chang Pu), 3 g of *Scorpio Pulverata* (Quan Xie Fen) (to be swallowed), 30 g of *Concha Haliotidis* (Shi Jue Ming) (to be decocted early), 30 g of *Mastodi Dentis Fossilia Cruda* (Sheng Long Chi) (to be decocted early) and 9 g of *Bumbusae Caulis in Taenia* (Dan Zhu Ru).

方药 安宫牛黄丸；常用药如牛黄粉（吞服）0.3 克，黄芩 9 克，黄连 9 克，栀子 9 克，石菖蒲 9 克，全蝎粉（吞服）3 克，石决明（先煎）30 克，生龙齿（先煎）30 克，淡竹茹 9 克。

Modification For occasional convulsion, *Ramulus Uncariae cum Uncis* (Gou Teng) and *Scorpio Pulverata* (Quan Xie Fen) are added. For syncope, 1 pill of *Crown Jewel Elixir* (Zhi Bao Dan) or 1 pill of *Styrax Pills* (Su He Xiang Wan) are added for oral taking, twice a day.

加减 有时抽搐者，加钩藤、全蝎粉；昏迷者，加服至宝丹 1 粒，或苏合香丸，每次 1 丸，每日 2 次。

3 Other therapeutic methods

3 其他疗法

3.1 Chinese patent drugs

3.1 中成药

(1) *Anemarrhena, Phellodendron, and Rehmannia Pill* (Zhi Bo Di Huang Wan): 10 g each time and twice a day, applicable to the treatment of vertigo due to yin asthenia and liver hyperactivity during pregnancy.

（1）知柏地黄丸：每次 10 克，每日 2 次，适用于阴虚肝旺型子晕。

(2) *Free Wanderer Pillin Addition* (Jia Wei Xi-

（2）加味逍遥丸：每次

ao Yao Wan): 6-9 g each time and twice a day, applicable to the treatment of vertigo in pattern of yin asthenia and liver hyperactivity during pregnancy.

6～9 克,每日 2 次,适用于脾虚肝旺型子晕。

(3) *Peaceful Palace Bovine Bezoar Pills* (An Gong Niu Huang Wan): 1 pill each time and twice a day, applicable to the treatment of eclampsia gravidarum in coma type.

(3) 安宫牛黄丸:每次 1 粒,每日 2 次,适用于昏迷型子痫。

(4) *Bovine Bezoar and Heart-Purifying Pills* (Niu Huang Qing Xin Wan): 9 g each time and twice a day, applicable to the treatment of eclampsia gravidarum in patterns of phlegm-fire attacking the brain.

(4) 牛黄清心丸:每次 9 克,每日 2 次,适用于痰火上扰型子痫。

(5) *Purple Snow Elixir* (Zi Xue Dan): 1.5-3 g each time and once or twice a day, applicable to the treatment of eclampsia gravidarum in pattern of internal disturbance of liver wind.

(5) 紫雪丹:每次 1.5～3 克, 每日 1～2 次,适用于肝风内动型子痫。

3.2 Empirical and folk recipes

3.2 单验方

(1) 9 g of *Rhizoma Gastrodiae* (Tian Ma) is decocted together with two eggs. The decoction is applicable to the treatment of premonitory signs of eclampsia gravidarum in pattern of yin asthenia and yang hyperactivity.

(1) 天麻 9 克,水煎炖鸡蛋 2 个,适用于阴虚阳亢型先兆子痫。

(2) 250 g of *White Flos Chrysanthemi* (Bai Ju Hua) is decocted. The decoction is taken orally as tea, applicable to the treatment of premonitory signs of eclampsia gravidarum in pattern of yin asthenia and liver hyperactivity.

(2) 白菊花 250 克,泡茶饮,适用于阴虚肝旺型先兆子痫。

(3) 15 ml of *Succus Phyllostachydis Henonis* (Zhu Li Shui) is mixed with water for oral taking, applicable to the treatment of eclampsia gravidarum in pattern of phlegm heat.

(3) 竹沥水 15 毫升,冲服,适用于痰热型子痫。

(4) 500 g of carp, 6 g of scallion and ginger, 15 g of *Poriae* (Fu Ling), 20 g of *Rhizoma Atractylodis Macrocephalae* (Bai Zhu) and 15 g of *Semen*

(4) 鲤鱼 500 克,葱姜 6 克,茯苓 15 克,白术 20 克,车前子(包煎)15 克,水煎服,适

Plantaginis (Che Qian Zi) (to be wrapped for decocting) are decocted in water for oral taking, applicable to the treatment of various types of edema during pregnancy.

用于各型妊娠水肿。

(5) 400 g of *Rice Root* (Zao Dao Gen) is decocted for oral taking, applicable to the treatment of edema in pattern of asthenia of spleen and kidney yang during pregnancy.

(5) 早稻根400克,水煎服,适用于脾肾阳虚证妊娠水肿。

Chapter 7 Puerperal diseases

第7章 产后病

Puerperal diseases refer to the diseases happening after new childbirth and in the puerperium in relation to delivery or puerperium. The etiology and pathogenesis of puerperal diseases are of body fluid by blood collapse, original qi depletion, vacuity fire tending to stir, and internal obstruction of static blood, frenetic movement of vanquished blood, and improper ingestion of food, overstress and external pathogens. Because the puerperal diseases happen due to deficiency and detriment in qi, blood and body fluid, the constitutional energy is deficient and the pathogenic factors are exberant, therefore leading to multiple deficiency and blood stasis.

产妇在新产后及产褥期内发生的与分娩或产褥有关的疾病，称为“产后病”。产后病的病因病机一是亡血伤津，元气亏损，虚火易动；二是瘀血内阻，败血妄行；三为饮食劳倦外邪所伤。由于产后病是在气血津液虚损的基础上发生的，正虚邪盛，故形成了多虚多瘀的特点。

According to the feature of multiple asthenia and blood stasis in the pathogenesis of the puerperal diseases, based upon the therapeutical principle of “not limited to postpartum, and remembering postpartum”, it is necessary in the clinical treatment to pay attention to the relationship between deficiency tonification and evil elimination, by circulating qi without its over consumption and distribution, and strengthening the spleen. In removing food retention, by using the warm and dry drugs carefully in treating cold pattern, and by preventing hiding of ice in treatng heat pattern. Although it is appropriate to treat deficiency and detriment by tonic drug,

根据产后多虚多瘀的病机特点，治疗本着“勿拘于产后，亦勿忘于产后”的原则，临证时应注意补虚与祛邪的关系，注意行气勿过耗散，消导需兼扶脾，治寒慎用温燥，疗热谨防冰伏。虽有虚损宜补，但不可过于温热滋腻厚味，以防碍胃助邪。同时，应掌握产后用药“三禁”：禁大汗、禁峻下、禁通利小便。禁大汗以防亡阳，禁峻下以防亡阴，禁通利小便以防亡津

it is advisable not to use the drugs in over warm, hot, greasy property, in order to avoid hindering the stomach and assisting the pathogens. At the same time, it is necessary to pay attention to three prohibitions "in using herbal drugs for postpartum to prohibit profuse sweating", "to prohibit harsh purgation" and "to prohibit freeing urine". To prohibit profuse sweating is to prevent yang depletion. To prohibit harsh purgation is to prevent yin depletion. To prohibit freeing urine is to prevent depletion of body fluid. For critical and serious puerperal diseases, it is advisable to seek the integrated therapy of Chinese medicine and Western medicine.

液。对产后危急重证，应中西医结合治疗。

Postpartum hemorrhage

产后出血

Postpartum hemorrhage refers to bleeding volume in or over 500 ml within 24 hours after labor. It is one of the important causes to induce maternal death and also one of the causes in puerperal infection. It is a severe and acute disease in obstetrics, which requires immediate and correct treatment.

产后出血是指胎儿娩出后 24 小时内出血量达到或超过 500 毫升者。本病是导致产妇死亡的重要原因之一，也是产褥感染的诱因之一，是产科的危重急症，必须及时抢救，正确处置。

This disease belongs to the scope of "puerperal metrorrhagia" and "postpartum blood dizziness" in TCM. It is usually caused by the constitutional weakness of the parturient, or overstrain and consumption of primordial qi due to prolonged labor, or by invasion of exogenous pathogenic cold, coagulating blood and turbid fluid in the Thoroughfare and Conception Vessels, or by injury of the birth canal.

本病属中医学"产后血崩""产后血晕"范畴。本病多因产妇素体虚弱，或因产程过长，疲劳过度，损伤元气，或感受寒邪，凝滞余血浊液，瘀阻冲任，或产道损伤所致。

1 Key points for diagnosis

1 诊断要点

1.1 Clinical manifestation

1.1 临床表现

Sudden massive bleeding from the vagina right

新产后突然阴道大量出

after labor, especially over 500 ml of bleeding volume from the vagina within 24 hours after labor.

血。特别是产后24小时内出血量达500毫升以上。

1.2 Examination

To see if placenta and fetal membrane is damaged; if the birth canal is injured; whether the uterus is poor in involution or soft and large or hard and painful. Examination: Routine blood test, blood platelet test, coagulation factors test and B ultrasonic examination are helpful for diagnosis of the illness.

1.2 检查

胎盘、胎膜有无缺损；软产道有无损伤；子宫复旧不良，或软而大，或硬而痛。检查血常规、血小板、凝血因子，查B超以帮助诊断。

2 Syndrome differentiation and treatment

Clinical postpartum hemorrhage is classified into qi asthenia syndrome, blood stasis syndrome and birth injury syndrome. The therapeutic principle is nourishing qi and resolving blood stasis. In addition to the treatment based upon syndrome differentiation between asthenia and sthenia, it is necessary to give the rescue therapy, and the integrated therapy of Chinese medicine and Western medicine if needed, in order to avoid delaying the pathological condition.

2 辨证论治

本病临床主要分为气虚证、血瘀证及产伤证。治疗以益气化瘀为原则，除按虚实辨证论治外，危重者均须立即抢救，必要时应予中西结合治疗，以免延误病情。

2.1 Syndrome of qi asthenia

Main manifestations Sudden massive bleeding from the vagina, in fresh red color right after labor, dizziness, blurred vision, palpitation, shortness of breath, no desire to speak, cold limbs, sweating, pale complexion, pale tongue, weak and rapid pulse.

Therapeutic methods Replenishing qi and strengthening the Thoroughfare Vessel, controlling blood and stopping bleeding.

Formulas and herbs *Uplifting and Major-Supplementing Decoction* (Sheng Ju Da Bu Tang), com-

2.1 气虚证

主要证候 新产后，突然阴道大量出血，色鲜红，头晕目眩，心悸怔忡，气短懒言，肢冷汗出，面色苍白，舌淡，脉虚数。

治法 补气固冲，摄血止崩。

方药 代表方为升举大补汤；常用药如黄芪20克，

posed of 20 g of *Radix Astragali* (Huang Qi), 10 g of *Rhizoma Atractylodis Macrocephalae* (Bai Zhu), 6 g of *Pericarpium Citri Tangerinae* (Chen Pi), 10 g of *Radix Ginseng* (Ren Shen) (to be decocted separately and then mixed up with the other ingredients), 6 g of *Radix Glycyrrhizae Praeparata* (Zhi Gan Cao), 6 g of *Rhizoma Cimicifugae* (Sheng Ma), 10 g of *Radix Angelicae Sinensis* (Dang Gui), 10 g of *Radix Rehmanniae Praeparata* (Shu Di Huang), 10 g of *Ophiopogon* (Mai Dong), 10 g of *Rhizoma Ligustici Chuanxiong* (Chuan Xiong), 10 g of *Radix Angelicae Dahuricae* (Bai Zhi), 10 g of *Flos Schizonepetae Carbonisata* (Hei Jie Sui), 10 g of *Radix Sanguisorbae Carbonisata* (Di Yu Tan) and 15 g of *Os Sepiellae seu Sepiae* (Wu Zei Gu).

白术 10 克，陈皮 6 克，人参（另炖，兑入）10 克，炙甘草 6 克，升麻 6 克，当归 10 克，熟地黄 10 克，麦冬 10 克，川芎 10 克，白芷 10 克，黑芥穗 10 克，地榆炭 10 克，乌贼骨 15 克。

Modification For coma, cold limbs, sweating and indistinct pulse, *Ginseng Solo Decoction* (Du Shen Tang) or *Pulse-Engendering Injection* (Sheng Mai Zhu She Ye) is used to nourish qi and stop bleeding. For incessant cold sweating and cold limbs, *Ginseng and Aconite Decoction* (Shen Fu Tang) or *Ginseng and Aconite Injection* (Shen Fu Qing Zhu She Ye) is used to restore yang and restore yang for resuscitation.

加减 若昏不知人，肢冷汗出，脉微细欲绝者，用独参汤或生脉注射液补气固脱；若冷汗淋漓，四肢厥逆者，用参附汤或参附青注射液回阳救逆。

2.2 Blood stasis syndrome

2.2 血瘀证

Main manifestations Sudden massive bleeding with blood clot from the vagina right after labor, pain aggravated by pressure in the lower abdomen, alleviation of abdominal pain after removal of blood clot, pale and dark tongue or with ecchymoses, deep and unsmooth pulse.

主要证候 新产后，突然阴道大量下血，挟有血块，小腹疼痛拒按，血块下后腹痛减轻，舌淡暗，或有瘀点瘀斑，脉沉细。

Therapeutic methods Activating blood and eliminating blood stasis, regulating blood and returning blood to the meridians.

治法 活血祛瘀，理血归经。

Formulas and herbs *Stasis-Resolving and Bleeding-Stopping Decoction* (Hua Yu Zhi Xue Tang), composed of 10 g of *Typhae Pollen Frictus* (Chao Pu Huang), 10 g of *Faeces Trogopterorum* (Wu Ling Zhi), 30 g of *Herba Leonuri* (Yi Mu Cao), 10 g of *Radix Adenophorae* (Nan Sha Shen), 10 g of *Radix Angelicae Sinensis* (Dang Gui), 6 g of *Rhizoma Ligustici Chuanxiong* (Chuan Xiong) and 1.5 g of *Notoginseng Radix Pulverata* (San Qi Fen) (to be swallowed).

方药　代表方为化瘀止血汤；常用药如炒蒲黄 10 克，五灵脂 10 克，益母草 30 克，南沙参 10 克，当归 10 克，川芎 6 克，三七粉（另吞）1.5 克。

Modification For accompanying chest oppression and vomiting, *Rhizoma Pinelliae Preparata* (Jiang Ban Xia) is added to descend adverse flow of qi and resolve phlegm.

加减　若兼胸闷呕吵者，加姜半夏以降逆化痰。

2.3 Birth injury syndrome

2.3 产伤证

Main manifestations Sudden massive and incessant bleeding from the vagina with fresh red blood after labor, laceration of the soft birth canal, pale complexion, pale tongue, thin tongue fur, thready and rapid pulse.

主要证候　新产后，突然阴道大量下血，血色鲜红，持续不止，软产道有裂伤，面色苍白，舌淡，苔薄，脉细数。

Therapeutic methods Invigorating qi and nourishing blood, promoting granulation and securing the menses.

治法　益气养血，生肌固经。

Formulas and herbs *Oyster Shell Powder* (Mu Li San), composed of 15 g of *Ostreae Concha Calcinata* (Duan Mu Li), 10 g of *Radix Rehmanniae Praeparata* (Shu Di Huang), 10 g of *Poriae* (Fu Ling), 10 g of *Mastodi Ossis Fossilia Calcinata* (Duan Long Gu) (to be decocted first), 10 g of *Radix Dipsaci* (Xu Duan), 10 g of *Radix Angelicae Sinensis* (Dang Gui), 10 g of *Folium Artemistae Argyi* (Chao Ai Ye), 10 g of *Radix Ginseng* (Ren Shen), 10 g of *Fructus Schisandrae* (Wu Wei Zi), 10 g of *Radix Sanguisorbae* (Di Yu) and 5 g of *Radix Glycyrrhizae*

方药　代表方为牡蛎散；常用药如煅牡蛎 15 克，熟地黄 10 克，茯苓 10 克，龙骨（先煎）10 克，续断 10 克，当归 10 克，炒艾叶 10 克，人参 10 克，五味子 10 克，地榆 10 克，甘草 5 克。

(Gan Cao).

Modification If the soft birth canal is evidently injured, it must be sutured immediately and then treated with Chinese medicinal herbs.

加减 若产道裂伤明显者,应及时缝合止血,继以中调治。

2 Other therapeutic methods

2 其他疗法

2.1 Chinese patent drugs

2.1 中成药

(1) *Chinese Angelica Blood-Supplementing Pill* (Dang Gui Bu Xue Wan): 9 g each time and twice or three times a day, applicable to the treatment of postpartum hemorrhage due to blood asthenia.

(1) 当归补血丸:每次9克,每日2～3次,适用于血虚型产后出血的调理。

(2) *Perfect Major Supplementation Pill* (Shi Quan Da Bu Wan): 9 g each time and twice a day, applicable to the treatment of postpartum hemorrhage due to qi asthenia.

(2) 十全大补丸:每次9克,每日2次,适用于气虚型产后出血的调理。

(3) *Motherwort Paste* (Yi Mu Cao Gao): One spoonful each time and twice or three times a day, applicable to the treatment of postpartum hemorrhage due to blood stasis.

(3) 益母草膏:每次1匙,每日2～3次,适用于血瘀型产后出血的调理。

2.2 Empirical and folk recipes

2.2 单验方

(1) *Radix Notoginseng Pulverata* (Shen San Qi Fen): 1.5 g each time and twice or three times a day, applicable to the treatment of postpartum hemorrhage due to blood stasis.

(1) 参三七粉:每次1.5克,每日2～3次,适用于血瘀型产后出血。

(2) *Ginseng Powder* (Ren Shen Fen): 1.5-2 g is taken when hemorrhage occurs, applicable to the treatment of postpartum hemorrhage due to blood asthenia and qi exhaustion.

(2) 人参粉:每次1.5～2克,失血时吞服,适用于血虚气脱型产后出血。

(3) 0.5 g of *Resina Draconis* (Xue Jie) powder is taken each time and three times a day, applicable to the treatment of postpartum hemorrhage due to blood stasis.

(3) 血竭末0.5克,每日3次冲服,适用于血瘀型产后出血。

(4) 15 g of *Pollen Typhae* (Pu Huang) is decocted for oral taking, applicable to the treatment of

(4) 蒲黄15克,水煎服,适用于血瘀型产后出血。

postpartum hemorrhage due to blood stasis.

(5) 6 g of *Pollen Typhae* (Chao Pu Huang), 15 g of *Herba Agrimoniae* (Xian He Cao) and 6 g of *Radix Angelicae Sinensis* (Dang Gui) are decocted for oral taking, applicable to the treatment of sudden postpartum and incessant hemorrhage.

(5) 炒蒲黄6克，仙鹤草15克，当归6克，水煎服，适用于产后血崩，出血不止之证。

postpartum fever

产后发热

Postpartum fever refers to persistent high or low fever, or sudden high fever and chills, accompanied by other symptoms during puerperium. If slight fever happens one or two days after labor due to sudden asthenia of yin-blood, disharmony between Ying-nutrient qi and Wei-defensive qi without other symptoms, it would disappear by itself and is a physiological fever. Low fever within 3 or 4 days after labor during lactation is commonly known as "steaming milk". It will disappear naturally, not a pathological range. Sudden high fever, or persistent fever, pertains to postpartum fever.

产褥期内，出现发热持续不退，或低热持续，或突然高热寒战，并伴有其他症状者，称为“产后发热”。如在产后一二日内，由于阴血骤虚，营卫失调，常有轻微的发热，不兼有其他的症状，一般能自行退热，属生理性发热；或产后三四日内，泌乳期间有低热，俗称“蒸乳”，这种现象以后会自然消失，亦不属病理范围。若突然高热，或持续性的低热不退者，均属产后发热。

The reproductive tract infections after delivery is called "puerperal infection", also known as "puerperal fever" in Western medicine. It is in the scope of this disease, a common serious postpartum disorder and one of the four major causes of maternal mortality. Evil toxin infection syndrome of this disease may be referred to in the treatment.

分娩后的生殖道感染，西医学称“产褥感染”，亦称“产褥热”，属本病范围，是产褥期常见的严重病症，是导致孕产妇死亡的四大原因之一，治疗和处理可参照本病的感染邪毒证。

The main symptoms are fever, abdominal pain and foul lochia. The causes of the disease are complex and the pathogenesis is different due to the physiological environment of "excessive asthenia

本病以发热、腹痛、恶露有臭气为主要症状。发生的原因较为复杂，病机各异，这是以产后“多虚多瘀”的生理

and blood stasis" after labor. Postpartum fever can be easily caused by excessive asthenia after delivery, insufficiency of right qi, interstices failing to close tightly, disharmony between Ying-nutrient qi and Wei-defensive qi, excessive blood stasis after labor, open blood chamber, incomplete elimination of left blood.

内环境为先决条件的。由于产后多虚，正气不足，腠理不密，营卫失调；产后多瘀，血室开放，余血未尽，容易因各种原因导致产后发热。

1 Key points for diagnosis

1 诊断要点

1.1 Clinical manifestation

Fever lingers for 10 days after labor and remains over 38 ℃, accompanied by abdominal pain and abnormal changes of the color, texture, quantity and odor of vaginal secreta or red swelling, distention and pain of perineal wound.

1.1 临床表现

产后 10 日内发热不解，连续 3 日体温在 38 ℃以上，并伴有腹痛及阴道分泌物的色、质、量、气味异常；或有会阴部伤口红肿胀痛。

1.2 Examination

Gynecological examination, blood and urine routine test as well as culture of cervical secret are made to determine the location of infection and the pathogenic bacteria.

1.2 检查

作妇科检查，血、尿常规检查，宫颈分泌物培养等，以明确感染部位及致病菌。

1.3 Identification

Puerperal infection should be differentiated from fever due to blood asthenia, infection of exogenous pathogenic factors and mammary inflammation.

1.3 鉴别

应与血虚、外感及乳腺炎所致发热相鉴别。

2 Syndrome differentiation and treatment

This disease is mainly characterized by postpartum fever, often accompanied by abnormal lochia and abdominal pain. Asthenia or sthenia, cold or heat are mainly differentiated according to the characteristics of fever, the amount, color, quality and odor of lochia, concurrent patterns, and tongue diagnosis. High fever, chills, foul lochia and pain aggravated by pressure in the lower abdomen, belong

2 辨证论治

本病以产后发热为主症，常伴有恶露异常及腹痛，辨证主要根据发热的特点，参照恶露的量、色、质、味及腹痛的性质，以及兼症、舌脉，辨其虚实寒热。若高热寒战，恶露臭秽，小腹疼痛拒按，则为感染邪毒；若发热恶

rapid and weak pulse.

Therapeutic methods Activating blood and resolving blood stasis.

Formulas and herbs *Production and Transformation Decoction* (Sheng Hua Tang), compose of 10 g of *Radix Angelicae Sinensis* (Dang Gui), 15 g of *Herba Leonuri* (Yi Mu Cao), 6 g of *Rhizoma Ligustici* Chuanxiong (Chuan Xiong), 6 g of *Rhizoma Zingiberis Praeparata* (Pao Jiang), 9 g of *Semen Persicae* (Tao Ren), 9 g of *Fructus Crataegi* (Shan Zha), 5 g of *Radix Glycyrrhizae* (Gan Cao), 10 g of *Flos Lonicerae* (Jin Yin Hua), 10 g of *Fructus Forsythiae* (Lian Qiao), 15 g of *Herba Patriniae* (Bai Jiang Cao) and 9 g of *Rhizoma Aspidii* (Guan Zhong).

Modification For intermittent fever and chills, *Radix Bupleuri* (Chai Hu), *Radix Scutellariae* (Huang Qin), *Rhizoma Zingiberis Recens* (Sheng Jiang), *Fructus Ziziphi Jujubae* (Da Zao), *Radix Paeoniae Rubra* (Chi Shao) and *Cortex Moutan Radicis* (Mu Dan Pi) are added. For infection due to retention of placenta, *Radix Cyathulae* (Chuan Niu Xi), *Herba Dianthi* (Qu Mai) and *Malvae Semen* (Dong Kui Zi) are added. For poor appetite and greasy and thick tongue fur, *Caulis Sargentodoxae* (Da Xue Teng), *Semen Coicis* (Yi Yi Ren) and *Rhizoma Atractylodis Praeparatum* (Zhi Cang Zhu) are added.

3 Other therapeutic methods

3.1 Chinese patent drugs

(1) *Bovine Bezoar and Heart-Purifying Pills* (Niu Huang Qing Xin Wan): 1 pill each time and twice a day, applicable to the middle stage of patho-

苔薄黄，脉数虚大无力。

治法 活血化瘀。

方药 代表方为生化汤；常用药如当归10克，益母草15克，川芎6克，炮姜6克，桃仁9克，山楂9克，甘草5克，金银花10克，连翘10克，败酱草15克，贯众9克。

加减 寒热往来者，加柴胡、黄芩、生姜、大枣、赤芍、牡丹皮；胎盘胎膜残留引起感染者，加川牛膝、瞿麦、冬葵子；纳欠、苔腻厚者，加红藤、薏苡仁、制苍术。

3 其他疗法

3.1 中成药

（1）牛黄清心丸：每次1丸，每日2次，适用于邪热火毒证中期。

genic heat and virulent fire.

(2) *Bovine Bezoar Heat-Clearing Powder* (Niu Huang Qing Re San): 1.5 g each time and three or four times a day, applicable to puerperal infection due to invasion of pathogenic heat in blood.

(2) 牛黄清热散：每次1.5克，每日3～4次，适用于热入营血证产褥期感染。

(3) *Qing Kai Ling Injection* (Qing Kai Ling Zhu She Ye): Each ampule in 2 ml, 2-4 ml each time for intramuscular injection and twice or three times a day. Or 5% GS 500 ml + 2-4 ml Qing Kai Ling Injection for intravenous drip, applicable to the treatment of puerperal infection due to invasion of heat into the pericardium.

(3) 清开灵注射液：每支2毫升，1次2～4毫升，肌肉注射，每日2～3次，或用5%葡萄糖注射液500毫升加2～4毫升清开灵注射液静脉滴注，适用于产褥感染热陷心包证。

(4) *Mulberry Leaf, Chrysanthemum, Lonicera and Forsythia Powder* (Sang Ju Yin Qiao San): 10 g each time and twice or three times a day, applicable to the treatment of postpartum infection of exogenous wind-heat or infection of toxin.

(4) 桑菊银翘散：每次10克，每日2～3次，适用于产后外感风热或感染邪毒。

3.2 Empirical and folk recipes

3.2 单验方

(1) *Heat-Abating Decoction* (Tui Re Yin), composed of 12 g of *Fructus Crataegi* (Shan Zha), 12 g of *Radix Rehmanniae Cruda* (Sheng Di Huang), 8 g of *Rhizoma Ligustici Chuanxiong* (Chuan Xiong), 15 g of *Herba Leonuri* (Yi Mu Cao), 9 g of *Flos Carthami* (Da Xue Hua) and 8 g of *Radix Scutellariae* (Huang Qin). These ingredients are decocted for oral taking, applicable to the treatment of postpartum retention of blood stasis marked by abdominal pain and lingering fever.

(1) 退热饮：山楂12克，生地黄12克，川芎8克，益母草15克，红花9克，黄芩8克，水煎服，适用于产后瘀郁，腹痛身热不退。

(2) 100 g of *Herba Portulacae* (Ma Chi Jian) and 50 g of *Herba Taraxaci* (Pu Gong Ying) are decocted for oral taking, applicable to the treatment of puerperal infection due to toxic factors.

(2) 马齿苋100克，蒲公英50克，水煎服，适用于感染邪毒证产褥感染。

3.3 External therapy

3.3 外治法

External application: 50 g of *Radix et Rhizoma*

大黄芒硝外敷：大黄50

Rhei (Da Huang) and 200 g of *Natrii Sulfas* (Mang Xiao) are mixed and wrapped in gauze and applied on the worst place of lower abdominal pain. It has a good effect to disperse swelling and relieve pain, clear away heat and dissolve blood stasis.

克，芒硝 200 克，两药匀和后以纱布包裹敷于下腹部疼痛最甚处，具有消肿止痛、清热化瘀的良好功效。

Lochiorrhea

Lochiorrhea refers to incessant discharge of lochia for over 10 days after labor or termination of pregnancy due to family planning. It is also called "persistent flow of lochia", etc.

Lochiorrhea is usually caused by constitutional weakness, exhaustion of qi with loss of blood during labor, or impairment of the spleen due to puerperal overstrain, sinking of the gastrosplenic qi, weakness of the Thoroughfare and Conception Vessels to control blood, or by excessive intake of pungent and dry foods after labor, or by transformation of heat from stagnation of liver qi, impairing the Thoroughfare and Conception Vessels as well as driving blood to flow abnormally, or by invasion of pathogenic cold after labor, leading to cold coagulation and blood stasis in the Thoroughfare and Conception Vessels as well as abnormal circulation of qi and blood. The treatment is given based upon the main symptoms of incessant lochiorrhea for over three weeks and distension or pain in the lower abdomen.

产后恶露不绝

产后恶露不绝是指产后血性恶露持续 10 日以上仍淋漓不尽或计划生育终止妊娠后，出血超过 10 日以上者。又称"恶露不尽""恶露不止""血露不尽"。

本病多因素体虚弱，产时气随血耗，或产后操劳过早伤脾，中气虚陷，冲任失固，血失统摄；或产后过食辛辣温燥之品，或肝气郁而化热，热伤冲任，破血妄行；或产后寒邪乘虚而入，寒凝血瘀，瘀阻冲任所致，主要是冲任为病，气血运行失常。临证以产后恶露逾 3 周仍淋漓不止，小腹或坠或胀或痛为主要症状。

1　Key points for diagnosis

1.1　Clinical manifestation

Small amount of vaginal bleeding over three

1　诊断要点

1.1　临床表现

产后 3 周以上，阴道仍

weeks after labor.

有少量出血。

1.2 Examination

Gynecological examination is necessary to detect poor involution, or mild infection of the uterus, or retention of placenta and fetal membrane.

1.2 检查

妇科检查可确诊子宫复旧不良，或子宫轻度感染，或胎盘、胎膜残留。

1.3 Identification

Choriocarcinoma and malignant mole should be excluded.

1.3 鉴别

应排除绒癌及恶性葡萄胎。

2 Syndrome differentiation and treatment

Syndrome differentiation for this disease is done according to the quantity, color, texture and odor of lochia, in order to decide whether it is cold, heat, asthenia or sthenia in nature. The therapeutic principles are to get rid of asthenia, purge stagnation and clear away heat. Syndrome differentiation should be done in light of disease differentiation. The therapeutic methods usually are checking blood, clearing away heat and resolving blood stasis. Lochiorrhea must be controlled as quickly as possible lest massive uterine bleeding ensues.

2 辨证论治

本病的辨证，应从恶露的量、色、质、气味等辨别寒、热、虚、实，治疗应宗虚者补之，瘀者攻之，热者清之的原则，且必须辨证与辨病相结合，分别采用摄血、清热、化瘀法。尽早控制恶露，严防血崩。

2.1 Qi asthenia syndrome

Main manifestations Postpartum incessant and profuse lochiorrhea with light color, thin texture and no odor, empty and prolapsing sensation in the lower abdomen, spiritual lassitude, shortness of breath, bright pale complexion, pale tongue with white fur, slow and weak pulse.

Therapeutic methods Boosting qi and nourishing blood, promoting the securing and containing ability in the Thoroughfare and Conception Vessels.

Formulas and herbs *Center-Supplementing Qi-Boosting Decoction* (Bu Zhong Yi Qi Tang), composed of 20 g of *Radix Codonopsis Pilosulae* (Dang

2.1 气虚证

主要证候 产后恶露逾期不止，量多，色淡，质稀，无臭气，小腹空坠，神疲倦怠，气短懒言，面色㿠白。舌淡苔白，脉缓弱。

治法 益气养血，固摄冲任。

方药 代表方为补中益气汤；常用药如党参 20 克，黄芪 20 克，白术 10 克，炙甘

Shen), 20 g of *Radix Astragali* (Huang Qi), 10 g of *Rhizoma Atractylodis Macrocephalae* (Bai Zhu), 6 g of *Radix Glycyrrhizae Praeparata* (Zhi Gan Cao), 5 g of *Pericarpium Citri Tangerinae* (Chen Pi), 6 g of *Rhizoma Cimicifugae* (Sheng Ma), 6 g of *Radix Bupleuri* (Chai Hu) and 10 g of *Colla Corii Asini* (E Jiao)(to be melted).

草6克,陈皮5克,升麻6克,柴胡6克,阿胶(烊化)10克。

Modification For lumbago due to kidney asthenia, *Cortex Eucommiae* (Chao Du Zhong) and *Radix Dipsaci Carbonisatum* (Xu Duan Tan) are added to nourish the liver and kidney and stanch bleeding. For light dark lochiorrhea with blood clot and lower abdominal pain due to qi asthenia and blood stasis, *Herba Leonuri* (Yi Mu Cao) and *Notoginseng Radix Pulverata* (San Qi Fen) are added to dissolve blood stasis and stanch blood. For dual depletion of qi and blood and profuse sweating, *Fossilia Ossis Calcinata* (Duan Long Gu), *Concha Ostreae Calcinata* (Duan Mu Li), *Radix Paeoniae Alba* (Bai Shao) and *Fructus Schisandrae* (Wu Wei Zi) are added to nourish blood, astringe yin, astringe blood to stanch bleeding.

加减　兼肾虚腰痛者,加炒杜仲、续断炭补益肝肾止血;兼气虚血瘀者,见恶露色淡暗,夹小血块,小腹疼痛,加益母草、三七粉化瘀止血;气血两亏多汗者,加煅龙骨、煅牡蛎、白芍、五味子养血敛阴,固涩止血。

Shanghai doctor HU Guohua's experience prescription, *Qi Boosting and Uterus Recovering Decoction* (Yi Qi Fu Gong Tang): 12 g of *Radix Codonopsis Pilosulae* (Dang Shen), 9 g of *Rhizoma Atractylodis Macrocephalae* (Chao Bai Zhu), 12 g of *Radix Astragali cum Liquido Fricta* (Zhi Huang Qi), 12 g of *Rhizoma Dioscoreae* (Huai Shan Yao), 12 g of *Cortex Eucommiae* (Chao Du Zhong), 12 g of *Radix Dipsaci* (Xu Duan), 9 g of *Colla Cornus Cervi* (Lu Jiao Jiao) (to be melted), 12 g of *Fructus Rosae Laevigatae* (Jin Ying Zi) and 12 g of *Rhizoma Cibotii* (Gou Ji).

上海医家胡国华经验方(益气复宫汤):党参12克,炒白术9克,炙黄芪12克,炒怀山12克,炒杜仲12克,续断12克,鹿角胶(烊冲)9克,金樱子12克,狗脊12克。

2.2 Blood heat syndrome

2.2 血热证

Main manifestations Postpartum incessant and

主要证候　恶露过期不

profuse lochiorrhea with soy paste-like color, sticky texture and foul odor, flushed cheeks and red lips, dry mouth and throat, or abdominal pain, retention of dry feces, or feverish sensation over the palms, soles and chest, red tongue with dry or scanty fur, rapid, slippery or thready pulse.

止，量较多，色红或深红，质稠，或色如败酱，有臭气，面红唇赤，口燥咽干，或有腹痛、便秘，或兼五心烦热。舌红，苔燥或少苔，脉滑数或细数。

Therapeutic methods Nourishing yin, clearing away heat and stanching bleeding.

治法 养阴清热止血。

Formulas and herbs *Yin-Protecting Decoction* (Bao Yin Jian), composed of 10 g of *Radix Rehmanniae Cruda* (Sheng Di Huang), 10 g of *Radix Paeoniae Alba* (Bai Shao), 10 g of *Rhizoma Dioscoreae* (Shan Yao), 10 g of *Radix Dipsaci* (Xu Duan), 6 g of *Radix Scutellariae* (Huang Qin), 10 g of *Cortex Phellodendri* (Huang Bo), 10 g of *Radix Rehmanniae Praeparata* (Shu Di Huang) and 6 g of *Radix Glycyrrhizae* (Gan Cao).

方药 代表方为保阴煎；常用药如生地黄 10 克，白芍 10 克，山药 10 克，续断 10 克，黄芩 6 克，黄柏 10 克，熟地黄 10 克，甘草 6 克。

Modification For asthenia of qi, *Radix Astragali cum Liquido Fricta* (Zhi Huang Qi) and *Radix Pseudostellariae* (Tai Zi Shen) are added. For transformation of fire from liver qi stagnation, distending pain in hypochondria, dysphoria, bitter taste in the mouth, taut and rapid pulse, *Moutan and Gardenia Free Wanderer Powder* (Dan Zhi Xiao Yao San) can be used. For attack by pathogenic heat with the complication of damp-heat, *Caulis Sargentodoxae* (Da Xue Teng), *Herba Patriniae* (Bai Jiang Cao) and *Radix Sanguisorbae* (Di Yu) are added.

加减 兼气虚者，加炙黄芪、太子参；肝郁化火，两胁胀痛，心烦口苦，脉弦数者，用丹栀逍遥散；感受邪热，兼挟湿热者，加红藤、败酱草、地榆。

2.3 Blood stasis syndrome

2.3 血瘀证

Main manifestations Postpartum incessant scanty or profuse lochiorrhea with purplish and darkish color and blood clot, pain aggravated by pressure in the abdomen, alleviation of pain after

主要证候 恶露过期不止，淋漓涩滞，量时多时少，色紫暗有块，腹痛拒按，块下痛减。舌紫暗，边尖有瘀斑

removal of the clot, purplish and blackish tongue or with ecchymoses, deep, taut and unsmooth pulse.

瘀点，脉沉弦涩。

Therapeutic methods Activating blood, resolving blood stasis and stanching bleeding.

治法 活血化瘀止血。

Formulas and herbs *Production and Transformation Decoction* (Sheng Hua Tang), composed of 10 g of *Radix Angelicae Sinensis* (Dang Gui), 6 g of *Rhizoma Ligustici Chuanxiong* (Chuan Xiong), 6 g of *Semen Persicae* (Tao Ren), 5 g of *Rhizoma Zingiberis Praeparata* (Pao Jiang), 10 g of *Radix Glycyrrhizae* (Gan Cao), 10 g of *Great Guffaw Powder* (Shi Xiao San) (to be wrapped) and 10 g of *Herba Leonuri* (Yi Mu Cao).

方药 代表方为生化汤；常用药如当归10克，川芎6克，桃仁6克，炮姜5克，甘草10克，失笑散(包)10克，益母草10克。

Modification For qi asthenia with empty and prolapsing sensation in the lower abdomen, *Radix Codonopsis Pilosulae* (Dang Shen) and *Radix Astragali* (Huang Qi) are added. For stagnation of liver qi with distending pain in the chest and hypochondria, and taut pulse, *Radix Curcumae* (Yu Jin), *Rhizoma Cyperi* (Xiang Fu) and *Fructus Meliae Toosendan* (Chuan Lian Zi) are added. For relative predominance of cold, alleviated with warmth, *Cortex Cinnamomi* (Rou Gui) and *Fructus Foeniculi* (Xiao Hui Xiang) are added, or *Lesser Abdomen Stasis-Expelling Decoction* (Shao Fu Zhu Yu Tang) is used. For downward migration of damp heat with sticky and foul lochiorrhea, *Caulis Sargentodoxae* (Da Xue Teng), *Herba Patriniae* (Bai Jiang Cao), *Herba Taraxaci* (Pu Gong Ying), *Herba Portulacae* (Ma Chi Jian) and *Semen Coicis* (Yi Yi Ren) are added.

加减 气虚，小腹空坠者，加党参、黄芪；肝气郁结，胸胁胀痛，脉弦者，加郁金、香附、川楝子；偏寒得热则舒者，加肉桂、小茴香，或用少腹逐瘀汤；兼有湿热下注，恶露黏稠，有秽臭味者，加红藤、败酱草、蒲公英、马齿苋、薏苡仁。

3 Other therapeutic methods

3 其他疗法

3.1 Chinese patent drugs

3.1 中成药

(1) *Herba Leonuri* (Yi Mu Cao): 20 ml each

(1) 益母草：每次20毫

time and three times a day, applicable to the treatment of blood stasis syndrome.

升，每日 3 次，适用于血瘀证。

(2) *Production and Transformation Decoction Pill* (Sheng Hua Tang Wan): 9 g each time and three times a day, applicable to the treatment of blood stasis and cold coagulation.

（2）生化汤丸：每次 9 克，每日 3 次，适用于血虚寒凝证。

(3) *Yunnan White Powder* (Yun Nan Bai Yao): 0.2-0.3 g each time and once every four hours, applicable to the treatment of blood stasis syndrome.

（3）云南白药：每次 0.2～0.3 克，每 4 小时 1 次，适用于血瘀证。

(4) *Chan Fu Kang Granules* (Chan Fu Kang Ke Li): 1 bag each time and three times a day, applicable to the treatment of syndrome of asthenia of qi and blood.

（4）产妇康颗粒：每次 1 袋，每日 3 次，适用于气血亏虚证。

3.2 Empirical and folk recipes

3.2 单验方

(1) *Compound Production and Transformation Decoction* (Fu Fang Sheng Hua Tang): 10 g of *Radix Angelicae Sinensis* (Dang Gui), 6 g of *Rhizoma Ligustici Chuanxiong* (Chao Chuan Xiong), 9 g of *Radix Rehmanniae Praeparata* (Shu Di Huang), 6 g of *Semen Persicae* (Tao Ren), 5 g of *Rhizoma Zingiberis Praeparata* (Pao Jiang), 10 g of *Herba Leonuri* (Yi Mu Cao), 9 g of *Cortex Moutan Radicis* (Mu Dan Pi) and 5 g of *Radix Glycyrrhizae Praeparata* (Zhi Gan Cao) are decocted for oral taking, applicable to the treatment of lochiorrhea due to faulty uterine contraction.

（1）复方生化汤：当归 10 克，炒川芎 6 克，熟地黄 9 克，桃仁 6 克，炮姜 5 克，益母草 10 克，牡丹皮 9 克，炙甘草 5 克，水煎服，适用于产后子宫收缩不良之恶露不绝。

(2) Cockscomb and Lonicera Decoction (Shuang Hua Tang): 15 g of *Flos Celosiae Cristatae* (Ji Guan Hua), 15 g of *Flos Lonicerae* (Jin Yin Hua), 10 g of *Radix Angelicae Sinensis* (Dang Gui) and 10 g of *Herba Lycopi* (Ze Lan) are decocted for oral taking, applicable to the treatment of lochiorrhea after artificial abortion or induced labor.

（2）双花汤：鸡冠花 15 克，金银花 15 克，当归 10 克，泽兰 10 克，水煎服，适用于人流或引产后恶露不绝。

(3) 15 g of *Fructus Crataegi Ustus* (Jiao Shan Zha), 5 g of *Herba Lycopi* (Ze Lan) and 10 g of *Herba Leonuri* (Yi Mu Cao) are decocted with proper amount of brown sugar and water for oral taking, applicable to the treatment of postpartum lochiorrhea due to blood asthenia and blood stasis.

(3) 焦山楂15克,泽兰5克,益母草10克,红糖适量,水煎服,适用于血虚血瘀证产后恶露不绝。

Postpartum hypogalactia

产后缺乳

Postpartum hypogalactia refers to very little milk or no milk of the parturient in the lactation period. In Chinese language, it is also described: "insufficient of milk", "no flow of milk", and "no milk".

This disease was earliest seen in *Origin and Outcome of Diseases* of the Sui Dynasty (Zhu Bing Yuan Hou Lun): "In women, the meridians of Hand Taiyin and Shaoyin work downward for menstruation and upward for milk. After labor, water and blood come down together. If body fluid is suddenly exhausted, and menstruation is insufficient, there will be no milk." This quotation gives a preliminary explanation about lack of lactation. In *On Inquiring the Properties of Things* (Ge Zhi Yu Lun), there is such a discussion that "If the mother of infant does not know how to nurse herself, while disturbed by anger, hindered by depressed mood, and induced by greasy food, leading to no circulation in Jueyin meridians. As a result, the orifice is obstructed and no milk would come out". This discussion develops the knowledge about the etiologyand pathogenesis of hypogalactia.

产后缺乳指产妇在哺乳期内,乳汁甚少或全无。又称"乳汁不足""乳汁不下""乳迟不来"。

本病最早见于隋代《诸病源候论》:"妇人手太阴少阴之脉,下为月水,上为乳汁……即产则水血俱下,津液暴竭,经血不足者,故无乳汁也。"初步提出了缺乳的病因。《格致余论》有"乳子之母,不知调养,怒气所逆,郁闷所遏,厚味所酿,以致厥阴之气不行,故窍不得通,而乳汁不得出"的论述,在缺乳的病因病机方面有了发展。

1 Key points for diagnosis

1 诊断要点

1.1 Clinical manifestation

1.1 临床表现

Scanty or no secretion of milk for feeding in-

产后排出的乳汁量少,

fant after labor.

甚或全无,不够喂养婴儿。

1.2 Examination

The breast is soft without distention and pain. By pressure, a few drops of thin milk are secreted. Or the breast is full, but the mammary gland appears in mass. By pressure, it is very painful and cannot secret milk.

1.2 检查

乳房检查松软,不胀不痛,挤压乳汁点滴而出,质稀。或乳房丰满乳腺成块,挤压乳汁疼痛难出。

1.3 Identification

Hypogalactia should be differentiated from obstruction of milk due to crater nipple, and rupture of nipple, and difficult in breast feeding.

1.3 鉴别

排除因乳头凹陷和乳头皲裂造成的乳汁壅积不通,哺乳困难。

2 Syndrome differentiation and treatment

Asthenia or sthenia is differentiated based on the conditions of the woman's milk, breasts, emotions, tongue and pulse. Clear thin milk, soft breast without distention or pain, and in low spirit are mostly due to insufficiency of qi and blood. Thick milk, hardness and distending pain in the breasts, mental depression, chest oppression and belching are mostly due to liver qi stagnation. For qi and blood asthenia, nourish qi and invigorate blood. For liver qi stagnation, course the liver and resolve mental depression. Both treatments should be assisted by promoting lactation.

2 辨证论治

辨证主要根据乳汁、乳房、情绪、舌脉来辨其虚实。乳汁清稀,乳房柔软,不胀不痛,精神萎靡者,多为气血不足;若乳汁较稠,乳房胀硬疼痛,精神抑郁,胸闷嗳气者为肝郁气滞。治疗气血虚弱者应补气养血,肝郁气滞者应疏肝解郁,二者均应佐以通乳。

2.1 Syndrome of asthenia of qi and blood

Main manifestations Insufficient or even no milk in postpartum milk, not enough to feed the baby, soft breasts without distention, clear and thin milk, lusterless complexion, spiritual lassitude, lack of strength, poor appetite, pale tongue with white fur, theady and weak pulse.

Therapeutic methods Nourishing qi and blood, promoting lactation.

2.1 气血虚弱证

主要证候 产后乳汁不充甚或全无,不够喂养婴儿,乳房柔软无胀感,乳汁清稀,面色无华,神疲乏力,食欲不振。舌淡苔白,脉细弱。

治法 补气养血通乳。

Formulas and herbs *Lactation-Promoting Elixir* (Tong Ru Dan), composed of 12 g of *Radix Codonopsis Pilosulae* (Dang Shen), 12 g of *Radix Astragali* (Huang Qi), 10 g of *Radix Angelicae Sinensis* (Dang Gui), 9 g of *Ophiopogonis Radix* (Mai Dong), 6 g of *Caulis Akebiae* (Mu Tong), 6 g of *Radix Platycodi* (Jie Geng), 5 g of *Radix Glycyrrhizae* (Gan Cao) and 2 pig trotters.

方药　代表方为通乳丹；常用药如党参 12 克，黄芪 12 克，当归 10 克，麦冬 9 克，木通 6 克，桔梗 6 克，甘草 5 克，猪蹄 1 对。

Modification For dizziness and palpitation, *Fructus Lycii* (Gou Qi Zi), *Radix Salviae Miltiorrhizae* (Dan Shen) and *Semen Ziziphi Spinosi* (Chao Zao Ren) are added. For anorexia and abdominal distension, *Pericarpium Citri Tangerinae* (Chen Pi) and *Radix Aucklandiae* (Mu Xiang) are added.

加减　头晕心悸者，加枸杞子、丹参、炒枣仁；纳呆腹胀者，加陈皮、木香。

2.2 Syndrome of liver qi stagnation

2.2 肝郁气滞证

Main manifestations Scanty secretion of milk or no secretion of milk after labor, or normal or scanty secretion of milk after labor, sudden decrease of milk or no milk after injury to emotion, milk in thick texture, distension, hardness and pain in the breasts, or slight fever, mental depression, distending pain in the chest and hypochondria, poor appetite, darkish and red tongue with thin and yellow fur, taut and thready or taut and rapid pulse.

主要证候　产后乳汁甚少或全无，或产后乳汁正常或偏少，伤于情志后，乳汁骤减或点滴全无，乳汁稠，乳房胀硬而痛，或有微热，精神抑郁，胸胁胀痛，食欲减退。舌暗红，苔薄黄，脉弦细或弦数。

Therapeutic methods Soothing the liver and relieving stagnation, activating collaterals and promoting secretion of milk.

治法　舒肝解郁，通络下乳。

Formulas and herbs *Milk Fountain-Promoting Powder* (Xia Ru Yong Quan San), composed of 10 g of *Radix Angelicae Sinensis* (Dang Gui), 10 g of *Radix Paeoniae Rubra* (Chi Shao), 10 g of *Radix Paeoniae Alba* (Bai Shao), 6 g of *Rhizoma Ligustici Chuanxiong* (Chuan Xiong), 9 g of *Radix Rehmanniae Cruda* (Sheng Di Huang), 6 g of *Radix*

方药　代表方为下乳涌泉散；常用药如当归 10 克，赤芍 10 克，白芍 10 克，川芎 6 克，生地黄 9 克，柴胡 6 克，青皮 6 克，陈皮 6 克，天花粉 9 克，漏芦 9 克，桔梗 5 克，白芷 5 克，木通 5 克，炙山甲片

Bupleuri (Chai Hu), 6 g of *Pericarpium Citri Reticulatae Viride* (Qing Pi), 6 g of *Pericarpium Citri Tangerinae* (Chen Pi), 9 g of *Radix Trichosanthis* (Tian Hua Fen), 9 g of *Radix Rhapontici* (Lou lu), 5 g of *Radix Platycodi* (Jie Geng), 5 g of *Radix Angelicae Dahuricae* (Bai Zhi), 5 g of *Caulis Akebiae* (Mu Tong), 9 g of *Squama Manis* (Zhi Shan Jia Pian), 9 g of *Semen Vaccariae* (Wang Bu Liu Xing) and 5 g of *Radix Glycyrrhizae* (Gan Cao).

9克,王不留行9克,甘草5克。

Modification For severe distension in the breasts, *Fructus Citri Reticulatae* (Ju Luo), *Fructus Luffae Retinervus* (Si Gua Luo) and *Rhizoma Cyperi* (Xiang Fu) are added to move qi, activate collaterals and promote secretion of milk. For slight fever, *Radix Scutellariae* (Huang Qin) and *Herba Taraxaci* (Pu Gong Ying) are added to clear away heat. For distention, hardness, heat and pain in the breasts with palpable masses due to blood stasis from qi stagnation and transformation of heat from accumulated milk, *Fructus Luffae Retinervus* (Si Gua Luo), *Spica Prunellae* (Xia Ku Cao) and *Radix Paeoniae Rubra* (Chi Shao) are added to clear away heat, activate blood and disperse stagnation, with local massage and hot pad massage to help disperse stagnation and promote secretion of milk. For breast lump with a tendency of transforming to pus, it may be treated as "mammary -abscess".

加减 若乳房胀甚者,加橘络、丝瓜络、香附以增强行气通络下乳之力;身有微热者,酌加黄芩、蒲公英以清热;若乳房胀硬热痛,触之有块者,为郁而成瘀,乳积化热,宜加丝瓜络、夏枯草、赤芍清热活血散结,同时配合局部按摩及热熨,以助散结通乳;若乳房结块,势欲成脓者,可按"乳痈"处理。

3 Other therapeutic methods

3 其他疗法

3.1 Chinese patent drugs

3.1 中成药

(1) *Lactation Granules* (Tong Ru Chong Ji): 30 g each time and three times a day, applicable to the treatment of hypogalactia due to dual depletion of qi and blood.

(1)通乳冲剂:每次30克,每日3次,适用于气血两亏型缺乳。

(2) *Lactation promoting pill* (Cui Ru Wan): 9 g each time and twice a day, applicable to the treatment of hypogalactia due to depletion of qi and blood.

(3) *Fountain Powder* (Yong Quan San): 3 g each time and three times a day, applicable to the treatment of hypogalactia due to accumulation of qi and blood.

3.2 Empirical and folk recipes

(1) *Milk-Adding Prescription* (Zeng Ru Fang): 10 g of *Squama Manis* (Zhi Shan Jia Pian), 1 carp and 10 g of *Semen Vaccariae* (Wang Bu Liu Xing Zi) are decocted for oral taking, applicable to the treatment of agalactia due to blood asthenia and liver qi stagnation.

(2) 250 g of *Semen Phaseoli* (Chi Xiao Dou) is decocted for oral taking, applicable to the treatment of agalactia due to asthenia of qi and blood.

(3) 6 g of *Roasted Semen Trichosanthis* (Chao Gua Lou Ren) is grounded into powder and taken orally with wine, applicable to the treatment of agalactia due to blood stasis and cold coagulation.

(2) 催乳丸：每次 9 克，每日 2 次，适用于气血亏损型缺乳。

(3) 涌泉散：每次 3 克，每日 3 次，适用于气血壅滞型缺乳。

3.2 单验方

(1) 增乳方：炙山甲片 10 克，鲫鱼(去鳞肠)1 尾，王不留行子 10 克，水煎服，适用于血虚肝郁型缺乳。

(2) 赤小豆 250 克煮服，适用于气血虚弱证缺乳。

(3) 炒瓜蒌仁 6 克，研末，酒送服，适用于血瘀寒凝乳汁不下。

Chapter 8 Tumor and other diseases of female genital organ

第8章 女性生殖器官肿瘤及其他

Hysteromyoma

Hysteromyoma, a most commonly encountered benign tumor of the female reproductive system, with the symptoms of enlarged uterus and abnormal menstruation, formed with hyperplasia of the smooth muscle and connective tissue, is often seen in women from the age of 30 to 50, rarely seen in women under 20 years old, accounting for over 90% of gynecological tumors. According to statistics, 20% of women over 30 years old suffer from hysteromyoma.

Hysteromyoma is usually caused by emotional upsets, stagnation of liver qi, dysfunction of qi activity, unsmooth flow of qi and inhibited circulation of blood, or by invasion of wind, cold and dampness into the uterus and struggle with blood, or by sexual activity during menstruation and after labor; or by insufficiency of the spleen and kidney, asthenia of yang-qi, dysfunction of the spleen in transformation, retention of dampness and water into phlegm in the uterus, stagnation of phlegm and

子宫肌瘤

子宫肌瘤是指以子宫增大，月经异常为主要症状的女性生殖道最常见的良性肿瘤，由平滑肌及结缔组织组成，常见于30～50岁妇女，20岁以下少见。占妇科良性肿瘤的90%以上，据统计，30岁以上妇女约20%患有子宫肌瘤。

本病多由情志不遂，肝气郁积，气机不畅，血行滞涩；或经期产后血室正开，风寒湿邪，侵袭胞宫，与血相搏结；或经期产后余血未净，伤于房劳，余血败精，交结内阻而成；亦有脾肾不足，阳气虚弱，脾运失健，水湿不化，凝聚成痰，痰瘀阻于胞脉，冲任失调，新血不得归经，而致月

blood stasis in the uterine collaterals, and dysfunction of the Thoroughfare and Conception Vessels as well as failure of newly produced blood to flow in the meridians, changing menstruation or leading sudden profuse uterine bleeding. Consequently, anemia may be caused. So, in TCM it pertains to the scopes of "abdominal mass", "profuse menstruation" and "sudden profuse uterine bleeding".

经改变，或崩中漏下。又可继发贫血。本病属中医学"癥瘕""月经过多""崩漏"之范畴。

1 Key points for diagnosis

1 诊断要点

1.1 Clinical manifestation

1.1 临床表现

Progressive increase of menstruation, prolonged menstruation, or irregular uterine bleeding and even secondary anemia as well as pressure symptoms of bladder and rectum when tumor is enlarged.

进行性月经增多，经期延长，或有不规则的子宫出血，甚者可继发贫血。肌瘤增大时可见膀胱和直肠压迫症状。

1.2 Gynecological examination

1.2 妇科检查

Irregular enlargement, hardening, normal movement and no tenderness of the uterus.

子宫不规则的增大，质地硬，活动度尚好，无触痛。

1.3 Auxiliary examination

1.3 辅助检查

B ultrasonic examination, hysteroscopy and abdominoscopy are helpful for accurate diagnosis.

B 超、宫腔镜、腹腔镜可协助明确诊断。

1.4 Identification

1.4 鉴别

It should be differentiated from gravid uterus, ovary tumor, metrauxe, adenomyosis, pelvic inflammatory mass and deformity of uterus.

与妊娠子宫、卵巢肿瘤、子宫肥大症、子宫腺肌病、盆腔炎性包块、子宫畸形鉴别。

2 Syndrome differentiation and treatment

2 辨证论治

Hysteromyoma is mainly classified into pattern of qi stagnation and blood stasis, kidney asthenia and blood stasis, pattern of mixture of phlegm and stasis, and pattern of yin asthenia and liver hyperactivity. The basic therapeutic principle is resolving stasis and dissipating stagnation. The therapeutic methods are regulating qi, resolving phlegm, nour-

本病临床表现主要为气滞血瘀证、肾虚血瘀证、痰瘀互结证及肝旺阴虚证。治疗以化瘀散结为基本治则，根据辨证及经期或非经期分别采用理气、化痰、滋阴、补气等法。必要时采用西医手术

ishing yin and replenishing qi according to different syndromes and treatment time, during menstruation or not. Treatment based on integrated traditional Chinese and western medicine can be used if necessary.

治疗。

2.1 Syndrome of qi stagnation and blood stasis

Main manifestations Mass in lower abdomen, pain or not when pressed, distention in lower abdomen, irregular, profuse and residual menstruation with blood clot and darkish color, mental depression, oppression in the chest, dry mouth with no desire for drinks, not moist in the skin, somber facial complexion, purplish and darkish tongue with ecchymosis on the edge and tip of tongue, deep and thready or deep and taut pulse.

Therapeutic methods Soothing the liver and eliminating stagnation, resolving blood stasis and dissipating retention.

Formulas and herbs *Sanguine Mansion Stasis-Expelling Decoction* (Xue Fu Zhu Yu Tang), composed of 10 g of *Radix Bupleuri* (Chai Hu), 10 g of *Rhizoma Cyperi* (Xiang Fu), 10 g of *Fructus Aurantii* (Zhi Qiao), 10 g of *Pericarpium Citri Tangerinae* (Chen Pi), 6 g of *Rhizoma Ligustici Chuanxiong* (Chuan Xiong), 10 g of *Radix Paeoniae Alba* (Bai Shao), 15 g of *Rhizoma Sparganii Stoloniferi* (San Leng), 15 g of *Rhizoma Zedoariae* (E Zhu), 6 g of *Fructus Meliae Toosendan* (Chuan Lian Zi), 10 g of *Fructus Crataegi* (Shan Zha) and 10 g of *Radix Curcumae* (Yu Jin).

Modification For hard mass, *Carapax Trionycis* (Zhi Bie Jia) and *Thallus Laminariae seu Eckloniae* (Kun Bu) are added. For severe pain, *Rhizoma Corydalis* (Yan Hu Suo) and *Rhizoma Curcumae*

2.1 气滞血瘀证

主要证候 下腹部结块，触之有形，按之痛或不痛，小腹胀满，月经先后不定期，经血量多有块，经行难净，经色暗；精神抑郁，胸闷不舒，口干不欲饮，肌肤不润，面色晦暗。舌紫暗，舌尖、边有瘀点或瘀斑，脉沉涩或沉弦。

治法 疏肝行滞，化瘀散结。

方药 代表方为血府逐瘀汤；常用药如柴胡 10 克，香附 10 克，枳壳 10 克，陈皮 10 克，川芎 6 克，白芍 10 克，三棱 15 克，莪术 15 克，川楝子 6 克，山楂 10 克，郁金 10 克。

加减 若积块坚牢者，加炙鳖甲、昆布；若疼痛剧烈者，加延胡索、姜黄；若小腹冷痛，加小茴香、炮姜；月经

Longae (Jiang Huang) are added. For cold pain in lower abdomen, *Fructus Foeniculi* (Xiao Hui Xiang) and *Rhizoma Zingiberis Praeparata* (Pao Jiang) are added. For profuse menstruation and incessant profuse uterine bleeding, *Radix Notoginseng Pulverata* (San Qi Fen), *Pollen Typhae* (Chao Pu Huang) and *Crinis Carbonisatus* (Xue Yu Tan) are added. For severe blood stasis, squamous skin and blackish complexion, *Rhubarb and Ground Beetle Pills* (Da Huang Zhe Chong Wan) is added. For prolonged mass, *Squama Manis* (Zhi Shan Jia) and *Whitmania pigra* (Shui Zhi) are added to resolve blood stasis and disperse concretions.

过多，崩漏不止，加三七粉、炒蒲黄、血余炭；若血瘀甚者，兼肌肤甲错，面目暗黑，加用大黄蟅虫丸。包块日久者，加炙山甲、水蛭以化瘀消癥。

Shanghai doctor SHEN Zhongli's experience prescription: composed of 10 g of *Radix Rehmanniae Cruda* (Sheng Di Huang), 15 g of *Radix Paeoniae Alba* (Bai Shao), 10 g of *Glycyrrhizae Radix* (Gan Cao), 6 g of *Cortex Moutan Radicis* (Mu Dan Pi), 15 g of *Herba Taraxaci* (Pu Gong Ying), 30 g of *Herba Scutellariae Barbatae* (Ban Zhi Lian), 20 g of *Rhizoma Sparganii Stoloniferi* (San Leng), 20 g of *Herba Salvia Chinensis* (Shi Jian Chuan), 30 g of *Sargassum* (Hai Zao), 30 g of *Radix Polyphylla Smith* (Zao Xiu) and 20 g of *Faeces Trogopterorum* (Wu Ling Zhi).

上海医家沈仲理经验方：生地黄 10 克，白芍 15 克，甘草 10 克，牡丹皮 6 克，蒲公英 15 克，半枝莲 30 克，三棱 20 克，石见穿 20 克，海藻 30 克，蚤休 30 克，五灵脂 20 克。

2.2 Syndrome of mixture of phlegm and blood stasis

2.2 痰瘀互结证

Main manifestations　Mass in lower abdomen, not hard, intermittent pain, profuse leukorrhea with white color, sticky and thick texture, chest oppression or desire to retch, delayed menstruation or amenorrhea, pale and bulgy tongue, white and greasy tongue fur, taut and slippery pulse.

主要证候　小腹有包块，按之不坚，时或作痛，带下量多，色白质黏稠，胸闷或欲呕，月经后错或闭经。舌淡胖，舌白腻，脉弦滑。

Therapeutic methods　Resolving phlegm and eliminating dampness, activating blood and disperse concretions.

治法　化痰除湿，活血消癥。

Formulas and herbs *Two Matured Ingredients Depression-Opening Decoction* (Kai Yu Er Chen Tang), composed of 10 g of *Rhizoma Pinelliae Praeparata* (Zhi Ban Xia), 10 g of *Pericarpium Citri Tangerinae* (Chen Pi), 15 g of *Poriae* (Fu Ling), 10 g of *Pericarpium Citri Reticulatae Viride* (Qing Pi), 10 g of *Rhizoma Cyperi* (Xiang Fu), 6 g of *Rhizoma Ligustici Chuanxiong* (Chuan Xiong), 10 g of *Rhizoma Zedoariae* (E Zhu), 6 g of *Radix Aucklandiae* (Mu Xiang), 10 g of *Semen Arecae* (Bing Lang), 10 g of *Rhizoma Atractylodis* (Cang Zhu) and 6 g of *Radix Glycyrrhizae* (Gan Cao).

方药 代表方为开郁二陈汤；常用药如制半夏10克，陈皮10克，茯苓15克，青皮10克，香附10克，川芎6克，莪术10克，木香6克，槟榔10克，苍术10克，甘草6克。

Modification For yellowish leukorrhea due to transformation of heat from accumulation of dampness, *Herba Patriniae* (Bai Jiang Cao), *Cortex Moutan Radicis* (Mu Dan Pi) and 15 g of *Caulis Sargentodoxae* (Da Xue Teng) are added. For evident asthenia of spleen, *Semen Arecae* (Bing Lang) is deleted while *Rhizoma Atractylodis Macrocephalae* (Bai Zhu) and *Radix Codonopsis Pilosulae* (Dang Shen) are added.

加减 若湿蕴化热，带下色黄者，加败酱草、牡丹皮、红藤15克；若脾虚明显者，上方去槟榔，加白术、党参。

2.3 Syndrome of liver hyperactivity and yin asthenia

2.3 肝旺阴虚证

Main manifestations Uterine mass, delayed and scanty menstruation, or early profuse menstruation with red color, scanty leukorrhea, or dry sensation in the vagina, dry mouth and irritating sensation in the eyes, feverish sensation in the palms, soles and chest, flushed cheeks, vertigo, purplish red tongue with thin and yellow fur, thready and taut pulse.

主要证候 胞中结块，月经后期，量少，或先期量多，色红，带下甚少，或阴中干涩，口干目涩，五心烦热，两颊潮红，头晕目眩，舌紫红，苔薄黄，脉细弦。

Therapeutic methods Calming the liver and nourishing the kidney, resolving mass and stopping menstruation.

治法 平肝滋肾，消瘤断经。

Formulas and herbs *Modified Anemarrhena, Phellodendron, and Rehmannia Decoction* (Zhi Bai Di Huang Tang), composed of 10 g of *Radix Angelicae Sinensis* (Dang Gui), 12 g of *Radix Rehmanniae* Cruda (Sheng Di Huang), 15 g of *Radix Adenophorae seu Glehniae* (Sha Shen), 12 g of *Fructus Lycii* (Gou Qi Zi), 10 g of *Ophiopogon* (Mai Dong), 6 g of *Fructus Meliae Toosendan* (Chuan Lian Zi), 15 g of *Thallus Laminariae seu Eckloniae* (Kun Bu), 12 g of *Radix Paeoniae Alba* (Bai Shao) and 10 g of *Spica Prunellae* (Xia Ku Cao).

方药 代表方为知柏地黄汤；常用药如当归10克，生地黄12克，沙参15克，枸杞子12克，麦冬10克，川楝子6克，昆布15克，白芍12克，夏枯草10克。

Modification For profuse early menstruation, *Herba seu Radix Cirsii Japonici* (Da Ji), *Herba Cephalanoploris* (Xiao Ji) and *Flos Sophorae* (Chao Huai Hua) are added. For dry mouth and throat, *Herba Dendrobii* (Shi Hu), *Fructus Schisandrae* (Wu Wei Zi) and *Rhizoma Polygonati Odorati* (Yu Zhu) are added.

加减 若月经先期量多者，加大蓟、小蓟、炒槐花；若口燥咽干者，加石斛、五味子、玉竹。

Shanghai doctor ZHU Nansun's experience prescription: *Puccoon and Oldenlandia Mass-Resolving and Menstruation-Stopping Prescription* (Zi She Xiao Liu Duan Jing Tang): 30 g of *Radix Arnebiae seu Lithospermi* (Zi Cao), 30 g of *Herba Hedyotis Diffusae* (Bai Hua She She Cao), 30 g of *Spica Prunellae* (Xia Ku Cao), 15 g of *Herba Ecliptae* (Han Lian Cao), 30 g of *Ostreae Concha* (Mu Li), 30 g of Calcitum Gypsum Rubrum (Han Shui Shi) 12 g of *Herba seu Radix Cirsii Japonici* (Da Ji), 12 g of *Herba Cephalanoploris* (Xiao Ji) and 15 g of *Herb Salvia Chinensis* (Shi Jian Chuan).

上海医家朱南孙经验方（紫蛇消瘤断经汤）：紫草30克，白花蛇舌草30克，夏枯草30克，旱莲草15克，牡蛎30克，塞水石30克，大小蓟各12克，石见穿15克。

3 Other therapeutic methods

3 其他疗法

3.1 Chinese patent drugs

3.1 中成药

(1) *Cinnamon Twig and Poria Pill* (Gui Zhi Fu Ling Wan): 1 pill each time and once or twice a day, applicable to the treatment of blood stasis syndrome.

（1）桂枝茯苓丸：每次1丸，每日1～2次，适用于血瘀证。

(2) *Rhubarb and Ground Beetle Pills* (Da Huang Zhe Chong Wan): 6 g each time and once or twice a day, applicable to the treatment of blood stasis syndrome.

(2) 大黄䗪虫丸：每次6克，每日1～2次，适用于血瘀证。

(3) *Uterine Tumour Capsule* (Gong Liu Ning Jiao Nang): 4 capsules each time and three times a day, 3 menstrual cycles as a course of treatment, applicable to the treatment of syndrome of qi stagnation and blood stasis.

(3) 宫瘤宁胶囊：每次4粒，每日3次，3个月经周期为1个疗程，适用于气滞血瘀证。

(4) *Minor Golden Elixir* (Xiao Jin Dan): 2-5 elixirs each time and twice a day, applicable to the treatment of syndrome of phlegm-stasis obstructing the collaterals.

(4) 小金丹：每次2～5丸，每日2次，适用于痰瘀阻络证。

(5) *Tangerine and Litchi Accumulation-Dispersing Pill* (Ju Li San Jie tablet): 6 g each time and three times a day, applicable to the treatment of various types of hysteromyoma.

(5) 橘荔散结丸：每次6克，每日3次，适用于各种类型子宫肌瘤。

3.2 Empirical and folk recipes

3.2 单验方

(1) Shanghai doctor LI Xiangyun's prescription (hysteromyoma with sterility): 9 g of *Rhizoma Sparganii Stoloniferi* (San Leng), 9 g of *Rhizoma Zedoariae* (E Zhu), 12 g of *Eupolyphaga seu Steleophaga* (Di Bie Chong), 9 g of *Whitmania pigra* (Shui Zhi), 30 g of *Epimedium davidii* (Xian Ling Pi), 15 g of *Herba Cistanchis* (Rou Cong Rong), 12 g of *Spica Prunellae* (Xia Ku Cao), 15 g of *Radix Astragali* (Huang Qi), 15 g of *Rhizoma Dioscoreae* (Shan Yao), 9 g of *Rhizoma seu Radix Notopterygii* (Qiang Huo), 9 g of *Radix Angelicae Pubescentis* (Du Huo), 12 g of *Radix Cyathulae* (Chuan Niu Xi) and 12 g of *Rhizoma Corydalis* (Yan Hu Suo) are decocted for oral taking, applicable to the treatment of hysteromyoma in kidney depletion stasis obstruction syndrome.

(1) 上海医家李祥云(子宫肌瘤伴不孕)：三棱9克，莪术9克，地鳖虫12克，水蛭9克，仙灵脾30克，肉苁蓉15克，夏枯草12克，黄芪15克，山药15克，羌活9克，独活9克，川牛膝12克，延胡索12克，水煎服适用于肾亏淤阻证子宫肌瘤。

(2) Shanghai doctor DAI Deying's experience prescription *No 1 hysteromyoma prescription* (Zi Gong Ji Liu Yi Hao Fang): 15 g of *Spica Prunellae* (Xia Ku Cao), 30 g of *Concha Ostreae* (Mu Li), 9 g of *Rhizoma Sparganii Stoloniferi* (San Leng), 9 g of *Rhizoma Zedoariae* (E Zhu), 15 gof *Radix Codonopsis Pilosulae* (Dang Shen), 9 g of *Rhizoma Atractylodis Macrocephalae*(Bai Zhu) and 30 g of *Fici Pumilae Flos* (Mu Man Tou).

（2）上海医家戴德英经验方（子宫肌瘤1号方）：夏枯草15克，牡蛎30克，三棱9克，莪术9克，党参15克，白术9克，木馒头30克。

(3) Shanghai doctor CAI Xiaosun's experience prescription, *Stasis-Resolving and Hardness-Dispersing Prescription* (Hua Yu Xiao Jian Fang): 12 g of *Poriae* (Fu Ling), 3 g of *Ramulus Cinnamomi* (Gui Zhi), 10 g of *Radix Paeoniae Rubra* (Chi Shao), 10 g of *Cortex Moutan Radicis* (Mu Dan Pi), 10 g of *Semen Persicae* (Tao Ren), 12 g of *Sargassum* (Hai Zao), 12 g of *Thallus Laminariae seu Eckloniae* (Kun Bu), 10 g of *Squama Manis* (Zhi Shan Jia Pian), 30 g of *Spina Gleditsiae* (Zao Jiao Ci), 20 g of *Ramulus Euonymi* (Gui Jian Yu) and 10 g of *Eupolyphaga seu Steleophaga* (Di Bie Chong).

（3）上海医家蔡小荪经验方（化瘀消坚方）：云茯苓12克，桂枝3克，赤芍10克，丹皮10克，桃仁10克，海藻12克，昆布12克，炙甲片10克，皂角刺30克，鬼箭羽20克，地鳖虫10克。

Oophoritic cyst

卵巢囊肿

Oophoritic cyst is a commonly encountered tumor in gynecology, either benign or malignant or borderline. The following discussion may focus on benign type. Oophoritic cyst belongs to the scopes of "Intestinal mass" and "Accumulation" in Chinese medicine and is usually caused by long-term anxiety, preoccupation, depression and anger, internal damage by the seven emotional factors, infection of six exogenous pathogenic factors, intermal attack of

卵巢囊肿是妇科常见肿瘤，有良性、恶性、交界性之分。本节主要对卵巢良性肿瘤加以叙述。本病属中医学"肠覃""积聚"范畴。多由长期忧思郁怒、内伤七情、外感六淫、湿（热）毒内攻，客于胞脉。正气虚衰，邪气羁留，日久气滞血结或痰湿凝聚，或

damp (heat) toxin in the uterine collaterals, deficiency of constitutional energy, retention of pathogens, and long-term qi stagnation and blood stasis or accumulation of phlegm and dampness, or retention of dampness (heat) toxin, struggling with blood.

湿(热)毒壅滞,与血相搏,而致本病。

1 Key points for diagnosis

1.1 Clinical manifestation

Mass in the lower abdomen, or accompanied by abdominal distension, abdominal pain, lumbago, pressure symptoms, pain and disturbance of menstruation.

1.2 Gynecological examination

Gynecological examination shows mass beside the uterus with evident margin or mobility.

1.3 Auxiliary examination

Cytological examination, biopsy by puncture with thin needle, ultrasonic examination, radiological examination, abdominoscopy and tumor biomarkers can be used as supplementary examinations to check benign and malignant tumor.

1.4 Identification

Benign ovarian tumor should be differentiated from oncological changes of ovary, oviduct and ovary cyst, hysteromyoma, gravid uterus and ascites. Malignant ovarian tumor should be differentiated from endometriosis, inflammation of pelvic connective tissue, tuberculous peritonitis, accidental tumor of birth canal and metastatic ovarian tumor.

1 诊断要点

1.1 临床表现

临证以下腹部肿块,或伴有腹胀、腹痛、腰痛、压迫症状、疼痛、月经紊乱等为主要症状。

1.2 妇科检查

妇科检查可及子宫旁肿块,边界清楚,或可活动。

1.3 辅助检查

细胞学检查,细针穿刺活检、B超、放射学诊断、腹腔镜检查、肿瘤标志物可辅助检查良、恶性肿瘤。

1.4 鉴别

良性卵巢肿瘤应与卵巢瘤样病变、输卵管卵巢囊肿、子宫肌瘤、妊娠子宫、腹水等相鉴别;恶性卵巢肿瘤须与子宫内膜异位症、盆腔结缔组织炎、结核性腹膜炎、生殖道意外的肿瘤、转移性卵巢等肿瘤相鉴别。

2 Syndrome differentiation and treatment

Clinically, oophoritic cyst is classified into pattern of qi stagnation and blood stasis, pattern of phlegm and dampness retention, and pattern of

2 辨证论治

本病临床主要分为气滞血瘀证、痰湿凝结证及湿热郁毒证。治疗以软坚消癥为

stagnation of virulent dampness and heat. The therapeutic principle is softening hardness and eliminating mass. The therapeutic methods used are promoting qi flow, resolving phlegm and clearing away heat and draining dampness.

原则，根据病情分别采用行气、化痰、清热利湿法。

2.1 Syndrome of qi stagnation and blood stasis

Main manifestations Cystic mass in the lower abdomen, abdominal distention and pain, dark complexion, spiritual lassitude, dry mouth without desire to drink water, dry lips, unsmooth urination and defecation, purplish tongue, taut and thready pulse.

Therapeutic methods Promoting qi and activating blood, softening hardness and eliminating mass.

Formulas and herbs *Sevenfold Processed Cyperus Pill* (Qi Zhi Xiang Fu Wan) combined with *Sanguine Mansion Stasis-Expelling Decoction* (Xue Fu Zhu Yu Tang), composed of 12 g of *Rhizoma Atractylodis* (Cang Zhu), 12 g of *Rhizoma Atractylodis Macrocephalae* (Bai Zhu), 9 g of *Radix Angelicae Sinensis* (Dang Gui), 10 g of *Radix Paeoniae Rubra* (Chi Shao), 10 g of *Semen Persicae* (Tao Ren), 0.5 g of *Succini Pulvis* (Hu Po Fen) (to be taken separately), 10 g of *Radix Aucklandiae* (Mu Xiang), 10 g of *Fructus Crataegi* (Shan Zha), 6 g of *Endothelium Corneum Gigeriae Galli* (Ji Nei Jin) and 5 g of *Fructus Aurantii* (Chao Zhi Qiao).

Modification For constipation, *Radix et Rhizoma Rhei* (Da Huang) is added. For red tongue with scanty fur, *Radix Rehmanniae Crnda* (Sheng Di Huang) and *Processed Plastrum Testudinis* (Zhi Gui Jia) are added.

2.1 气滞血瘀证

主要证候 下腹有囊性肿块，巨大囊肿可见腹胀腹痛，面色晦暗，神疲乏力，口干不欲饮，唇燥，二便不畅，舌紫暗，脉弦细。

治法 行气活血，软坚消癥。

方药 代表方为七制香附丸合血府逐瘀汤；常用药如苍术 12 克，白术 12 克，当归 9 克，赤芍 10 克，桃仁 10 克，琥珀粉（吞）0.5 克，木香 10 克，山楂 10 克，鸡内金 6 克，炒枳壳 5 克。

加减 大便秘结者，加大黄；舌红苔少者，加生地黄、炙龟甲。

2.2 Syndrome of phlegm and dampness coagulation

Main manifestations Mass in lower abdomen,

2.2 痰湿凝结证

主要证候 小腹有包

not hard, occasional pain, profuse leukorrhea with white color, sticky and thick texture, chest oppression or desire to retch, delayed menstruation or amenorrhea, pale and bulgy tongue, white and greasy tongue fur, taut and slippery pulse.

块，按之不坚，时或作痛，带下量多，色白质黏稠，胸闷或欲呕，月经后错或闭经。舌淡胖，舌白腻，脉弦滑。

Therapeutic methods Resolving phlegm and softening hardness, activating blood and eliminating symptoms.

治法 化痰软坚，活血消癥。

Formulas and herbs *Sargassum Jade Flask Decoction* (Hai Zao Yu Hu Tang), compose of 12 g of *Sargassum* (Hai Zao), 12 g of *Thallus Laminariae seu Eckloniae* (Kun Bu), 12 g of *Spica Prunellae* (Xia Ku Cao), 9 g of *Rhizoma Acori Graminei* (Shi Chang Pu), 9 g of *Arisaema cum Bile* (Dan Nan Xing), 30 g of *Concha Ostreae* (Mu Li) (to be decocted early), 9 g of *Rhizoma Atractylodis* (Cang Zhu), 6 g of *Pericarpium Citri Tangerinae* (Chen Pi), 9 g of *Rhizoma Zedoariae* (E Zhu), 9 g of *Rhizoma Sparganii Stoloniferi* (San Leng), 10 g of *Semen Persicae* (Tao Ren), 10 g of *Radix Paeoniae Rubra* (Chi Shao), 10 g of *Fructus Crataegi Ustus* (Jiao Shan Zha), 10 g of *Massa Medicata Fermentata Usta* (Jiao Liu Qu) and 3 g of *Cortex Cinnamomi* (Rou Gui) (to be decocted later).

方药 代表方为海藻玉壶汤；常用药如海藻 12 克，昆布 12 克，夏枯草 12 克，石菖蒲 9 克，胆南星 9 克，牡蛎(先煎)30 克，苍术 9 克，陈皮 6 克，莪术 9 克，三棱 9 克，桃仁 10 克，赤芍 10 克，焦山楂 10 克，焦六曲 10 克，肉桂(后下)3 克。

Modification For distending abdomen and loose stool, *Radix Aucklandiae* (Mu Xiang), *Rhizoma Dioscoreae* (Shan Yao), *Cortex Fraxini* (Qin Pi) and *Pericarpium Granati* (Shi Liu Pi) are added. For restless sleep, *Semen Biotae* (Bai Zi Ren), *Caulis Polygoni Multiflori* (Ye Jiao Teng), *Radix Polygalae* (Yuan Zhi) and *Fructus Schisandrae* (Wu Wei Zi) are added. For scanty menstruation, *Ophicalcitum* (Hua Rui Shi), *Herba Pyrolae* (Lu Xian Cao) and *Flos Sophorae* (Chao Huai Hua)

加减 腹胀便溏者，加木香、山药、秦皮、石榴皮；夜寐不安者，加柏子仁、夜交藤、远志、五味子；经量偏多者，加花蕊石、鹿衔草、炒槐花；瘀块多者，加三七。

are added. For more masses, *Radix Notoginseng* (San Qi) is added.

Shanghai doctor SHEN Zhongli's experience prescription: composed of 15 g of *Radix Rehmanniae Cruda* (Sheng Di Huang), 6 g of *Radix Paeoniae Rubra* (Chi Shao), 6 g of *Radix Paeoniae Alba* (Bai Shao), 15 g of *Herba Artemisiae Anomalae* (Liu Ji Nu), 20 g of *Herba Scutellariae Barbatae* (Ban Zhi Lian), 20 g of *Caulis Sargentodoxae* (Da Xue Teng), 20 g of *Herba Patriniae* (Bai Jiang Cao), 10 g of *Radix Angelicae Sinensis* (Dang Gui), 12 g of *Herba Euphorbiae Helioscopiae* (Ze Qi), 20 g of *Herb Monochasma savatierii* (Sha Shi Lu Rong Cao), 20 g of *Spica Prunellae* (Xia Ku Cao), 20 g of *Sargassum* (Hai Zao) and 6 g of *Radix Glycyrrhizae* (Gan Cao).

上海医家沈仲理经验方：生地黄15克，赤白芍各6克，刘寄奴15克，半枝莲20克，红藤20克，败酱草20克，当归10克，泽漆12克，沙氏鹿茸草20克，夏枯草20克，海藻20克，甘草6克。

2.3 Syndrome of stagnation of virulent dampness and heat

2.3 湿热郁毒证

Main manifestations Lower abdominal mass, abdominal distention or pain or fullness, or irregular vaginal bleeding, even accompanied by ascites, dry stool, brown urine, burning sensation in urination, dry mouth, bitter taste in the mouth and no desire to drink water, deep-red tongue with thick and greasy fur, taut and slippery or rapid and slippery pulse.

主要证候 小腹部肿块，腹胀或痛或满，或不规则阴道出血，甚至伴有腹水，大便干燥，尿黄灼热，口干口苦不欲饮，舌暗红，苔厚腻，脉弦滑或滑数。

Therapeutic methods Clearing away heat and draining dampness, eliminating toxin and dissipating mass.

治法 清热利湿，解毒散结。

Formulas and herbs *Heat-Clearing Dampness-Draining and Toxin-Eliminating Decoction* (Qing Re Li Shi Jie Du Tang), composed of 30 g of *Herba Scutellariae Barbatae* (Ban Zhi Lian), 30 g of *Herba Solani Nigri* (Long Kui), 30 g of *Herba Hedyotis Diffusae* (Bai Hua She She Cao), 10 g of *Fructus Meliae Toosendan* (Chuan Lian Zi), 30 g of *Herba Plantaginis* (Che Qian Cao), 30 g of *Rhizoma Smilacis*

方药 代表方为清热利湿解毒汤；常用药如半枝莲30克，龙葵30克，白花蛇舌草30克，川楝子10克，车前草30克，土茯苓30克，瞿麦15克，败酱草30克，鳖甲30克，大腹皮10克。

Glabrae (Tu Fu Ling), 15 g of *Herba Dianthi* (Qu Mai), 30 g of *Herba Patriniae* (Bai Jiang Cao), 30 g of *Carapax Trionycis* (Bie Jia) and 10 g of *Pericarpium Arecae* (Da Fu Pi).

Modification For predominant virulent heat, *Gentianae Radix* (Long Dan Cao), *Radix Sophorae Flavescentis* (Ku Shen) and *Herba Taraxaci* (Pu Gong Ying) are added.

加减 若热毒盛者，加龙胆草、苦参、蒲公英。

3 Other therapeutic methods

3 其他疗法

3.1 Chinese patent drugs

3.1 中成药

(1) *Cinnamon Twig and Poria Pill* (Gui Zhi Fu Ling Wan): 6 g each time and twice a day, applicable to the treatment of syndrome of phlegm and dampness retention.

（1）桂枝茯苓丸：每次 6 克，每日 2 次，适用于痰湿凝结证。

(2) *Rhubarb and Ground Beetle Pills* (Da Huang Zhe Chong Wan): 1 pill each time and twice a day, applicable to the treatment of blood stasis syndrome.

（2）大黄䗪虫丸每次 1 粒，每日 2 次，适用于血瘀证。

(3) *Concretion-Transforming Return-to-Life Elixir* (Hua Zheng Hui Sheng Dan): 1 elixir each time and twice a day, applicable to the treatment of blood stasis syndrome.

（3）化癥回生丹：每次 1 粒，每日 2 次，适用于血瘀证。

3.2 Empirical and folk recipes

3.2 单验方

(1) *Squama Manitis Powder* (Chuan Shan Jia San): *Squama Manitis* (Chuan Shan Jia), *Rhizoma Zedoariae* (E Zhu), *Rhizoma Sparganii Stoloniferi* (San Leng), *Semen Pharbitidis Atrum* (Hei Chou), *Faeces Trogopterorum* (Wu Ling Zhi), *Rhizoma Corydalis* (Yan Hu Suo), *Radix Achyranthis Bidentatae* (Niu Xi), *Radix Angelicae Sinensis* (Dang Gui), *Rhizoma Ligustici Chuanxiong* (Chuan Xiong), *Rhizoma Rhei* (Da Huang), *Radix Salviae Miltiorrhizae* (Dan Shen) and *Cortex Cinnamomi*

（1）穿山甲散：穿山甲、莪术、三棱、黑丑、五灵脂、延胡索、牛膝、当归、川芎、大黄、丹参、肉桂等，研末，每次 3 克，每日 2 次，适用于卵巢良性肿瘤。

(Rou Gui) etc. are grounded in the powder, 3 g each time and twice a day, applicable to the treatment of ovarian tumor.

(2) 9 g of *Radix Angelicae Sinensis* (Dang Gui), 9 g of *Radix Paeoniae Alba* (Bai Shao), 9 g of *Fructus Meliae Toosendan* (Chuan Lian Zi), 9 g of *Rhizoma Corydalis* (Yan Hu Suo), 9 g of *Radix Dipsaci* (Xu Duan), 12 g of *Caulis Sargentodoxae* (Da Xue Teng), 6 g of *Radix Bupleuri* (Chai Hu) and 6 g of *Radix Curcumae* (Yu Jin) are decocted in water for oral taking, applicablee to the treatment of syndrome of qi stagnation and blood stasis.

（2）当归 9 克，白芍 9 克，川楝子 9 克，延胡索 9 克，续断 9 克，红藤 12 克，柴胡 6 克，郁金 6 克，水煎服，适用于气滞血瘀证。

(3) 9 g of *Radix Angelicae Sinensis* (Dang Gui), 6 g of *Rhizoma Ligustici Chuanxiong* (Chuan Xiong), 6 g of *Herba Lycopi* (Ze Lan), 6 g of *Rhizoma Sparganii Stoloniferi* (San Leng), 6 g of *Rhizoma Zedoariae* (E Zhu), 6 g of *Rhizoma Corydalis* (Yan Hu Suo), 12 g of *Amethyst* (Zi Shi Ying), 9 g of *Semen Persicae* (Tao Ren), 9 g of *Faeces Trogopteri* (Chao Wu Ling Zhi), 9 g of *Pollen Typhae* (Chao Pu Huang), 9 g of *Rhizoma Cyperi Praeparata* (Zhi Xiang Fu), 9 g of *Semen Litchi* (Li Zhi He), 4. 5 g of *Radix et Rhizomai Rhei* (Shu Da Huang) and 4. 5 g of *Rhizoma Zingiberis* (Gan Jiang) are decocted in water for oral taking, applicable to the treatment of lower abdominal mass in women.

（3）当归 9 克，川芎 6 克，泽兰 6 克，三棱 6 克，莪术 6 克，延胡索 6 克，紫石英 12 克，桃仁 9 克，炒五灵脂 9 克，炒蒲黄 9 克，制香附 9 克，荔枝核 9 克，熟大黄 4.5 克，干姜 4.5 克，水煎服，适用于妇女小腹癥瘕。

Vaginal protrusion

阴　挺

Vaginal protrusion means that the uterus descends or even comes out of the vaginal orifice, or protrusion of vaginal wall after labor. The former is prolapsed of uterus, the latter is prolapse of vaginal

妇女子宫下脱，甚则挺出阴户之外，或阴道壁膨出。前者为子宫脱垂，后者为阴道壁膨出，统称阴挺，又称

wall. There are different Chinese characters for it. Because it happens mostly after labor, it is also described as "no restoration of birth canal".

"阴菌""阴脱"。因多发在产后,故又有"产肠不收"之称。

Hysteroptosis means that the uterus descends along the vagina from the normal position or even completely comes out of the vaginal orifice, often complicated by protrusion of the posterior and anterior walls of the vagina.

子宫脱垂是指子宫从正常位置沿阴道下降,宫颈外口达坐骨棘水平以下,甚至子宫全部脱出于阴道口外,常合并有阴道前壁或后壁膨出。

Hysteroptosis is usually caused by early labor, dystocia, prolonged labor, overstrain in labor and increase of long-term abdominal pressure; or by excessive sexual life, multiparity, damaging the uterine collaterals, or by weak constitution and asthenia of qi and blood to maintain the organs in the original position; or by asthenia-cold in uterus, or by downward migration of liver fire and damp-heat. The treatment is given based upon the main clinical symptoms of aching pain and prolapsing sensation in the lumbosacral region and protrusion of something out of the vaginal orifice.

本病多因临盆过早,难产,产程过长,产中用力太过,及长期腹压增加;或房劳多产,损伤胞络;或体质较差,气血虚弱,不能收摄;或子脏虚冷;或肝火湿热下注等所致。临证以腰骶部酸痛和下坠感,阴道口有物脱出等为主要症状。

The main pathogenesis of this disease is injury of uterine collaterals due to qi collapse, insecurity kidney due to asthenia, unable to uplift uterus. The disease pertains to "vaginal protrusion" category in TCM.

本病的主要病机是气虚下陷与肾虚不固致胞络损伤,不能提摄子宫。本病属中医学"阴挺"范畴。

1 Key points for diagnosis

1 诊断要点

1.1 Medical history

1.1 病史

A history of birth injury, or early physical exertion after labor, or chronic cough, constipation.

有分娩损伤史,或产后过早操劳负重,或长期咳嗽、便秘史。

1.2 Symptoms

1.2 症状

Something descends invagina or even comes out

阴道有物下坠,甚则脱

of vaginal orifice, aggravated after standing too long or overwork, self retracted after bed rest. It is accompanied by lumbosacral pain in varying degrees or a sense of falling, often accompanied by severe difficult urinating, constipation, enuresis in severe cases. Bleeding ulcer, or purulent discharge may occur inexposed cervical and vaginal walls.

出阴道口外，站立过久或劳累后加重，卧床休息后多可回纳。伴有不同程度的腰骶部酸痛或下坠感，严重者常伴有排尿困难、便秘、遗尿。暴露在外的宫颈和阴道壁可发生溃疡出血，或有脓性分泌物。

1.3 Gynecological examination

Uterus comes out of vaginal orifice. Uterus may go back after bed rest in mild cases, but it can not go back in severe cases. The severe degree of prolapse should be judged after diagnosis. Also, it is necessary to note whether there are the local ulceration, infection and stress urinary incontinence.

1.3 妇科检查

子宫脱垂于外阴，轻者卧床休息后可回纳，重者难以回纳，确诊后应判断脱垂的严重程度，并予以分度。同时注意有无局部溃疡、感染及压力性尿失禁存在。

2 Syndrome differentiation and treatment

Asthenia is the root cause of this syndrome, either qi asthenia, kidney asthenia, or damp-heat syndrome. The therapeutic principle is to get rid of asthenia, elevate the sinking and stop prolapsing. The therapeutic methods are mainly nourishing qi and promoting the lifting ability, nourishing the kidney and stopping prolapse. For damp-heat, clear away heat and disinhibit dampness, combine with local external treatment. After dispelling damp-heat, nourish qi and support the body so as to secure the constitution.

2 辨证论治

本病以虚为本，有气虚、肾虚之别，可兼有湿热之标证。在治法上应按“虚者补之，陷者举之，脱者固之”的原则，以益气升提，补肾固脱为主。兼湿热者，佐以清热利湿，并配合局部外治。去湿热后，仍需补气扶正以固本。

2.1 Qi asthenia syndrome

Main manifestations　Downward migration of uterus, or protrusion of uterus from the vaginal orifice, aggravation after overstrain, prolapsing sensation in the lower abdomen, weak limbs, shortness of breathing and no desire to speak, pale complex-

2.1 气虚证

主要证候　子宫下坠或脱出于阴道口外，劳则加剧，小腹下坠，四肢无力，气少懒言，面色少华，小便频数，带下量多，质稀色白。舌淡苔

ion, frequent urination, profuse leukorrhea with thin texture and white color, pale tongue with thin fur, vacuous and thready pulse.

薄，脉虚细。

Therapeutic methods Supplementing the center and boosting qi, upbearing yang and raising the falling.

治法 补中益气，升阳举陷。

Formulas and herbs *Center-Supplementing Qi-Boosting Decoction* (Bu Zhong Yi Qi Tang), composed of 30 g of *Radix Astragali* (Huang Qi), 30 g of *Radix Codonopsis Pilosulae* (Dang Shen), 15 g of *Rhizoma Atractylodis Macrocephalae* (Bai Zhu), 10 g of *Radix Angelicae Sinensis* (Dang Gui), 5 g of *Radix Glycyrrhizae Praeparata* (Zhi Gan Cao), 5 g of *Pericarpium Citri Tangerinae* (Chen Pi), 5 g of *Processed Rhizoma Cimicifugae* (Zhi Sheng Ma), 5 g of *Radix Bupleuri* (Chai Hu), 3 slices of *Rhizoma Zingiberis Recens* (Sheng Jiang) and 5 *Fructus Ziziphi Jujubae* (Da Zao).

方药 代表方为补中益气汤；常用药如黄芪 30 克，党参 30 克，白术 15 克，当归 10 克，炙甘草 5 克，陈皮 5 克，炙升麻 5 克，柴胡 5 克，生姜 3 片，大枣 5 枚。

Modification For profuse leukorrhea with whitish color and thin texture, *Rhizoma Dioscoreae* (Shan Yao), *Semen Euryales* (Qian Shi) and *Ootheca Mantidis* (Sang Piao Xiao) are added.

加减 若带下量多，色白质稀者，酌加山药、芡实、桑螵蛸。

2.2 Kidney asthenia syndrome

2.2 肾虚证

Main manifestations Downward migration of uterus, prolapsing sensation in the lower abdomen, frequent urination especially in the night, vertigo and tinnitus, slight red tongue, deep and weak pulse.

主要证候 子宫下脱，腰膝酸软，小腹下坠，小便频数，夜间尤甚，头晕耳鸣。舌淡红，脉沉弱。

Therapeutic methods Nourishing the kidney and stopping prolapse, nourishing qi and elevating the collapse.

治法 补肾固脱，益气升提。

Formulas and herbs *Major Yuan (Primary) Qi-Reinforcing Decoction* (Da Bu Yuan Jian), composed of 10 g of *Radix Ginseng* (Ren Shen), 10 g of *Rhizoma Dioscoreae* (Shan Yao), 10 g of *Radix Rehmanniae Praeparata* (Shu Di Huang), 10 g of

方药 代表方为大补元煎；常用药如人参 10 克，山药 10 克，熟地黄 10 克，杜仲 10 克，炒当归 10 克，山茱萸 10 克，枸杞子 9 克，炙甘草 6

Cortex Eucommiae (Du Zhong), 10 g of *Radix Chinese Angelica* (Chao Dang Gui), 10 g of *Fructus Corni* (Shan Zhu Yu), 9 g of *Fructus Lycii* (Gou Qi Zi), 6 g of *Radix Glycyrrhizae Praeparata* (Zhi Gan Cao), 12 g of *Fructus Rosae Laevigatae* (Jin Ying Zi), 12 g of *Semen Cuscutae* (Tu Si Zi) and 12 g of *Placenta Hominis* (Zi He Che).

克,金樱子12克,菟丝子12克,紫河车12克。

Modification For protrusion of uterus from the vaginal orifice, contusion, secondary damp-heat symptoms, local swelling and ulceration, profuse leukorrhea with yellow color like pus and foul odor, *Cortex Phellodendri* (Huang Bo), *Rhizoma Atractylodis* (Cang Zhu), *Rhizoma Smilacis Glabrae* (Tu Fu Ling) and *Semen Plantaginis* (Che Qian Zi) are added. For severe case, *Gentian Liver-Draining Decoction* (Long Dan Xie Gan Tang) is used.

加减 若子宫脱出阴道口外,摩擦损伤,继发湿热证候,局部红肿溃烂,黄水淋漓,带下量多,色黄如脓,有臭秽气味,轻者加黄柏、苍术、土茯苓、车前子,重者用龙胆泻肝汤。

3 Other therapeutic methods

3 其他疗法

3.1 Chinese patent drugs

3.1 中成药

(1) *Center-Supplementing Qi-Boosting Pills* (Bu Zhong Yi Qi Wan): 6-9 g each time and three times a day, applicable to the treatment of spleen asthenia and qi sinking syndrome.

(1) 补中益气丸:每次6～9克,每日3次,适用于脾虚气陷证。

(2) *Major Yuan (Primary) Qi-Reinforcing Decoction Pill* (Da Bu Yuan Jian Wan): 1 pill each time and three times a day, applicable to the treatment of syndrome of insufficiency of liver and kidney, dual depletion of qi and blood.

(2) 大补元煎丸:每次1丸,每日3次,适用于用于肝肾不足,气血两亏证。

(3) *Golden Chamber Kidney Qi Pills* (Jin Kui Shen Qi Wan): 4-5 g each time and twice a day, applicable to the treatment of kidney asthenia syndrome.

(3) 金匮肾气丸:每次4～5克,每日2次,适用于肾虚证。

3.2 Empirical and folk recipes

3.2 单验方

(1) 60 g of *Radix Gossypii* (Mian Hua Gen)

(1) 棉花根60克,枳壳

and 30 g of *Fructus Aurantii* (Zhi Qiao) are decocted in water for oral taking, applicable to the treatment of hysteroptosis of qi asthenia and sinking syndrome.

30 克，水煎服，适用于气虚下陷证子宫脱垂。

(2) 15 g of *Fructus Aurantii* (Zhi Qiao) and 15 g of *Fructus Leonuri* (Chong Wei Zi) are decocted in water for oral taking, applicable to the treatment of various types of hysteroptosis.

(2) 枳壳 15 克，茺蔚子 15 克，水煎服，适用于各证子宫脱垂。

3.3 External therapy

3.3 外治法

(1) 50 g of *Fructus Aurantii* (Zhi Qiao), 25 g of *Radix Astragali* (Huang Qi), 25 g of *Herba Leonuri* (Yi Mu Cao) and 10 g of *Rhizoma Cimicifugae* (Sheng Ma) are decocted in water for fumigation and washing or rinsing and washing, one dose a day and applicable to the treatment of qi asthenia syndrome.

(1) 枳壳 50 克，黄芪 25 克，益母草 25 克，升麻 10 克，水煎，每日 1 剂，分早晚熏洗或浸洗，用于气虚证。

(2) 50 g of *Fructus Aurantii* (Zhi Qiao), 25 g of *Herba Leonuri* (Yi Mu Cao), 10 g of *Rhizoma Cimicifugae* (Sheng Ma) and 50 g of *Fructus Rosae Laevigatae* (Jin Ying Zi) are decocted in water for fumigation and washing or rinsing and washing, one dose a day and applicable to the treatment of kidney asthenia syndrome.

(2) 枳壳 50 克，益母草 25 克，升麻 10 克，金樱子 50 克，水煎，每日 1 剂，分早晚熏洗或浸洗，用于肾虚证。

(3) 60 g of *Fructose Aurantii* (Sheng Zhi Qiao) and 10 g of *Receptaculum Nelumbinis* (Lian Peng Ke) are decocted in water for fumigation and washing, applicable to the treatment of hysteroptosis in various types.

(3) 生枳壳 60 克，莲蓬壳 10 克，煎水熏洗，适用于各证子宫脱垂。

(4) 15 g of *Radix Salviae Miltiorrhizae* (Dan Shen), 9 g of *Galla Chinensis* (Wu Bei Zi) and 9 g of *Fructose Chebulae* (Ke Zi Rou) are decocted in water for fumigation and washing, applicable to the treatment of hysteroptosis of various types.

(4) 丹参 15 克，五倍子 9 克，诃子肉 9 克，煎水趁热熏洗，适用于各证子宫脱垂。

(5) 30 g of *Flos Lonicerae* (Jin Yin Hua), 30 g

(5) 金银花 30 克，紫花

of *Herba Violae* (Zi Hua Di Ding), 30 g of *Herba Taraxaci* (Pu Gong Ying), 30 g of *Fructus Cnidii* (She Chuang Zi), 6 g of *Rhizoma Coptidis* (Huang Lian), 15 g of *Radix Sophorae Flavescentis* (Ku Shen), 10 g of *Cortex Phellodendri* (Huang Bo) and 10 g of *Alumen Dehydratum* (Ku Fan) are decocted in water for fumigation and washing, applicable to the treatment of hysteroptosis of damp-heat syndrome.

地丁30克，蒲公英30克，蛇床子30克，黄连6克，苦参15克，黄柏10克，枯矾10克，煎水熏洗坐浴，适用于湿热证子宫脱垂。

(6) 20-50 *Semen Ricini* (Bi Ma Zi) are ground into paste, spread over a piece of white cloth and applied to Baihui (GV 20). If the uterus begins to ascend, the paste over the cloth is taken off and applied to the region 1-3 cun below the navel, applicable to the treatment of hysteroptosis of various types.

（6）蓖麻子20～50粒，捣如泥，摊于白布上，贴百会穴。如子宫上收时，将药膏揭下贴脐下1～3寸处，适用于各证子宫脱垂。

Shanghai Pujiang Education Press (Former Shanghai University of Traditional Chinese Medicine Press)
1550 Haigang Haigang Ave, Shanghai, P.R.China 201306

图书在版编目(CIP)数据

中医妇科学/张婷婷主编. —上海：上海浦江教育出版社有限公司，2018.11
((英汉对照)精编实用中医文库/陈凯先，李其忠，何星海总主编)
ISBN 978-7-81121-578-6

Ⅰ.①中…　Ⅱ.①张…　Ⅲ.①中医妇科学—英、汉　Ⅳ.①R271.1

中国版本图书馆 CIP 数据核字(2018)第257097号

上海浦江教育出版社出版
社址：上海海港大道 1550 号上海海事大学校内　　邮政编码：201306
分社：上海蔡伦路 1200 号上海中医药大学内　　邮政编码：201203
电话：(021)38284910(12)(发行)　38284923(总编室)　38284916(传真)
E-mail：cbs@shmtu.edu.cn　URL：http://www.pujiangpress.cn
上海盛通时代印刷有限公司印装　上海浦江教育出版社发行
幅面尺寸：170 mm×240 mm　印张：18.75　字数：357 千字
2018 年 11 月第 1 版　2018 年 11 月第 1 次印刷
责任编辑：黄　健　封面设计：赵宏义
定价：85.00 元